Radionuclide Imaging of the Breast

Radionuclide Imaging of the Breast

edited by

Raymond Taillefer

Centre Hospitalier de l'Université de Montreal
Montreal, Quebec, Canada

Iraj Khalkhali

Harbor-UCLA Medical Center
Torrance, California

Alan D. Waxman

Cedars-Sinai Medical Center and
University of Southern California School of Medicine
Los Angeles, California

Hans J. Biersack

University of Bonn
Bonn, Germany

MARCEL DEKKER, INC.   NEW YORK · BASEL · HONG KONG

Library of Congress Cataloging-in-Publication Data

Radionuclude imaging of the breast / [edited by] Raymond Taillefer...[et al.]
    p. cm.
    Includes index.
    ISBN 0-8247-0202-6 (alk. paper)
       1. Breast—Cancer—Radionuclide imaging. 2. Breast—radionuclide
imaging. 3. Taillefer, Raymond.
      [DNLM: 1. Breast—radionuclide imaging. 2. Breast Diseases—diagnosis.
    3. Diagnostic Imaging—methods. WP 815R1295 1998]
    RC280.B8R34 1998
    616.994'4907575—dc21
    DNLM/DLC
    for Library of Congress   98-29128
                                                              CIP

Headquarters
Marcel Dekker, Inc.
270 Madison Avenue, New York, NY 10016
tel: 212-696-9000; fax: 212-685-4540

Eastern Hemisphere Distribution
Marcel Dekker AG
Hutgasse 4, Postfach 812, CH-4001 Basel, Switzerland
tel: 44-61-8482; fax: 44-61-261-8896

World Wide Web
http://www.dekker.com

The publisher offers discounts on this book when ordered in bulk quantities. For more information, write to Special Sales/Professional Marketing at the address below.

Current printing (last digit):
10 9 8 7 6 5 4 3 2 1

PRINTED IN THE UNITED STATES OF AMERICA

Preface

Breast cancer is the second leading cause of cancer death in North American women and a serious health problem around the world. Incidence of breast cancer continues to rise. For many years the mortality rate from this disease was stable; for the first time, in 1995, the mortality rate decreased slightly due at least in part to the increased utilization of screening mammography.

Despite mammography's overall success, it has had its limitations over the past decade. However, during that time the rate of lesion detection by mammography has been significantly improved. Dedicated mammography units, film processors, efficiently matched film-screen combinations, improved education of radiologists and mammography technologists, and tighter regulation by the Food and Drug Administration and the American College of Radiology have all contributed to the improvement. However, mammography still has problems with its sensitivity and specificity. In the U.S. trials, mammography has had specificities and positive predictive value for the detection of breast cancer on the order of 20–30%. Thus, only one out of every four to six "mammographically suspicious" lesions biopsied will prove to be malignant.

Therefore, there is a critical need for an accurate, safe, and noninvasive imaging technique to improve the sensitivity and specificity of conventional mammography.

In recent years, emerging nuclear medicine technology, both single-photon emission computed tomography (SPECT) and positron tomography (PET), has made significant progress worldwide. A variety of radiopharmaceuticals are availabe in both clinical and research settings for breast cancer imaging. These are summarized in Table 1. The preliminary results of trials using different radiopharmaceuticals are encouraging and we believe that in the near future scintimammography, or radionuclide imaging of the breast, will have a significant impact on work-ups of women with breast problems.

This book was written as a comprehensive volume for nuclear medicine-

TABLE I   Radiopharmaceuticals Used in Detection of Primary Breast Cancer

Planar or SPECT imaging radiopharmaceuticals
   Radiolabeled monoclonal antibodies and peptides
      several types of antibodies labeled with ^{131}I, ^{123}I, ^{111}In, or [99m]Tc
      ^{99m}Tc-pentadecapeptide α-M2

   Perfusion imaging agents
      201-thallium
      99mTc-sestamibi
      99mTc-tetrofosmin

   Receptors imaging
      ^{111}In-DTPA-octreotide (somatostatin receptors)
      ^{131}I-E-17α-iodovinyl estradiol (estrogen receptors)
      [123]I-16α-estradiol (estrogen receptors)

   Non-specific uptake mechanisms
      ^{99m}Tc-MDP
      ^{99m}Tc-DTPA
      ^{99m}Tc-Sulfur colloid
      [67]Gallium-citrate
      ^{99m}Tc-pertechnetate
      [32]Phosphorus
      [197]Hg-chlormerodrin

PET imaging radiopharmaceuticals
   Glucose metabolism
      2-[^{18}F]Fluoro-2-deoxy-D-glucose

   Receptor imaging
      21-[^{18}F]Fluoro-16α-ethyl-19-norprogesterone (progestin receptors)
      16β-[^{18}F]Fluoromoxestrol (estrogen receptors)
      16β-[^{18}F]Fluoroestradiol (estrogen receptors)

   Methionine metabolism
      L-methyl-^{11}C-methionine

physicians, radiologists, primary care physicians, and surgeons to demonstrate the role of nuclear medicine as a complementary technique to mammography and other imaging modalities for diagnosis of breast cancer.

    The authors describe their own experiences and review the medical literature on how the use of different radiopharmaceuticals and technology can improve the sensitivity and specificity of conventional mammography. There are also two chapters that deal with surgeon and pathologist points of view for the work-up and diagnosis of breast cancer. The specific indications and clinical utility of nuclear medicine breast imaging are fully described in several chapters, with attention to the detailed technical aspect of scintimammography.

We are encouraged that there will be dedicated nuclear medicine cameras available for breast imaging in the near future. We hope that the emerging technology will permit us to diagnose early preclinical premammographic breast cancers that have shown positive results with these biological markers.

Dr. Taillefer would like to thank his wife Christiane and their children Élisabeth, Alexandra, and Nicolas, who make it all worthwhile. He would also like to acknowledge his colleagues for their support.

Dr. Khalkhali wishes to thank Fred S. Mishkin, M.D. and Ismeal G. Mena, M.D. for their professional support and encouragement; Linda E. Diggles, C.N.M.T., for her outstanding technical assistance; Mr. Ali Massodi for his outstanding artwork; Dorothea Jones for her secretarial assistance; and Brenda Lee Richardson, R.T. for her technical assistance. Dr. Khalkhali would also like to dedicate this book to his family Janita, Ali, and Anita Khalkhali for their support and patience and to his patients whom he has learned from throughout the years.

Raymond Taillefer
Iraj Khalkhali
Alan D. Waxman
Hans J. Biersack

Contents

Contributors

WILLIAM L. ASHBURN, M.D.   Medical Director, Digirad Corporation, San Diego, California

NAOMI P. ALAZRAKI, M.D.   Professor, Emory University School of Medicine, Chief, Nuclear Medicine Service, Veterans Affairs Medical Center, Atlanta, Georgia

BRUCE J. BARRON, M.D.   Associate Professor, Department of Radiology, University of Texas Medical School, Houston, Texas

HANS BENDER, M.D.   Senior Instructor, Department of Nuclear Medicine, University of Bonn, Bonn, Germany

HANS J. BIERSACK, M.D.   Professor and Chairman, Department of Nuclear Medicine, University of Bonn, Bonn, Germany

MARCO BRESCIANI, M.S.   Medicina Nucleare Istituto di Scienze Radiologiche, Second University of Naples, Naples, Italy

DECIO CAPOBIANCO, M.D.   Medicina Nucleare Istituto di Scienze Radiologiche, Second University of Naples, Naples, Italy

JOSEPH CHIAO, M.D.   Assistant Professor, Department of Pathology, University of Florida Health Science Center, Jacksonville, Florida

VINCENZO CUCCURULLO, M.D.   Medicina Nucleare Istituto di Scienze Radiologiche, Second University of Naples, Naples, Italy

MARION DE JONG, M.D.   Associate Professor, Department of Nuclear Medicine, University Hospital Rotterdam, Rotterdam, The Netherlands

ENRICO DEL VECCHIO, M.D. Associate Professor, Medicina Nucleare Istituto di Scienze Radiologiche, Second University of Naples, Naples, Italy

LINDA DIGGLES, B.S., C.N.M.T. Supervising Technologist and Research Coordinator, Division of Nuclear Medicine, Harbor-UCLA Medical Center, Torrance, and Instructor, School of Health, California State University, Dominiguez Hills, California

PATRICIA J. EUBANKS, M.D. Assistant Professor, Department of Surgery, University of Nevada School of Medicine and Veterans Affairs Medical Center, Reno, Nevada

ANDRÉ GAGNON, C.N.M.T. Department of Nuclear Medicine, Centre Hospitalier de l'Université de Montreal, Montreal, Quebec, Canada

RAGHUVEER K. HALKUR, M.D. Assistant Professor, Department of Radiology, Emory University School of Medicine, and Veterans Affairs Medical Center, Atlanta, Georgia

SAEED IRANIHA, M.D. Surgical Resident, Department of Surgery, Harbor-UCLA Medical Center, Torrance, California

IRAJ KHALKHALI, M.D., F.A.C.R. Professor, Department of Surgery and Radiology, Harbor-UCLA Medical Center, Torrance, California

STANLEY R. KLEIN, M.D. Associate Professor, Department of Surgery, Harbor-UCLA Medical Center, Torrance, California

ERIC P. KRENNING, M.D., PH.D. Professor, Department of Nuclear and Internal Medicine, University Hospital Rotterdam, Rotterdam, The Netherlands

LAMK M. LAMKI, M.D., F.R.C.P.C., F.A.C.R. Professor, Department of Radiology, University of Texas Medical School, Chief, Hermann Hospital at Houston, Houston, Texas

SECONDO LASTORIA, M.D. Associate to the Chief, Department of Nuclear Medicine, National Cancer Institute, Naples, Italy

LUIGI MANSI, M.D. Associate Professor, Medicina Nucleare Istituto di Scienze Radiologiche, Second University of Naples, Naples, Italy

SHAHLA MASOOD, M.D., F.C.A.P., M.I.A.C. Professor and Associate Chair, Department of Pathology, Univeristy of Florida Health Science Center, Jacksonville, Florida

JEAN MAUBLANT, M.D., PH.D.   Professor, Division of Nuclear Medicine, Centre Jean Perrin, Clermont-Ferrand, France

PIETRO MUTO, M.D.   Associate Chief, Department of Nuclear Medicine, National Cancer Institute, Naples, Italy

HOLGER PALMEDO, M.D.   Physician, Clinic of Nuclear Medicine, University of Bonn, Bonn, Germany

FRANK J. PAPATHEOFANIS, M.D., PH.D.   Assistant Professor, The Institute for Biomedical Engineering, and Director, The Advanced Medical and Technology Assessment Program, University of California School of Medicine, La Jolla, California

BIAGIO PECORI, M.D.   Medicina Nucleare Istituto di Scienze Radiologiche, Second University of Naples, Naples, Italy

SERGIO PICCOLO, M.D.   Associate Chief, Department of Nuclear Medicine, National Cancer Institute, Naples, Italy

MARIO QUARANTELLI, M.D.   Medicina Nucleare Istituto di Scienze Radiologiche, Second University of Naples, Naples, Italy

PIER FRANCESCO RAMBALDI, M.D.   Medicina Nucleare Istituto di Scienze Radiologiche, Second University of Naples, Naples, Italy

ANTON SCHARL, M.D.   Department of Gynecology, University Hospital, Cologne, Germany

KLEMENS MARIA SCHEIDHAUER, M.D.   Department of Nuclear Medicine, University Hospital, Cologne, Germany

AXEL SCHOMBURG, M.D.   Department of Nuclear Medicine, Roentgeninstitut, Dusseldorf, Germany

RAYMOND TAILLEFER, M.D., F.R.C.P.(C), A.B.N.M.   Professor, Department of Nuclear Medicine, Centre Hospitalier de l'Université de Montreal, Montreal, Quebec, Canada

JORGE TOLMOS, M.D.   General Surgery Resident, Department of Surgery and Radiology, Harbor-UCLA Medical Center, Torrance, California

ROELF VALKEMA, M.D.   Physician, Department of Nuclear Medicine, University Hospital Rotterdam, Rotterdam, The Netherlands

CASPER H. J. VAN EIJCK, M.D., PH.D.   Surgical Oncologist, Department of General Surgery, University Hospital Rotterdam, Rotterdam, The Netherlands

HERNAN I. VARGAS, M.D.   Assistant Professor, Department of Surgery, Harbor-UCLA Medical Center, Torrance, California

ALAN D. WAXMAN, M.D.   Director, Department of Nuclear Medicine, Cedars-Sinai Medical Center and Clinical Professor of Radiology, University of Southern California School of Medicine, Los Angeles, California

1
Pathology of Breast Cancer

SHAHLA MASOOD and JOSEPH CHIAO
University of Florida Health Science Center, Jacksonville, Florida

I. INTRODUCTION

In recent years, improved mammographic techniques have resulted in a better recognition of subtle radiologic abnormalities and an earlier diagnosis of breast cancer [1]. The radiologic detection of in situ abnormalities and cancers <1 cm in size has resulted in better overall survival [2,3]. Controversy, however, remains in the cost-effectiveness of the widespread use of mammography as a screening procedure because of the relatively high cost of identification of each breast cancer patient [4,5]. Mammography suffers from relatively low specificity since only up to one-third of mammographically suspicious lesions are found to be malignant [6–8]. Thus, it is essential to obtain tissue diagnosis for all suspicious lesions noted at mammography. The occult lesions which are most amenable to cure offer the greatest dilemma for the physicians, since these are difficult to localize clinically for diagnostic biopsy.

Introduced in 1974, percutaneous needle localization biopsy procedure has provided an effective means of accurately and safely sampling clinically occult breast abnormalities [2,3,9,10]. These surgical biopsies, however, represent a large percentage of induced costs of screening for lesions that are frequently benign [11,12].

To avoid unnecessary surgical biopsies for women with an abnormal mammogram and benign breast disease, a less invasive sampling alternative, i.e., needle biopsy, has been introduced. Breast needle biopsy can be performed either as a fine needle aspiration biopsy or a core biopsy. These procedures can expedite patient diagnosis and treatment and may potentially reduce costs [13,14].

Controversy, however, remains as to the choice of needle, as well as the localizing device, for sampling of occult breast lesions. Similarly, there are still unresolved issues surrounding the precise diagnosis of radiologically detected breast lesions [15]. This overview is designed to address the issues that are commonly encountered in pathology practice.

II. HISTORY OF NEEDLE BIOPSY

Breast lesions can be sampled by a needle via clinical guidance or through one of three image guidance modalities—grid coordinate system, ultrasound, and stereotaxy. These modalities provide different degrees of accuracy and require varying degrees of training and experience.

Fine needle aspiration biopsy (FNAB) is the oldest procedure. The use of FNAB in evaluation of patients with palpable breast lesions dates back to 1930. Since then, FNAB has been viewed as a valid and challenging procedure that can provide valuable diagnostic and prognostic information [16–20]. Similarly, in nonpalpable breast lesions, when used in conjunction with appropriate radiologic guidance and in experienced hands, FNAB has improved the specificity of mammography [13,21–24]. Fine needle aspiration biopsy is known to provide several advantages over surgical biopsy. First, a woman is given an opportunity to have her breast lesion sampled and examined without significant morbidity and the associated costs. Second, it eliminates the need for short-term follow-up mammography of an indeterminate mass. Third, it provides minimal physical or psychological discomfort to the patient and leaves neither skin deformity nor parenchymal scar, which could interfere with subsequent follow-up study. In addition, the established diagnosis of breast cancer by needle biopsy provides more flexibility for treatment planning [25].

The diagnostic accuracy of palpable and nonpalpable breast lesions are similar. In review of the literature with analysis of data on 3000 cases of FNAB of nonpalpable breast lesions with histologic biopsy follow-up, we have demonstrated that the results are comparable to FNAB of palpable breast lesions. FNAB of palpable lesions has shown a sensitivity of 72% to 99% (average 87%) and specificity of 98% to 100% (average 97%). FNAB of nonpalpable lesions has shown a sensitivity of 68% to 100% (average 87%) and specificity of 82% to 100% (average 96%). The rate of insufficient samples in nonpalpable breast lesions is higher than those of palpable breast lesions. In contrast, this rate ranges between 4% and 3% in palpable breast lesions. FNAB of nonpalpable breast lesions carries an insufficient rate of 2% to 36% [26].

The high insufficient rate in breast FNAB, together with advances in radiological breast imaging, have focused interest in the use of stereotactic localization for sampling of nonpalpable breast lesions and the acquisition of core biopsy specimens with larger cutting needles [27,28].

Reports in the radiology literature have shown reductions in the number of insufficient cases by the use of stereotactic core biopsy. In addition, the agreement between stereotactic core biopsy and surgical biopsy diagnosis in these studies has been good to excellent, ranging from 87% to 100% [28,29].

The superiority of core biopsy versus FNAB in nonpalpable breast lesions has not been established and requires further controlled and well-designed studies. Dowlatshahi et al. [13] have compared the results of the two modalities in 250 patients with mammographically detected nonpalpable breast abnormalities suspicious for malignancy. They demonstrated that FNAB and core biopsy complement each other in the diagnosis of nonpalpable breast lesions. Complementing use of these procedures is now being practiced in some institutions [31]. However, it appears that the trend now is to use core needle biopsy for the initial assessment of nonpalpable breast lesions.

III.   GENERAL CONSIDERATIONS

To obtain a representative sample from an abnormal breast lesion, by either FNAB or core biopsy, it is important to develop a multidisciplinary team approach among the pathologist, the radiologist, and the clinician. The experience of the operator, the nature of the abnormality, the accuracy of needle placement, and the number of samples obtained are important factors to consider [27].

The presence of a cytopathologist or a pathologist for the assessment of the adequacy of the specimen and an immediate interpretation is of value in reducing the number of insufficient cases and also in decreasing the number of false-negative cases in FNAB [32,33]. It is also important to provide imprint preparation of the core needle biopsy samples to maximize the diagnostic accuracy of this procedure.

The effect of multiple passes and the size of the needle in nonpalpable breast sampling has remained controversial. While Parker et al. [29] conclude that 14-gauge needles provide more specific and sensitive results, there are other investigators who suggest that multiple passes with a 14-gauge needle an unacceptable for patient comfort and increased potential for complications [27].

Inappropriate sampling may lead to tissue fragmentation and extensive hemorrhage. This may cause difficulties in pathologic interpretation of the core biopsy. In these scenarios, scattered individual cells and clusters of epithelial cells may appear atypical and ultimately lead to an uncertain diagnosis (Figs. 1, 2).

Another major problem in nonsurgical sampling procedures is when a radiologically suspicious abnormality is missed or partially sampled (Fig. 3). Breast

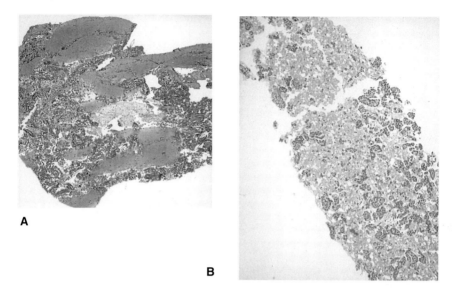

A

B

FIGURE I   Proliferative fibrocystic changes with artifacts that may render a differential diagnosis ranging from ductal carcinoma in situ (A) to invasive well-differentiated ductal carcinoma (B) [hematoxylin and eosin, (A) 4×, (B) 10×].

abnormalities are often heterogeneous, comprising benign, as well as malignant, components.

Sampling of such an abnormality may lead to a false-negative result. Sampling error may also occur when malignancy is not associated with the abnormality seen on the mammogram. As an example, lobular carcinoma in situ is a common incidental finding in tissue adjacent to but not within the abnormality for which the biopsy is performed [34,35].

The magnitude of the problems associated with sampling error has been heavily emphasized in FNAB procedure. This has had an adverse effect on the use of FNAB alone in sampling of nonpalpable breast lesions. Sampling error, however, also remains a concern for core needle biopsy. As an example, in situ lesions diagnosed by means of core biopsy often show areas of invasion at follow-up lumpectomy. Similarly, atypical hyperplasias diagnosed by core biopsy frequently demonstrate evidence of ductal carcinoma in situ on rebiopsy [36]. The rate of discovery of carcinoma in wider surgical excision of a lesion previously diagnosed as atypical hyperplasia by core biopsy has ranged between 50% and 60% [37,38].

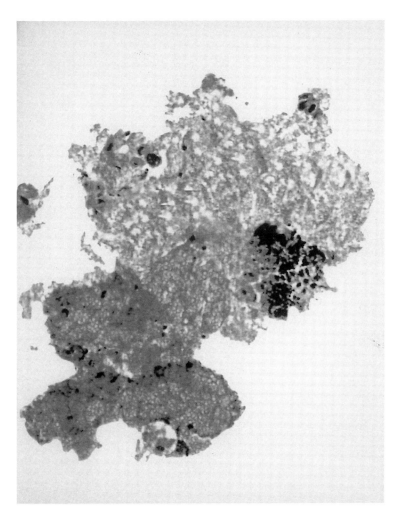

FIGURE 2   Ductal carcinoma that has extensive crush artifact that may render the core biopsy non-diagnostic (hematoxylin and eosin, 10×).

To overcome this problem, the radiologic abnormality should be correlated with tissue biopsy. The information should be incorporated in the communication process between the physician performing the biopsy and the pathologist. It is almost essential to confirm the presence of microcalcification by imaging the core biopsy specimen. For the pathologist sampling the specimen, a diligent search for microcalcification may be in order. This may include specimen radiography and extrasectioning of the specimen [39].

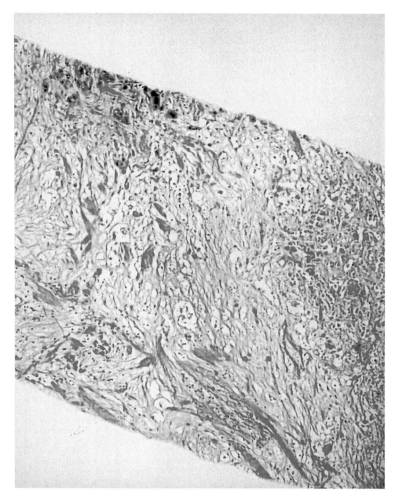

FIGURE 3   Core biopsy of a ductal carcinoma with only a few epithelial cells at the edge of the core tissue sample (hematoxylin and eosin, 10×).

It is equally important to realize that in nonsurgical biopsy procedures, the possibility of sampling error can never be completely excluded. Thus, it is essential to recommend further workup and/or close follow-up if the radiologic and pathologic findings do not correlate.

Aside from technical and sampling issues, there are inherent diagnostic difficulties in the interpretation of samples obtained by nonsurgical procedures. Smears from nonpalpable abnormalities are often of low cellularity [40]. This may lead to an impression of benignity or inadequacy and ultimately result in misinterpretation. Scant cellularity in mammography-detected abnormalities may sometimes be related to the small size of the lesions.

Some cases will always have a very scant cellularity, regardless of the size or localizing device. Hann et al. [40] reported that 40% of inadequate cases were from fibrotic and hypocellular abnormalities from which a low cellular yield would be anticipated. The histologic type and the nature of the lesion also play an important role in a diagnostic yield. Typically, medullary, mucinous, and comedo-carcinomas are more cellular than infiltrating lobular and scirrhous ductal carci-nomas. Benign lesions such as sclerosing adenosis and hyalinized fibroadenoma may be associated with a low yield.

In core biopsy, fragmentation and small size of the specimen may create diagnostic difficulty. Occasional artifactual distortion of the tissue may lead to misplacement of epithelial cells, making it difficult to assess whether the mis-placed epithelium represents a hyperplastic process, a ductal carcinoma in situ, or an invasive process [41]. Malignant seedling from the needle track in stereotaxic core biopsy is another issue to consider [42].

The level of complexity involved in the interpretation of a breast FNAB is different from core biopsy. Fine needle aspiration biopsy requires the availability of an interested pathologist with special training in breast cytopathology who also recognizes the limitations of breast FNAB. The diagnosis in FNAB is based on cellular elements only (Fig. 4). In contrast, aside from a smaller sample size, the morphologic criteria used in interpretation of a core biopsy are similar to those that have been well described for surgical pathology of the breast (Fig. 5). This may explain why core biopsy is preferred by many pathologists to FNAB.

IV. SPECIAL CONSIDERATION

Nonsurgical breast sampling usually results in a specimen that is significantly smaller than those obtained by traditional excisional breast biopsy. The handling of these specimens should comply with the recommended standardized guide-lines specifically developed for FNAB and core biopsies [43–45].

Adequacy of samples may be assessed via immediate microscopic evalua-tion of aspirated material or through visual examination of the cores of tissues [25,31,43]. Samples from each breast lesion must be identified and separately submitted for morphologic evaluation.

In order to accurately assess the presence or absence of calcification and to optimize histopathologic-radiographic correlation, the pathologist must have appropriate information about the location, size, number or type of calcification, and the mammographic abnormality in a given patient [46].

It is advisable to refrain from frozen-section preparation of tissue obtained

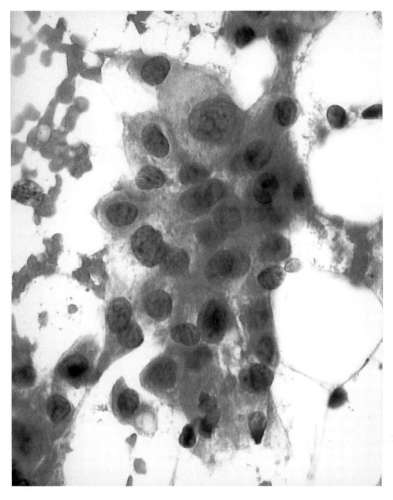

FIGURE 4   Fine needle aspiration biopsy of a ductal carcinoma showing a group of malignant ductal epithelial cells with pleomorphic and large nuclei with irregular nuclear membrane borders (papanicolaou stain, 40×).

from nonpalpable microcalcification [45,47]. The commonly seen nonpalpable lesions, such as atypical ductal hyperplasia, radial scar, and complex papillary breast lesions, are difficult to interpret in frozen-section preparations. Foci of in situ lesions or small sites of microinvasion may be lost in frozen-section preparation. Imprint preparations for immediate cytologic examination of a suspicious mammographic lesion provide an attractive alternative in providing adequate information.

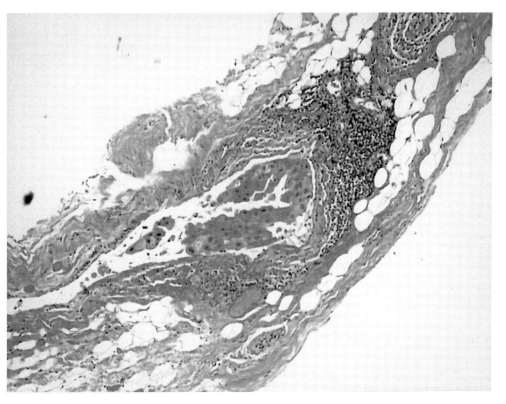

FIGURE 5   Core needle biopsy of nonproliferative fibrocystic change. The center of the biopsy shows apocrine changes surrounded by chronic inflammatory cells (lymphocytes) (hematoxylin and eosin, 10×).

In core biopsy, the pathologist should examine carefully for small but significant lesions and should identify the lesion for which the biopsy was performed. It is also important to recognize lesions that may require repeat biopsy or surgical excision, such as atypical ductal hyperplasia [48].

Occasionally, if calcification is not identified in the initial histologic sections, deeper levels should be examined. In the search for microcalcification, it may be necessary to radiograph the paraffin blocks or to use polarized light microscopy to identify calcium axalate crystals. These crystals are colorless in routinely stained tissue section, and may be overlooked [49].

Pathology reports for core biopsies should include information about the histologic grade and about special types, including the presence or absence of coexistent ductal carcinoma in situ as well as blood vessel and/or lymphatic vessel invasion. In cases of ductal carcinoma in situ, it is important to incorporate the architectural type, the nuclear grade, and the presence or absence of necrosis [44,50–52].

Samples from FNAB or core biopsy can be effectively utilized for ancillary studies to provide prognostic information. These include the study of the status of estrogen and progesterone receptor protein, p-glycoprotein, oncogenes, tumor suppressor genes by immunocytochemistry and DNA analysis, and proliferation rate by flow cytometry or image analysis (Figs. 6–9) [53–57].

Prognostic testing should only be performed in circumstances when a subsequent surgical specimen (lumpectomy or mastectomy) may not be available. This is to avoid possible false-negative results due to the small samples and the presence of intramural antigenic heterogeneity [58].

The small size of the samples obtained from mammographically detected lesions, and the inherent nature of specific lesions in the breast, such as atypical hyperplasia, occasionally preclude rendering a definite diagnosis by a pathologist. There are also benign lesions, such as radial scar, that have high incidence of coexisting cancer. In these scenarios, it is important to consider rebiopsy or wider surgical excision of a lesion (Fig. 10) [48,59,60].

V.   DIAGNOSTIC DILEMMAS IN PATHOLOGY OF NONPALPABLE BREAST LESIONS

With increasing use of screening mammography, more cases of high-risk proliferative breast diseases and carcinoma in situ are being detected. This is exemplified by the incidence of ductal carcinoma in situ (DCIS). As a palpable mass, DCIS accounted for <3% of breast cancers [61,62]. As detected by mammography, this incidence has increased to 30% [63]. There are also specific benign and malignant breast diseases that are commonly encountered by abnormal mammographic findings.

A.   Fibrocystic Change

Fibrocystic change is the most commonly diagnosed benign breast disease. This refers to a spectrum of changes that range from cysts, fibrosis, apocrine metaplasia, and sclerosing adenosis to varying degrees of proliferative changes, including atypical hyperplasia [64]. These changes with and without microcalcifications can be recognized on core biopsy (Fig. 11). The presence of microcalcification in the histologic sections helps to assure that the appropriate area is sampled [65].

Assessment of the degree of proliferative changes is of clinical significance and allows stratification of a lesion into nonproliferative and proliferative breast disease. There is a correlation between proliferative breast disease and subsequent development of breast cancers [66,67].

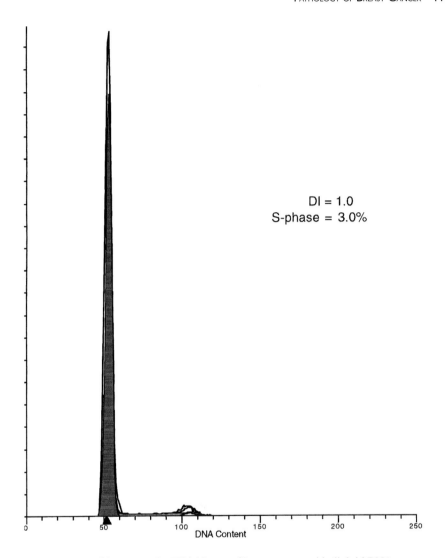

DI = 1.0
S-phase = 3.0%

DNA Content

Figure 6   DNA histogram of a FNA biopsy of breast cancer with diploid DNA pattern.

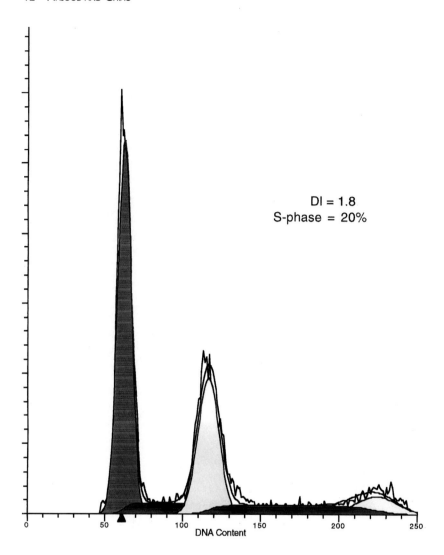

FIGURE 7   DNA histogram of a core biopsy of breast cancer with aneuploid DNA pattern.

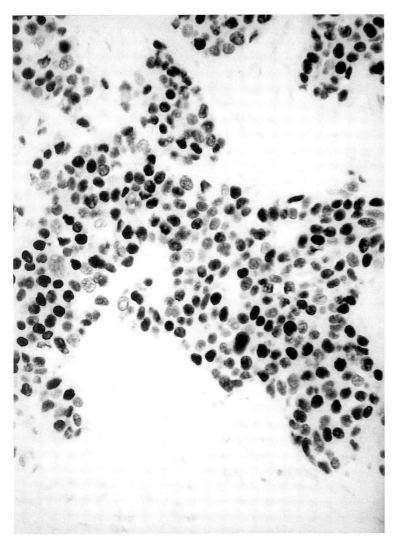

FIGURE 8 Cancer cells immunoreactive (nuclear staining) to estrogen (ER-positive) (immunoperoxidase, 20×).

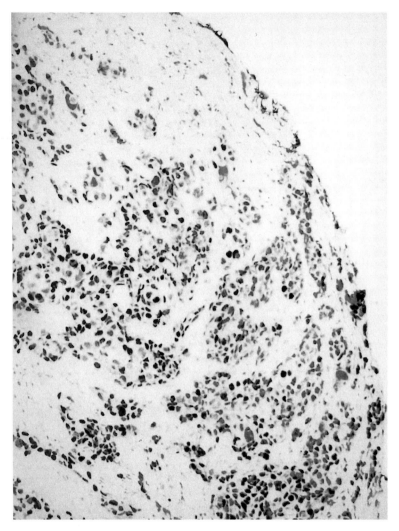

FIGURE 9   Reactive immunostaining to p53 protein, a tumor suppressor gene product (immunoperoxidase, 10×).

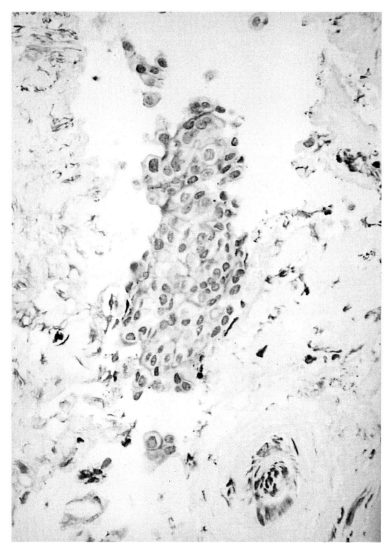

FIGURE 10   Cytoplasmic immunoreactivity to HER-2/neu oncogene (immunoperoxidase, 20×).

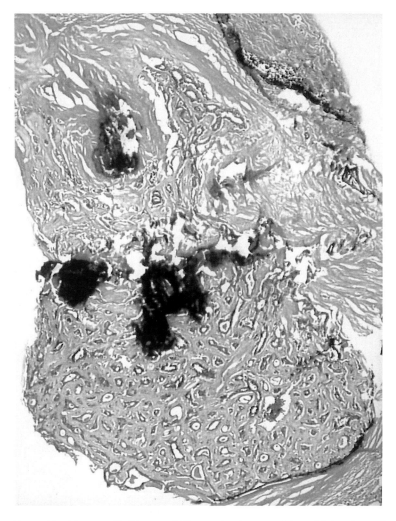

FIGURE 11   Core needle biopsy of fibrocystic changes with multiple microcalcifications seen here as dark gray to black irregular amorphous structures (hematoxylin and eosin, 4×).

The criteria for the diagnosis of proliferative breast disease have been defined in breast FNAB. In a prospective study of mammographically guided FNAB of 100 palpable breast lesions, my colleagues and I assessed the reliability of a cytologic grading system in defining the cytologic features of proliferative breast disease. We developed a cytologic grading system to evaluate smears for cellular arrangement, the degree of cellular pleomorphism and anisonucleosis,

TABLE 1   Cytologic Criteria/Grading System for Interpretation of Mammographically Guided Fine Needle Aspiration Biopsy

Cellular arrangement	Cellular pleomorphism	Myoepithelial cells	Anisonu-cleosis	Nucleoli	Chromatin clumping	Score[a]
Monolayer	Absent	Many	Absent	Absent	Absent	1
Nuclear overlapping	Mild	Moderate	Mild	Micronucleoli	Rare	2
Clustering	Moderate	Few	Moderate	Micro- and/ or rare macronucleoli	Occasional	3
Loss of cohesion	Conspicuous	Absent	Conspicuous	Predominantly micronucleoli	Frequent	4

Source: Masood S, Frykeberg ER, McLellan GL, et al. Prospective evaluation of radiologically detected fine needle aspiration biopsy of nonpalpable breast lesions. Cancer 66:1480–1487, 1990.
[a]Total score: nonproliferative breast disease, 6–10; proliferative breast disease without atypia, 11–14; proliferative breast disease with atypia, 15–18; carcinoma in situ and invasive cancer, 19–24.

the presence of myoepithelial cells and nuclei, and the chromatin pattern. Values ranging from 1 to 4 were assigned to each criterion, and a score based on the sum of individual values was calculated for each case (Tables 1, 2). When we compared the cytologic diagnosis with the histologic diagnosis obtained from follow-up needle localizing excisional biopsies, we found a high concordance between the results (Table 3) (Figs. 12–14) [22].

The significance of our study is in the introduction of a cytologic grading system that could enable us to define the spectrum of cytological changes seen in benign, high-risk, and proliferative breast disease. The recognition of atypical proliferative changes via breast FNAB cytology also provides an opportunity to identify high-risk breast cancer patients. This is particularly important for sampling and monitoring of surrogate endpoint biomarkers in chemoprevention trials [68–71].

Fibrocystic change can be seen adjacent to an in situ and/or an invasive carcinoma. Thus, it is necessary to confirm that the suspicious area on the mammogram is well sampled. Another concern in the use of FNAB and core biopsy in the diagnosis of fibrocystic change is the inherent limitation in the interpretation of these lesions. As in surgical biopsy, there is still significant confusion in the differentiation of atypical ductal hyperplasia from low-grade DCIS. This is reflected in the significant interobserver variability reported among pathologists in the diagnosis of these borderline lesions [72]. This problem is compounded in nonsurgical biopsy because of the small size of the samples, as well as the occasional artifactual distortion of the core biopsy. Thus, as in FNAB, when the diagnosis of

TABLE 2   Cytologic Findings Compared with Histologic Diagnosis in 100 Mammographically Suspicious Cases

| | | Histologic diagnosis | | | | | |
| | | | | | Carcinoma in situ | | Invasive |
Cytology	No. of cases	Non proliferative breast disease	Proliferative without atypia	Proliferative with atypia	LCIS	DCIS	cancer
Insufficient cellular material	9	7	2	—	—	—	—
Nonproliferative breast disease	34	29	4	—	1[a]	—	—
Proliferative without atypia	17	—	15	2	—	—	—
Proliferative with atypia	23	—	—	21	1[a]	1[a]	—
Carcinoma	17	—	—	—	—	5	12
Total	100	36	21	23	2	6	12

Source: Masood S, Frykeberg ER, McLellan GL et al. Prospective evaluation of radiologically detected fine needle aspiration biopsy of nonpalpable breast lesions. Cancer 66:1480–1487, 1990.

[a]False-negative cytologic interpretations.

LCIS, lobular carcinoma in situ; DCIS, ductal carcinoma in situ.

TABLE 3   Concordance Between Cytologic Evaluation and Histologic Diagnosis in 100 Mammographically Guided Fine Needle Aspirates

Diagnosis	No. of cases	Concordance (%)
Nonproliferative breast disease	29/34	85
Proliferative breast disease without atypia	15/17	88
Proliferative breast disease with atypia	21/23	91
Cancer	17/20	85

Source: Masood S, Frykberg ER, McLellan GL, et al. Cytologic differentiation between proliferative and nonproliferative breast disease in mammographically guided fine needle aspirates. Diagn Cytopathol 7:581–590, 1991.

atypical hyperplasia is suggested, it is advisable to recommend follow-up surgical biopsy [68].

Atypical hyperplasia is indeed a diagnostic challenge for a pathologist. This entity defines a noninfiltrating breast abnormality with some, but not all, of the features of cancer. Atypical hyperplasia occupies an intermediate position between

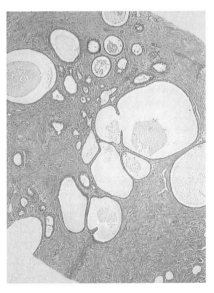
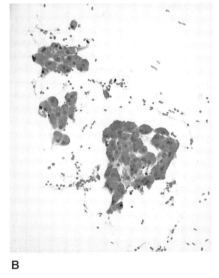

B

A

FIGURE 12   Core needle biopsy and fine needle aspiration biopsy of nonproliferative fibrocystic change. (A) The core biopsy shows cysts with apocrine epithelial lining cells. (B) The cytology sample shows apocrine metaplastic epithelial cells [(A) hematoxylin and eosin, 4×; (B) papanicolaou, 10×].

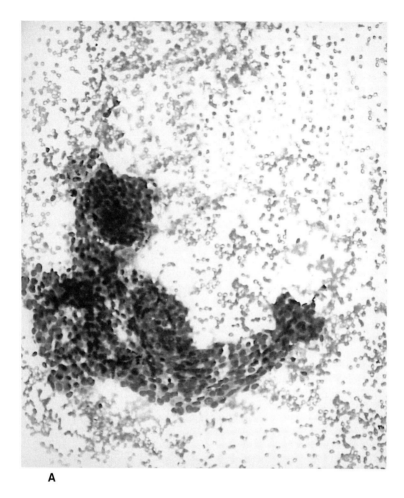

A

FIGURE 13   Core biopsy and FNAB (A) cytology of proliferative fibrocystic changes without atypia. (B) The biopsy is from a sclerosing adenosis which is an example of proliferative changes when the intraductal fibrosis becomes more prominent [(B) hematoxylin and eosin, 10×; (A) Diff-Quik, 20×].

benign and malignant lesions. The differentiation between atypical hyperplasia and low-grade ductal carcinoma in situ has major clinical implications, and yet truly reproducible morphologic criteria to ascertain the correct diagnosis are not present.

Attempts have been made to utilize ancillary studies to distinguish between atypical ductal hyperplasia and DCIS. We have observed that immunostaining for muscle-specific actin highlights the myoepithelial cells in atypical ductal hyper-

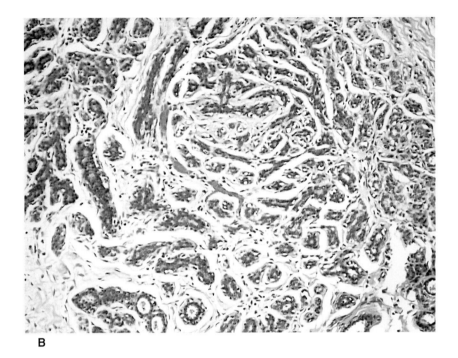

B

FIGURE 13   Continued

plasia and can be used as a useful diagnostic adjunct [73–75]. Our experience and others' reported in the literature, however, have concluded that other ancillary studies such as the study of HER-2/neu oncogene expression, DNA ploidy and/or nuclear measurements do not provide or substantiate evidence to differentiate between atypical hyperplasia and carcinoma [76–79]. Thus, until we design a long-term prospective study monitoring the natural history of atypical hyperplasias and ductal carcinoma in situ, the unresolved diagnostic issues will continue and create confusion for the patients, pathologists, and clinicians.

B.   Fibroadenomas

As a biphasic tumor, characterized by stromal proliferation which compresses adjacent ductal structures, a typical fibroadenoma, in a well-represented sample, can be easily recognized in FNAB and core biopsy (Fig. 15a,b). Technical difficulties in sampling may arise since fibroadenomas are typically firm and mobile [29]. In cases where the stroma is extremely hyalinized, it is difficult to recognize the biphasic stromal and epithelial features (Fig. 16).

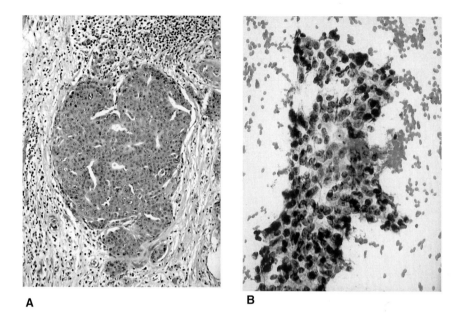

A
B

FIGURE 14 Core biopsy (A) and FNAB (B) cytology of proliferative fibrocystic changes with atypia [(A) hematoxylin and eosin, 10×; (B) papanicolaou, 30×].

Occasionally, extensive proliferative changes may occur in ductal elements of a fibroadenoma and create diagnostic difficulty in the interpretation of smears obtained from a fine needle aspirate. Other conditions such as squamous metaplasia, inflammatory processes, pregnancy, and hormonal changes may create cytologic atypia in a fibroadenoma (Fig. 17). In these circumstances, age, clinical presentation, and mammographic features may help to render a correct diagnosis.

The distinction between fibroadenoma and benign phyllodes tumor poses another diagnostic challenge in nonsurgical sampling of breast lesions. Malignant phyllodes tumors often present with mitoses and nuclear atypia. Benign phyllodes tumor has an unpredictable clinical outcome and often occurs at an older age than fibroadenomas. It is advisable to recommend surgical excision if a breast lesion shows increased stromal cellularity in both FNAB and core biopsy [25].

C. Intraductal Papilloma

Intraductal papilloma is a benign papilliform proliferation of ductal epithelium which is characterized by a prominent fibrovascular core lined by a two-cell ductal epithelial/myoepithelial layer (Fig. 18) [80,81]. The size varies from a few mil-

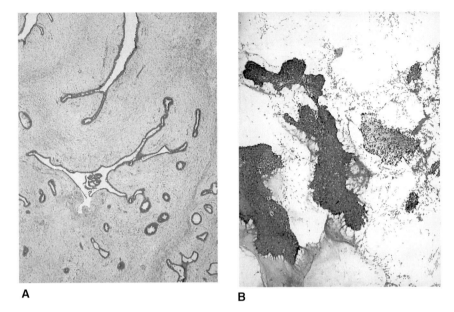

A   **B**

FIGURE 15   Histology and cytology of a fibroadenoma. The histologic section (A) consists of stroma with fibroblastic proliferation and epithelial ducts distorted into leaf or slit-like structures (intracanalicular pattern). The FNAB (B) cytology specimens are cellular with a biphasic pattern consisting of epithelial and stromal elements; with the ductal elements forming monolayered sheets resembling antler horns [(A) hematoxylin and eosin, 2×; (B) papanicolaou, 4×].

limeters to a few centimeters in diameter. Mammography following galactography helps to identify and localize small intraductal papillomas. The distinction between intraductal papilloma and intraductal carcinoma is difficult and may require demonstration of myoepithelial cells by immunostaining for muscle-specific actin [82,83]. It is best to recommend surgical biopsy of the entire lesion if there is any doubt in the exact nature of a papillary lesion [25].

D.   Ductal Carcinoma In Situ

The distinction between invasive versus DCIS and precise subtyping of in situ carcinoma is important for appropriate management of patients with breast cancer [84,85]. The morphologic features of these entities are well described. However, there is a limitation in differentiation between invasive and in situ breast carcinomas by FNAB [25,69,79]. This distinction requires assessment of the integrity of the basement membrane and the architectural pattern that only histopathology can provide.

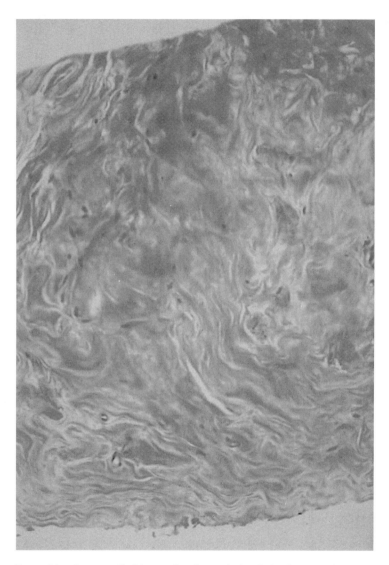

FIGURE 16 Core needle biopsy showing only hyalinized stroma from a fibroadenoma (hematoxylin and eosin, 10×).

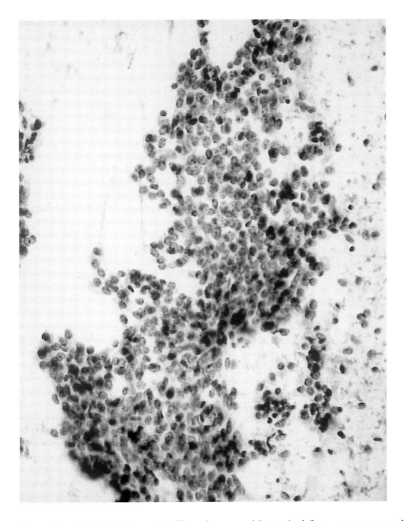

FIGURE 17   FNAB cytology of a fibroadenoma with atypical features represented here as discohesion, slight nuclear enlargement and nuclear overlapping (papanicolaou, 30×).

Nevertheless, if coupled with clinical presentation and mammographic features, FNAB can reliably distinguish between an in situ and an invasive breast cancer. This includes recognition of special subtypes of ductal carcinoma such as mucinous, medullary, sarcomatoid, and small-cell carcinoma. These tumors most often present as an invasive lesion. Similarly, association with skin retraction, ulceration, nipple fixation, inflammatory carcinoma, and/or evidence of metastasis indicates an advanced breast carcinoma.

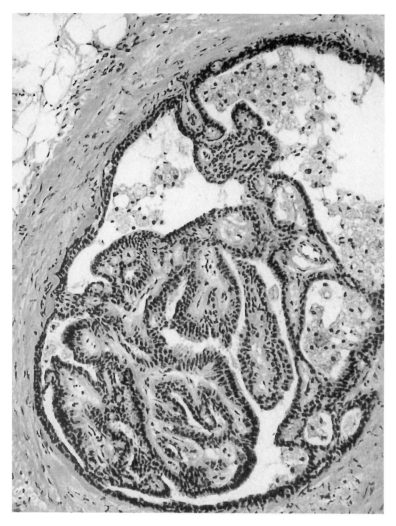

FIGURE 18   Histologic example of an intraductal papilloma (hematoxylin and eosin, 10×).

In contrast to FNAB, in a well-sampled core biopsy, it is possible to reliably distinguish between DCIS and invasive cancer (Figs. 19, 20). However, there are occasional cases when sampling error may result in misrepresentation of a breast lesion and lead to a misdiagnosis. As previously mentioned, core biopsy can miss an area of invasion adjacent to an in situ cancer. Similarly, carcinoma in situ with early stromal invasion may be underdiagnosed. In addition, distortion of the ducts involved with DCIS may lead to false-positive diagnosis of cancer.

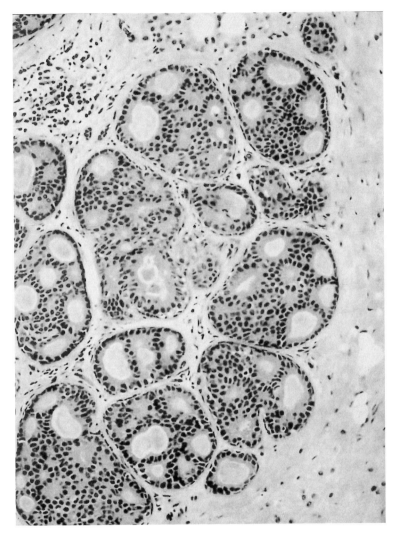

FIGURE 19   Ductal carcinoma in situ with cribriform features (hematoxylin and eosin, 10×).

If the clinical management of DCIS is similar to that of an invasive ductal carcinoma, the distinction between the two entities may not be critical. Otherwise, it is essential to recommend confirmatory surgical biopsy to precisely assess the presence or absence of tumor invasion. This is particularly important for patients selected for preoperative chemotherapy or radiotherapy.

Subtyping of DCIS is also important prognostically. DCIS has been tradi-

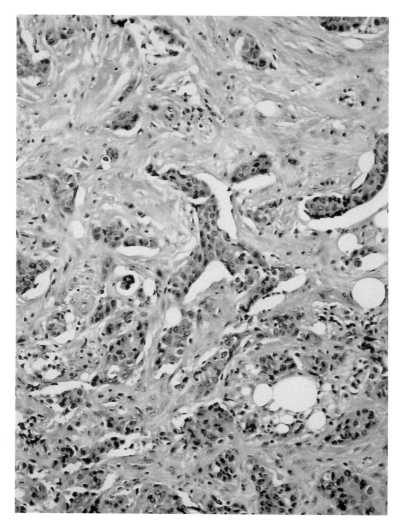

FIGURE 20   Infiltrating ductal carcinoma (hematoxylin and eosin, 20×).

tionally subtyped on the basis of architectural features. These include comedo, cribriform, papillary, micropapillary, and solid types with distinct differences in multiplicity and tendency toward microinvasion. Various types of treatment have been preposed based on histologic subtype [86,87].

Lagios et al. [88], in 1989, were the first to suggest another classification based on nuclear grade and presence or absence of necrosis. This was a clear departure from the traditional classification. The new classification also stratified DCIS into a group with a high risk of local recurrence (i.e., those with high nuclear grade) and a group with a very low rate of local recurrence (i.e., those with low nuclear grade). Subsequently, Silverstein et al. [89] demonstrated that the high nuclear grade and presence of necrosis are significant predictors of local recurrence after breast conservation therapy in patients with DCIS.

Since then, several other classification systems for DCIS have been introduced [90–92]. Three main subtypes of DCIS are recognized: high, intermediate, and low grade. This is also based on the study of biological markers in DCIS. Studies have shown that high-grade lesions are typically hormone receptor-negative, have a high proliferation rate, are aneuploid, and often show expression of HER-2/neu oncogene and tumor suppressor gene p53. In contrast, low-grade lesions are hormone receptor-positive, are diploid, and have a low proliferation rate and rare expression of HER-2/neu oncogene, bcl-2 and p53. The intermediate group shows biological marker profiles that are intermediate between those of high- and low-grade lesions [93].

Despite all the efforts to introduce a practical classification scheme for DCIS, difficulty remains in the reproducibility. Lack of consensus on these very important issues has significant clinical and therapeutic implications.

E. Radial Scar

Radial scar is a fibroelastic core surrounded by radiating ducts and lobules displaying various amounts of epithelial hyperplasia, adenosis, or ectasia. The central core often shows entrapped tubular structures (Fig. 21) [94]. Radial scar typically presents as small, nonpalpable lesions that measure only a few millimeters. Radial scar is strongly associated with bilaterality and multiplicity [95]. Radiographically, radial scar appears as small, spiculated structures that mimic cancer. Grossly, this lesion appears firm with a satellite pattern that characteristically has central puckering and creamy white streaks of elastica that may be indistinguishable from carcinoma.

Microscopically, radial scar is difficult to diagnose by frozen section. The appearance of the lesion depends on the degree of sclerosis and the nature of proliferative changes [96]. Women with biopsy-treated tubular carcinoma do not have an increased risk of subsequent development of breast cancer [97]. However, the presence of intraductal carcinoma or lobular neoplasia within the radial scar are associated with an unfavorable prognosis [98].

Precise diagnosis of radial scar by FNAB and core biopsy is difficult. The cytologic differential diagnosis includes low-grade carcinomas such as non-comedo type DCIS and lobular and tubular carcinomas [99]. Similarly, radial scar

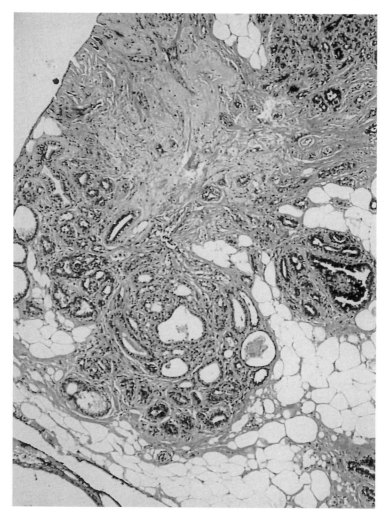

FIGURE 21   Biopsy sample of a radial scar with a "pseudoinfiltrative" appearance (hematoxylin and eosin, 4×).

often has a "pseudoinfiltrative" appearance in tissue sections which can only be distinguished in the context of the architecture of the entire abnormality. Thus, it is difficult to assume that this lesion can be completely sampled and accurately diagnosed by core biopsy. In addition, radial scar has been found to have coexistent carcinoma in 20% of the cases [100]. This may explain why it is advisable to recommend an open surgical biopsy when the diagnosis of radial scar is being entertained by either FNAB or core biopsy.

VI. INVASIVE BREAST CARCINOMA

A. Infiltrating Duct Cell Carcinoma

The most common breast carcinoma is infiltrating duct cell carcinoma which can be detected clinically or by the use of mammography. The clinical presentation, radiological features, and the gross and microscopic appearance of infiltrating duct cell carcinoma vary among different patients. Morphologically, infiltrating duct cell carcinoma is characterized by a spectrum of changes that vary according to the degree of differentiation, extent of stromal reaction, and presence or absence of necrosis and inflammatory cells.

The diagnosis of infiltrating duct cell carcinoma by FNAB or core biopsy in a well-sampled lesion is not difficult (Fig. 22a,b). However, there are lesions, such as sclerosing adenosis or radial scar, that can simulate the infiltrative pattern of a cancer and lead to false-positive diagnosis on core biopsy. Increased cellularity and atypia in fibroadenomas, pregnancy-associated changes, treatment-induced changes, and atypical ductal hyperplasia are potential causes of false-positive diagnosis in FNAB [25].

To avoid false-negative diagnosis, repeat sampling by FNAB, core biopsy, or an open surgical biopsy is necessary when there is nonconcordance of the pathology results with the differential diagnosis for the imaging abnormalities. Liberman et al. have shown that with nonconcordance, carcinoma may be found in 47% of cases upon repeat biopsy [36].

B. Infiltrating Lobular Carcinoma

The next most common breast carcinoma is infiltrating lobular carcinoma which characteristically presents with a deceptively bland morphology. Infiltrating lobular carcinoma is the most common cause of false-negative diagnosis in breast FNAB [101]. In core biopsy, the typical infiltrative pattern of lobular carcinoma helps to suggest the correct diagnosis (Fig. 23a, b).

Infiltrating lobular carcinoma may be mixed with ductal carcinoma. This may result in a discrepancy between the report on core biopsy versus the result on the lumpectomy or mastectomy specimen. This distinction, however, has no clinical significance, since the treatment of these two entities is similar.

It should be remembered that a diagnosis of lobular carcinoma in situ should not be accepted as consistent with mammographic findings requiring biopsy. This entity has no characteristic imaging findings. Thus, in the presence of diagnosis of lobular carcinoma in situ in a core biopsy, a repeat biopsy should be considered to sample the exact site of abnormality seen by mammography.

C. Low-Grade Carcinomas

Aside from common breast carcinomas, several histologic subtypes of invasive carcinomas are viewed as low-grade tumors and are associated with

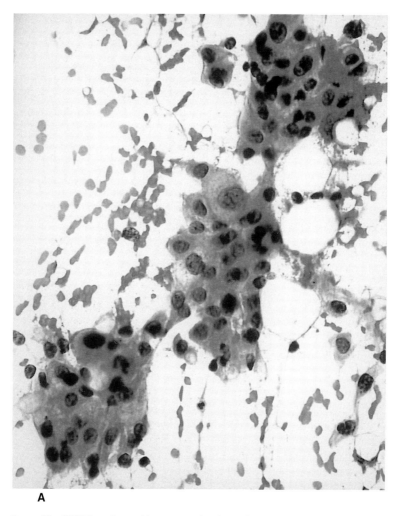

A

FIGURE 22   FNAB and core biopsy samples from the same case of an infiltrating duct cell carcinoma [(B) hematoxylin and eosin, 4×; (A) papanicolaou, 30×].

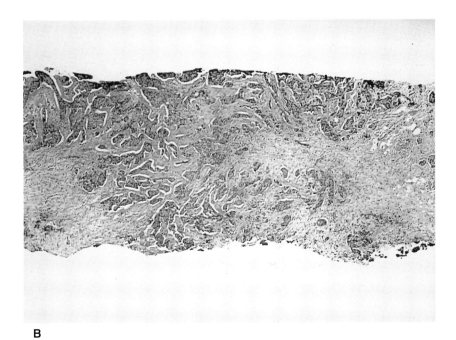

B

Figure 22   Continued

a good prognosis. These include tubular, colloid, papillary, and medullary carcinoma [102].

D. Tubular Carcinoma

Tubular carcinoma is a distinct variant of breast carcinoma which constitutes about 20% of nonpalpable breast lesions [103]. It occurs in younger age groups than infiltrating duct cell carcinoma, and is associated with a higher incidence of bilaterality and multiplicity [104]. A family history of breast carcinoma has been found in 40% of patients with tubular carcinoma [105]. Mammographically, tubular carcinoma presents as a small spiculated abnormality or as an early ductal carcinoma [106].

The diagnosis of tubular carcinoma by FNAB or core biopsy is difficult since there is minimal nuclear abnormality and the architectural pattern of breast tissue is well maintained. Tubular carcinoma can be mistaken for a variety of conditions such as radial scar or complex sclerosing abnormality with a "pseudoinfiltrative" appearance. The presence of one cell layer in the ducts and lack of

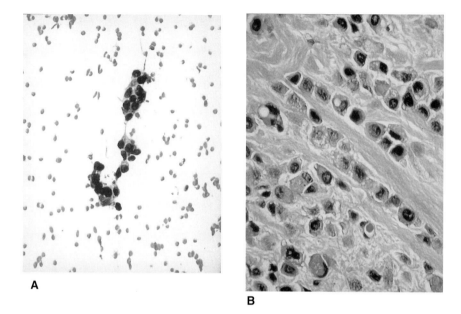

A

B

FIGURE 23A,B   FNAB and core biopsy from a lobular carcinoma. The histologic sample (B) shows the classic "single-file" growth pattern. The cytology (A) of a lobular carcinoma often has scant cellularity with cells singly or in small groups composed of uniform small cells with mild atypia. [(B) hematoxylin and eosin, 40×; (A) papanicolaou, 30×].

myoepithelial cells in ducts may differentiate tubular carcinoma from other entities (Fig. 24a, b).

E.   Mucinous (Colloid) Carcinoma

Another prognostically good variant of ductal cell carcinoma is mucinous (colloid) carcinoma. Mucinous carcinoma occurs in older age groups and has a distinct appearance characterized by a soft, gelatinous consistency. Microscopically, isolated epithelial cells and cell clusters are seen scattered within lakes of mucin (Fig. 25a, b).

The diagnosis of mucinous carcinoma in FNAB and core biopsy is usually not difficult. The clinical information on the age of the patient can easily exclude the possibility of mucocele as a differential diagnosis [25]. However, in the presence of a mixed mucinous carcinoma, FNAB or core biopsy can potentially miss

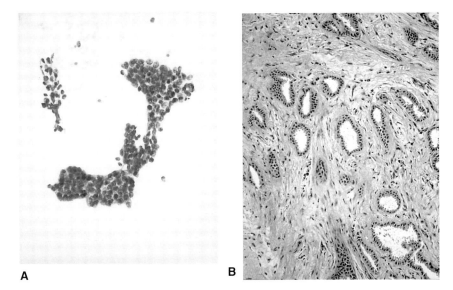

A   B

FIGURE 24   (A) FNAB and core biopsy (B) from a tubular carcinoma [(B) hematoxylin and eosin, 10×; (A) papanicolaou, 20×].

the infiltrating component. This is prognostically important, since mixed forms of mucinous carcinoma behave the same as an infiltrating duct cell carcinoma [107]. Therefore, it may be necessary to perform a surgical biopsy to assess the patient prognosis on evaluation of the entire lesion.

F. Medullary Carcinoma

Medullary carcinoma is also viewed as another subtype of breast cancer which carries a good prognosis. It presents as a well-defined soft lesion and may resemble a fibroadenoma clinically and mammographically. Medullary carcinoma has a distinct gross appearance of a fleshy lesion and contrasts with the typical shrunken and firm appearance of the other breast cancers. Microscopically, medullar carcinoma is characterized by a syncytial growth pattern in which anastomosing cords and sheets are separated by small amounts of loose connective tissue and surrounded by a conspicuous lymphocytic infiltrate. The tumor cells are large and pleomorphic and have prominent nucleoli (Fig. 26a, b) [108,109].

The diagnosis of medullary carcinoma can only be suggested by FNAB or core biopsy, since the final diagnosis of medullary carcinoma is based on gross

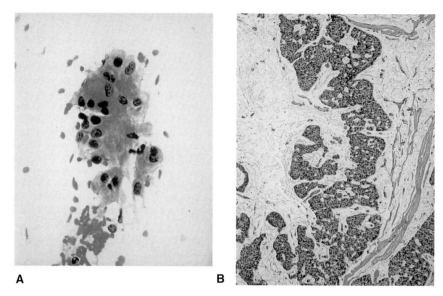

A   **B**

FIGURE 25   FNAB (A) and core biopsy (B) samples of mucinous (colloid) carcinoma. The histology (B) shows groups of tumor cells surrounded by abundant extracellular mucin [(B) hematoxylin and eosin, 4×; papanicolaou, 30×].

and microscopic assessment of the border of the tumor and its relation with the surrounding breast tissue. In addition, it may be difficult to differentiate a medullary carcinoma from a poorly differentiated duct cell carcinoma with lymphocytic infiltrate. Associated with sampling error, the representative specimen may also only display the lymphoid component and lead to a misdiagnosis of malignant lymphoma. In this case, immunophenotypic analysis of aspirated material or core biopsy specimen by either flow cytometry or immunocytochemistry may substantiate the diagnosis [25].

G.   Papillary Carcinoma

Papillary carcinoma is also associated with a good prognosis. It often occurs in postmenopausal women and may also develop in male breast [110,111]. As a variant of an intraductal carcinoma, papillary carcinoma may cause bloody nipple discharge, skin dimpling, and nipple retraction or deviation.

Papillary carcinoma presents as a palpable mass in 90% of patients. Therefore, our experience is limited in relation to the diagnosis of papillary carcinoma

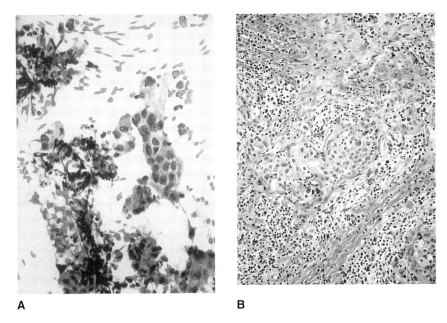

A   B

FIGURE 26   FNAB (A) and biopsy (B) of medullary carcinoma. Note the close association of lymphocytes and the malignant epithelial component [(B) hematoxylin and eosin,10×; (A) papanicolaou, 30×].

as a nonpalpable lesion sampled by FNAB or core biopsy. Nevertheless, based on our information on FNAB of palpable breast lesions, as well as surgical pathology, we recognize the same dilemma in the distinction between intraductal papilloma and papillary carcinoma of the breast. Thus, a surgical excisional biopsy including a rim of normal surrounding breast tissue is essential for any case suspicious of a papillary lesion of the breast by FNAB or core biopsy.

VII.   REPORTING, MANAGEMENT, AND FOLLOW-UP

Similar to an excisional biopsy, it is the responsibility of pathologists to provide pertinent information to the clinician and to the patient via his/her report and to follow the national guidelines [43,45,112]. The importance of the accuracy of the pathology report cannot be overemphasized, since it defines the nature of a lesion as being benign or malignant, and dictates therapy. In addition, when a nonsurgical biopsy shows benign features, there might be an associated change in the risk status of a patient for subsequent development of breast cancer (Table 4) [113]. Furthermore, the report gives a message as how a patient should be managed and

TABLE 4   Benign Breast Disease and Relative Risk for Subsequent Development of Invasive Breast Cancer

No increased risk	Slight risk (1.5- to 2.0-fold)	Moderate (4-to 5-fold)	High (8- to 10-fold)
Nonproliferative breast disease	Proliferative breast disease without atypia	Proliferative breast disease with atypia	In situ carcinomas
Cyst	Florid sclerosing adenosis	Atypical hyperplasia, ductal or lobular	Lobular carcinoma in situ
Duct ectasis	Moderate or florid ductal hyperplasia		Ductal carcinoma in situ
Fibroadenoma	Papilloma with fibrovascular core		
Mild epithelial hyperplasia			
Mild sclerosing adenosis			
Fibrosis			
Mastitis			
Metaplasia, squamous, or apocrine			

monitored (Figs. 27, 28). The report also influences other issues such as compliance and the cost associated with nonsurgical sampling of nonpalpable breast lesions. As an example, awareness of the risk factors has already shown to enhance the compliance rate for screening mammography [112–116]. This further emphasizes the role of communication in the practice of medicine.

VIII.   SUMMARY

Nonsurgical sampling of nonpalpable breast lesions is a potentially effective means of providing diagnostic and prognostic information. Aside from technical and diagnostic issues, measures should be taken to incorporate adequate training and quality control measures to justify the use of these procedures. It is equally important to recognize the limitations of these procedures and the necessity for rebiopsy or wider excision of specific lesions. It should also be realized that we need further well-designed and well-controlled prospective studies to address long-term patient outcome and the emerging economic issues.

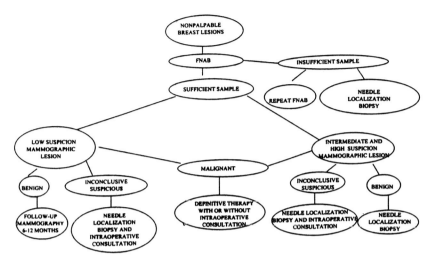

FIGURE 27   Management of patients with nonpalpable breast lesions following fine needle aspiration biopsy.

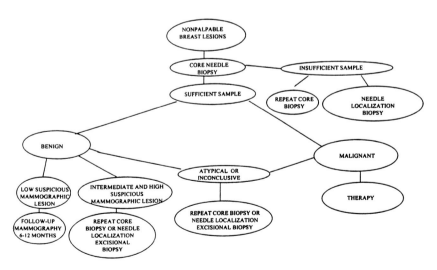

FIGURE 28   Management of patients with nonpalpable breast lesions following core needle biopsy.

REFERENCES

1. Feig SA. Decreased breast cancer mortality through mammographic screening. Results of clinical trials. Radiology 1988;167:659–665, 1988.
2. Werlheimer MD, Castanza ME, Dodson TF, D'Ars C, Pastides H, Zapka JG. Increasing the effort toward breast cancer detection. JAMA 255:1131–1315, 1986.
3. Azavedo E, Fallenius A, Svane G, Auer G. Nuclear DNA content, histological grade and clinical course in patient with nonpalpable mammographically detected breast adenocarcinoma. Am J Clin Oncol 13(1):23–27, 1990.
4. Eddy DM. Screening for breast cancer. Ann Intern Med 111:389–399, 1989.
5. Hall F. Screening mammography, potential problems on the horizon. NEJM 31:53–55, 1986.
6. Marrujo G, Jolly PC, Hall MH. Nonpalpable breast cancer: needle localized biopsy for diagnosis and consideration for treatment. Am J Surg 151:599–602, 1987.
7. Hermann G, Janns C, Schwartz IS, Krivisky B, Bier S, Robinowitz JG. Nonpalpable breast lesions. Accuracy of pre-biopsy mammographic localization. Radiology 165:323–326, 1987.
8. Hall WC, Aust JB, Gaskill HV, Polter JM, Flourney JG, Cruz AB. Evaluation of nonpalpable breast lesions: experience in a training institution. Am J Surg 151:467–496, 1986.
9. Leis Jr HP, Cammarata A, La Raja R, Higgins H. Breast biopsy and guidance for occult lesions. Int Surg 70(2):115–118, 1985.
10. Threatt B, Appleman H, Dow R, O'Rourke J. Percutaneous localization of clustered mammary microcalcification prior to biopsy. Am J Roentgenol 121:839–842, 1974.
11. Norton L, Zeligman B, Pearlman N. Accuracy and cost of needle localization breast biopsy. Arch Surg 123:947–950, 1988.
12. Weinster SJ, Whitehouse GH, McDicken I. The biopsy of impalpable lesions of the breast. Surg Gynecol Obstet 164(3):269–271, 1987.
13. Dowlatshahi K, Gent HJ, Schmidt R, Jokick PM, Bibbo M, Sprenger E. Nonpalpable breast tumors: diagnosis with stereotaxic localization and fine needle aspiration. Radiology 170:427–433, 1989.
14. Lindfors K, Rosenquist J. Needle core biopsy guided with mammography: a study of cost effectiveness. Radiology 190:217–222, 1994.
15. Masood S. Occult breast lesions and aspiration biopsy. Editorial. Diagn Cytopathol 9(6):613–614, 1994.
16. Martin HE, Ellis EB. Biopsy of needle puncture and aspiration. Ann Surg 92:169–181, 1930.
17. Saphir O. Early diagnosis of breast lesions. JAMA 150:859–861, 1952.
18. Franzen S, Zajicek J. Aspiration biopsy in diagnosis of palpable lesions of the breast. Critical review of 3,479 consecutive biopsies. Acta Radiol 7:241–262, 1968.
19. Berg JW, Robbins GF. A late look at the safety of aspiration biopsy. Cancer 15:826–827, 1962.
20. Masood S. Use of monoclonal antibody for assessment of estrogen receptor content in

fine needle aspiration biopsy specimen from patients with breast cancer. Arch Pathol Lab Med 113:26, 30, 1989.

21. Svane G, Silfversward C. Stereotaxic needle biopsy of nonpalpable breast lesions. Acta Radiol Diagn 24:283–288, 1983.

22. Masood S, Frykeberg ER, Mitchum DG, McLellan GL, Scalapino MC, Bullard JB. Prospective evaluation of radiologically directed fine needle aspiration biopsy of nonpalpable breast lesions. Cancer 66:1480–1487, 1990.

23. Fajardo LL, Davis JR, Weins JL. Mammographically guided stereotactic fine needle aspiration cytology of nonpalpable breast lesions. Prospective comparison of surgical biopsy results. Am J Radiol 155:977–981, 1990.

24. Sullivan DC. Needle core biopsy of mammographic lesions. Am J Radiol 162:601–608, 1994.

25. Masood S. Cytopathology of the Breast. Chicago: American Society of Clinical Pathology Press, 1996, pp 1–10.

26. Masood S. Fine needle aspiration biopsy of nonpalpable breast lesions. In: WS Williams, ed. Cytopathology Annual 1994. Baltimore: William and Wilkins 1994, pp 33–63.

27. Jackson VP, Reynolds HE. Stereotaxic needle core biopsy and fine needle aspiration cytologic evaluation of nonpalpable breast lesions. Radiology 181:633–634, 1991.

28. Parker SH, Lovin JDF, Jobe WE, Burke NJ, Hopper KD, Yakes WF. Nonpalpable breast lesions: stereotactic automated large core biopsies. Radiology 180:403–407, 1991.

29. Parker SH, Lovin JD, Jobe WE, et al. Stereotactic breast biopsy with a biopsy gun. Radiology 176:741–744, 1990.

30. Parker SH, Jobe WE, Dennis MA, et al. US guided automated large core breast biopsy. Radiology 187:507–511, 1993.

31. Schmidt RA. Stereotactic breast biopsy. CA Cancer J Clin 44:172–191, 1994.

32. Cohen MB, Rogers C, Hales MS, et al. Influence of training and experience in fine needle aspiration biopsy of breast: receiver operating characteristic cure analysis. Arch Pathol Lab Med 111:518–520, 1987.

33. Lee KR, Foster RS, Papillo JL. Fine needle aspiration of the breast. Importance of the aspirator. Acta Cytol 31:281–284, 1987.

34. Fisher ER, Fisher B. Lobular carcinoma of the breast: an overview. Am Surg 185:377–385, 1988.

35. Schwartz GF, Feig SA, Patchefsky AS. Significance of nonpalpable carcinomas of the breast. Surg Gynecol Obstet 166:6–10, 1988.

36. Liberman L, Cohen MA, Dershaw DD, Abramson AF, Hann LE, Rosen PP. Atypical ductal hyperplasia diagnosed at stereotaxic core biopsy of breast lesions: An indication for surgical biopsy. AJR 164:1111–1113, 1995.

37. Hall FM, Sotvella JM, Silverstone DZ, Wyshak G. Nonpalpable breast lesions. Recommendation for biopsy based on suspicion of carcinoma at mammography. Radiology 167:252–258, 1988.

38. Jackman RJ, Nowels KW, Shepard MJ, Finkelstein SI, Marzoni FA. Stereotaxic large

core needle biopsy of 450 nonpalpable breast lesions with surgical correlation in lesions with cancer or atypical hyperplasia. Radiology 193:91–95, 1994.

39. Liberman L, Evans III WP, Dershaw DD, et al. Radiography of microcalcification in stereotaxic mammary core biopsy specimens. Radiology 190:223–225, 1994.

40. Hann L, Ducatman BS, Wang HH, Fein V, McIntire JM. Nonpalpable breast lesions: evaluation by means of fine needle aspiration cytology. Radiology 171:375–376, 1989.

41. Youngson BJ, Liberman L, Rosen PP. Epithelial displacement in surgical breast specimens following stereotaxic core biopsy. Mod Pathol 8:29A, 1995.

42. Harter LP, Curtis JS, Ponto G, Craig PH. Malignant seeding of the needle track during stereotaxic biopsy. Radiology 185:713–717, 1992.

43. Final version: the uniform approach to breast fine needle aspiration biopsy. National Cancer Institute sponsored conference. Breast J 4:149–168, 1997.

44. Association of Directors of Anatomic and Surgical Pathology. Recommendations for the reporting of breast carcinoma. Mod Pathol 9:77–81, 1996.

45. Association of Directors of Anatomic and Surgical Pathology. Immediate management of mammographically detected breast lesions. Hum Pathol 24:689–690, 1993.

46. Holland R, Hendriks JH. Microcalcifications associated with ductal carcinoma in situ: mammographic-pathologic correlation. Semin Diagn Pathol 11:181–192, 1994

47. Fechner RE. Frozen section examination of breast biopsies. Practice parameters. Am J Clin Pathol 103:6–7, 1995.

48. Gisvold JJ, Goellner JR, Grant CS, et al. Breast biopsy: a comparative study of stereotaxically guided core and excisional techniques. AJR 162:813–820, 1994.

49. Schnitt SJ, Connolly JL. Processing and evaluation of breast excision specimens: a clinically oriented approach. Am J Clin Pathol 98:125–137, 1992.

50. Henson DE, Oberman HA, Hutter RV. Practice protocol for the examination of specimens removed from patients with breast cancer. Arch Pathol Lab Med 121:27–33, 1997.

51. Lagios MD. Ductal carcinoma in situ controversies in diagnosis, biology and treatment. Breast J 1(2):68–78, 1995.

52. Silverstein MJ, Lagios MD, Craig PH, et al. The Van Nuys Prognostic Index for carcinoma in situ. Breast J 2(1):38–40, 1996.

53. Masood S, Frykberg ER, McLellan G, et al. Application of estrogen receptor immunocytochemical assay to aspirates from mammographically guided fine needle biopsy of nonpalpable breast lesions. South Med J 84:857–861, 1991.

54. Masood S. Prognostic factors in breast cancer: use of cytologic preparations. Diagn Cytopathol 13:388–395, 1995.

55. Masood S, Hardt N. Use of fine needle aspiration biopsy specimens in DNA flow cytometry study. AJCP 92:535(A), 1989.

56. Masood S, Lu L, Rodenroth N. Potential value of estrogen receptor immunocytochemical assay in formalin fixed breast tumors. Modern Pathol 3(6):724–728, 1990.

57. Masood S, Dee S, Goldstein JD. Immunocytochemical analysis of progesterone receptors in breast cancer. AJCP 96(1):59–63, 1991.

58. Esteban JM, Battifora H, Warsiz, et al. Quantification of estrogen receptors on paraffin-embedded tumors by image analysis. Mod Pathol 4:53–57, 1991.
59. Hann LE, Liberman L, Dershaw DD, et al. Mammography immediately after stereotaxic breast biopsy: Is it necessary? AJR 165:59–52, 1995.
60. Parker SH, Burbank F, Jackman RJ, et al. Percutaneous large-core breast biopsy: a multi-institutional study. Radiology 193:359–364, 1994.
61. Rosen PP, Braun DW, Kinne DE. The clinical significance of preinvasive breast carcinoma. Cancer 46:919–925, 1980.
62. Smart CR, Meyers MH, Gloeckler LA. Implications from SEER data on breast cancer management. Cancer 41:787–789, 1978.
63. Silverstein MJ, Gamagami P, Roser RJ, et al. Hooked-wire directed breast biopsy and over penetrated mammography. Cancer 59:715–722, 1987.
64. Page DL, Anderson TJ, Rogers LW. Epithelial hyperplasia. In: Page DL, Anderson TJ, eds. Diagnostic Histopathology of the Breast. New York: Churchill Livingstone, 1987, pp 120–156.
65. Meyer JE, Lester SC, Frenna JH, White FV. Occult breast calcifications sampled with large core biopsy confirmation with radiography of the specimen. Radiology 188:581–582, 1993.
66. Dupont WD, Page DL. Risk factors for breast cancer in women with proliferative breast disease. NEJM 312:146–151, 1985.
67. Dupont WD, Parl FF, Hartman WH, et al. Breast cancer risk associated with proliferative breast disease and atypical hyperplasia. Cancer 71:1258–1265, 1993.
68. Masood S, Frykberg ER, McLellan GL, Dee S, Bullard JB. Cytologic differentiation between proliferative and nonproliferative breast disease in mammographically guided fine needle aspirates. Diagn Cytopathol 7:581–590, 1991.
69. Masood S. Cytomorphology of fibrocystic change, high risk and premalignant breast lesions. Breast J 4:210–221, 1995.
70. Masood S. Standardization of immunoassays on surrogate endpoints. J Cell Biochem 9(suppl):28–35, 1994.
71. Fabian CJ, Kamel S, Kimler BF, et al. Potential use of biomarkers in breast cancer with assessment and chemoprevention trials. Breast J 1:235–242, 1995.
72. Rosai J. Borderline epithelial lesions of the breast. Am J Surg Pathol 15:599–603, 1991.
73. Masood S, Sim SJ, Lu L. Immunohistochemical differentiation of atypical hyperplasia versus carcinoma in situ of the breast. Cancer Detect Prev 16(4):223–225, 1997.
74. Masood S. The value of muscle specific actin immunostaining in differentiation between atypical hyperplasia and carcinoma in breast fine needle aspirates. Acta Cytol 38:860–861, 1994.
75. Masood S, Lu L, Assaf-Munasifi N, McCaulley K. Application of immunostaining for muscle specific actin in detection of myoepithelial cells in breast fine needle aspirates. Diagn Cytopathol 13:71–74, 1995.
76. Crissman JD, Visscher DW, Kubus J. Image cytophotometric DNA analysis of atypical hyperplasia and intraductal carcinoma of the breast. Arch Pathol Lab Med 114:1249–1253, 1990.

77. Teplitz RL, Butler BB, Tesluk H, et al. Quantitative DNA pattern in human preneoplastic breast lesions. Anal Quant Cytol Histol 12:98–120, 1990.

78. Masood S. HER-2/neu oncogene expression in atypical ductal hyperplasia, carcinoma in situ and invasive breast cancer. Modern Pathol 4(1):12(A), 1991.

79. Masood S. Cytomorphology in Ductal Carcinoma of the Breast. Baltimore: Williams and Wilkins, 1997, pp 181–187.

80. Carter D. Intraductal papillary tumors of the breast. A study of 78 cases. Cancer 39:1689–1692, 1977.

81. Kraus FT, Neubecker RD. The differential diagnosis of papillary tumors of the breast. Cancer 15:444–455, 1962.

82. Papotti M, Gugliotta P, Chivingello B, Bussolatti G. Association of breast carcinoma and multiple intraductal papillomas on histological and immunohistochemical investigation. Histopathology 8:963, 1984.

83. Raju VB, Lee MW, Zarbo RJ, Crissman JD. Papillary neoplasia of the breast. Immunocytochemically defined myoepithelial cells in the diagnosis of benign and malignant papillary breast neoplasms. Mod Pathol 2:569–576, 1989.

84. Lennington WJ, Jensen RA, Dalton LW, Page DL. Ductal carcinoma in situ of the breast. Heterogeneity of individual lesions. Cancer 73:118–124, 1994.

85. Bellamy COC, McDonald C, Salter DM, Chetty U, Anderson TJ. Noninvasive ductal carcinoma of the breast: the relevance of histologic categorization. Hum Pathol 24:16–23, 1993.

86. Bestil WL Jr, Roen PP, Lieverman PH, Robbins GF. Intraductal carcinoma: long term treatment by biopsy alone. JAMA 239:1863–1867, 1978.

87. Muir R. The evaluation of carcinoma of the mamma. J Pathol Bacteriol 52:155–172, 1941.

88. Lagios, MD, Westdahl PR, Margolin FR, Ross MR. Duct carcinoma in situ: relationship of the extent of noninvasive disease to the frequency of occult invasion, multicentricity, lymph node metastasis and short-term treatment failures. Cancer 50:1309–1314, 1982.

89. Silverstein MD, Lagios MD, Craig PH, et al. The Van Nuys Prognostic Index for ductal carcinoma in situ. Breast J 2(1):38–40, 1996.

90. Millis RR. Classification of ductal carcinoma in situ of the breast. Adv Anat Pathol 3:114–129, 1996.

91. Scott MA, Lagios MD, Axelsson K, et al. Ductal carcinoma in situ of the breast: reproducibility of histologic subtype analysis. Hum Pathol 28:967–973, 1997.

92. Tavassoli FA, Man Y. Morphofunctional features of intraductal hyperplasia, atypical intraductal hyperplasia and various grades of intraductal carcinoma. Breast J 1:155–162, 1995.

93. Mack L, Kerkvliet N, Doig G, et al. Relationship of a new histologic categorization of DCIS of the breast with size and the immunohistochemical expression of p53, c-erbB2, and Ki-67. Hum Pathol 28:974–979, 1997.

94. Anderson JA, Carter D, Linell F. A symposium on sclerosing duct lesions of the breast. Pathol Ann 21:145–179, 1986.

95. Nielsen M, Jensen J, Anderson JA. An autopsy study of radial scar in the female breast. Histopathology 9:287–295, 1985.

96. Anderson TJ, Battersby S. Radial scar of benign and malignant breast: comparative features and significance. J Pathol 147:23–32, 1985.
97. Fenoglio C, Lattes R. Sclerosing papillary proliferations in the female breast. A benign lesion often mistaken for carcinoma. Cancer 33:691–700, 1974.
98. Tavassoli FA. Pathology of the Breast. Norwalk, CT: Appleton and Lange, 1992, pp 107–114.
99. Masood S. Pathological interpretation of fine needle aspiration cytology. In: L Fajardo, KM Willison, RJ Pizzutiello, eds. A Comprehensive Approach to Stereotactic Breast Biopsy. Cambridge: Blackwell Science, pp 225–239.
100. Linell F. Precursor lesions of breast carcinoma. Breast 2:202–223, 1993.
101. Kline TS, Joshi LP, Neal HS. Fine needle aspiration of the breast. Diagnostic pitfalls. Cancer 44:1458, 1979.
102. Early Breast Cancer Trialists' Collaborative Group: Effects of adjuvant tamoxifen and of cytotoxic therapy on mortality in early breast cancer: an overview of 61 randomized trials among 28,896 women. N Engl J Med 319:1681, 1988.
103. Patchefsky AS, Shaver GS, Schwartz GF, et al. The pathology of breast cancer detected by mass screening mode. Radiology 132:273–276, 1979.
104. Carstens PHB. Tubular carcinoma of the breast: A study of frequency. Am J Clin Pathol 70:204–210, 1978.
105. Lagios MD, Rose MR, Margolin FR. Tubular carcinoma of the breast. Association with multicentricity, bilaterality and family history of mammary carcinoma. Am J Clin Pathol 73:25–30, 1981.
106. Parl FF, Richardson LD. The histological and biological spectrum of tubular carcinoma of the breast. Human Pathol 14:694–698, 1983.
107. Rasmussen BB, Rose C, Christensen I. Prognostic factors in primary mucinous carcinoma of the breast. Am J Clin Pathol 87:155–160, 1987.
108. Moore OS Jr, Foote FW Jr. The relatively favorable prognosis of medullary carcinoma of the breast. Cancer 2:635–642, 1949.
109. Ridolfi RE, Rosen PP, Post A, et al. Medullary carcinoma of the breast. A clinical pathological study with 10-year follow-up. Cancer 40:1365–1385, 1977.
110. Ramos CV, Doeghart, C, Restrapo GL. Intracystic papillary carcinoma of the male breast. Arch Pathol Lab Med 109:858–861, 1985.
111. Carter D. Intraductal papillary tumors of the breast. A study of 78 cases. Cancer 39:1689–1692, 1977.
112. Bassett L, Winchester DP, Caplan RB, et al. Stereotactic core-needle biopsy of the breast: a report of the Joint Task Force of the American College of Radiology, American College of Surgeons, and College of American Pathologists. Cancer J Clin 47(3):171–190, 1997.
113. Sickles EA, Park SLT. An appropriate role of core breast biopsy in the management of probably benign lesions. Radiology 188:315, 1993. Editorial.
114. Head JF, Bruce TL, Haynes AE, et al. Two year follow-up of a prospective study of patients with abnormal mammograms who had stereotaxic localization and needle biopsy of nonpalpable breast lesions. Proc Am Soc Clin Oncol 12:56(A), 1993.
115. Jackman RJ, Finklestein SI, Marzoni FA Jr. Stereotaxic large core needle biopsy of

histologically benign nonpalpable breast lesions: false negative results and failed follow-up. Radiology 197(suppl):203(A), 1995.

116. Pal S, Ikeda DM, Birdwell RL. Retrospective study of compliance with recommended follow-up after fine needle aspiration biopsy of nonpalpable breast lesions. Radiology 195(suppl):407(A), 1995.

2
Breast Cancer: Surgical Perspectives

Patricia J. Eubanks
University of Nevada School of Medicine and Veterans Affairs Medical Center, Reno, Nevada

Hernan I. Vargas and Stanley R. Klein
Harbor-UCLA Medical Center, Torrance, California

I. INTRODUCTION

Thirteen out of 100 women in the United States will develop breast cancer in their lifetime [1]. This incidence has increased over the last few decades [2–5]. While the incidence in other countries has modestly increased, in the United States the growing numbers of women with breast cancer are staggering. Since millions of women are at risk, breast cancer captures a considerable amount of patient anxiety as well as medical cost. No other cancer has captured as much media attention or undergone as much evolution in management issues as breast cancer. In fact, public opinion has been important in changing the entrenched Halsteadian concepts of surgical treatment.

Classic surgical principles of breast cancer treatment invoke Halstead's concept of lymphatic clearance at the time of mastectomy. This belief led to wide surgical extirpation of the breast, underlying musculature, and axillary lymphatics. The relatively recent embracement of breast-conserving surgery has only been made possible by well-designed studies that demonstrate near equivalent results of lumpectomy with axillary node dissection to modified radical mastectomy [6–8]. The trend to less "radical" surgery has proven successful in patient outcome. But this evolution has also sparked inquiry into the need for any axillary dissection. More cancers are being diagnosed in the early stages (via mammography) before the development of axillary metastases. As the criteria expand to treat more patients with chemotherapy, there is less need for staging studies to dictate therapy. Moreover, the routine use of screening mammography has resulted in increased survival in breast cancer patients [9], principally because these cancers are being diagnosed earlier. Core and stereotactic biopsy specimens are being scrutinized as possible treatment options. Therefore, in the era of earlier cancer diagnoses and systemic-designed therapy, the available testing and treatment modalities array themselves in a confusing line-up.

The genetic environment in tumorigenesis has received attention recently. Identifying the BRCA 1 and BRCA 2 genes has impacted our screening methods as well as our surgical treatment arms. Women identified as high risk patients by family history and genetic testing are offered aggressive and even prophylactic surgery. While the role of surgery in the treatment of breast cancer is often minimized, the goal of this chapter is to clarify the importance of surgery in the multi-modality treatment of breast cancer.

II. DIAGNOSIS

Although mammography accounts for an increasing number of new breast cancer diagnoses, the workup of a palpable mass remains relevant [10]. Much effort has been put forth in educating women in breast self-exam, such that women will present themselves to a physician's office having noted a mass. Examination of the breasts by an experienced clinician is an important screening tool. Careful breast exam should separate dominant masses from the surrounding breast architecture. Every palpable mass should be assessed with aspiration cytology. Aspirating the mass can distinguish cystic lesions from solid ones. The aspiration of a cyst with resolution of the mass is sufficient therapy if the patient is given close follow-up. Aspirating the solid mass is an important first step in the diagnostic paradigm.

A. Fine Needle Aspiration (FNA) Cytology

Fine needle aspiration cytology to diagnose breast cancer has been shown to have a high specificity and sensitivity [11]. In a series of 1311 cases over a 5-year period, no false-positive FNAs were found [12]. A recent study comparing core needle biopsy (or Tru-cut biopsy) with FNA showed FNA to be more sensitive than core needle biopsy [13]. However, they classified "suspicious" FNA results as being true positives when confirmed with excised specimens. A "suspicious" result is not adequate to dictate therapy that does not involve subsequent excision (i.e., neoadjuvant chemotherapy). Of note in this study, the only false negatives on FNA (3/124) were also found to be false negative by core needle biopsy. FNA sensitivity and specificity from this study were 97.5% and 100% respectively. Clearly, FNA is cost-effective and simple. Previous studies have attested to the improved sensitivity and specificity of FNA [14]. The advantages of FNA over core needle biopsy are ease of multidirectional sampling, improved tactile guidance (as compared to the automative core needle guns), as well as decreased expense and potential complications. In addition, FNA has also been shown to be reliable when used by inexperienced clinicians. Hindle et al. reported results of fine needle aspirations performed by obstetrics-gynecology residents. They report unsatisfactory aspirations in only 86 of 810 aspirations performed in the outpatient clinic [15]. Although FNA has excellent specificity, it is not able to definitively distinguish in situ cancer from invasive cancer [16]. FNA is most valuable when interpreted within the clinical and mammographical context. Butler et al. showed that when clinical, mammographical, and cytological findings are combined the accuracy is as high as 97% [17].

B.   Core Needle Biopsy (CNB)

We recommend proceeding to core needle biopsy (CNB) in patients with a "suspicious" or nondiagnostic FNA. CNB with five to eight passes will often lead to the pathological diagnosis of a breast mass [18]. In the previously cited study [13], four patients with "suspicious" FNA results were subsequently diagnosed by CNB. Core needle biopsy is important in making the diagnosis of cancer in patients with large primary tumors who are candidates for preoperative chemotherapy. Moreover, open biopsy can be avoided if the diagnosis is made by core needle biopsy [19]. It can be just as difficult to distinguish in situ carcinomas from infiltrating ductal carcinomas on core needle biopsies as it is on FNA. In a recent series, eight of 43 cases (19%) diagnosed as ductal carcinoma in situ (DCIS) by core needle biopsy were subsequently found to have invasive carcinoma after excision [20]. The shortcomings of CNB or FNA to diagnose DCIS may be clinically insignificant since treatment of in situ lesions requires subsequent excision.

C.   Surgical Biopsy

If FNA and CNB fail to diagnose a palpable mass, we then proceed with excisional or incisional biopsy. We favor incisional biopsy if the lesion is >5 cm in size. An incisional biopsy may be performed on smaller lesions if the patients breast size is small relative to the size of the mass. Open biopsies are the gold standard to which all other minimally invasive biopsy techniques are compared [21–23]. A margin of grossly normal tissue is taken with the mass. Of note, there have been reports of subsequent carcinoma occurring in the site of a previously benign biopsy. Therefore, a recurrent mass or persistent mass in the site of a previous biopsy should prompt excision [24].

The paradigm of FNA followed by core needle biopsy followed by excisional biopsy is not always applicable. If a woman presents with a large breast mass that is highly suspicious for malignancy, then we will consider core needle biopsy as the primary diagnostic test. A core biopsy specimen can often provide enough tissue and architecture to distinguish between DCIS (high grade) and infiltrating ductal carcinoma as well as allowing receptor status determination. If the diagnosis can be made by core needle biopsy, then the patient can undergo neoadjuvant chemotherapy to allow potential for breast conservation surgery in the future.

An important surgical concept that is often overlooked is that a normal mammogram in a patient with a palpable mass does not preclude diagnostic workup of this mass. We have seen several cases of large breast cancers with "normal" mammograms secondary to dense architecture seen on mammography. Thus, regardless of mammography or other imaging test results, a palpable breast mass should be assessed with aspiration cytology or core needle biopsy.

D.   Biopsy of Mammographic Lesions

The use of screening mammography has been shown to contribute to decreased breast cancer mortality. Results from a Swedish trial during 13 years of follow-up show reduction in breast cancer mortality with the use of mammography every 2 years [9]. Approximately 500,000 breast biopsies are performed yearly based on mammographic abnormalities, of which 60% to 90% may be benign [25].

Recent experience with stereotactic breast biopsy machines has altered the surgical paradigm. Under stereotactic guidance, an FNA or core needle biopsy can be obtained [26]. A patient with an abnormal mammogram can undergo a stereotactic biopsy and avoid a needle localization procedure (thus avoiding two operations). Large core biopsy using stereotactic imaging (up to 2 cm cores) can be used to obtain a diagnosis as well as obtain clear margins. Certainly, most needle localization biopsies are benign. Avoiding an operation, the use of smaller incisions and the lower attendant morbidity for a probably "benign" lesion are quite attractive.

Also, use of this modality can simplify mammographic follow-up, simplify or expedite definitive surgery, and allow expeditious initiation of adjuvant therapy. The stereotactic procedure is particularly useful in diagnosing indeterminate mammographic lesions. Yim et al. compared stereotactic core needle biopsy with needle localization biopsy in a retrospective study [27]. They reviewed records from 52 consecutive patients diagnosed with invasive breast cancer over a 2-year period and evaluated surgical margins and cost. They found that in the stereotactic needle biopsy group there were no positive margins, as opposed to the needle-localized biopsy group. In other words, a preoperative diagnosis of infiltrating cancer (prior to a trip to the operating room) saved the patient a procedure (reexcision) since all of those patients had clear margins. In contrast, the needle-localized biopsy group (no preoperative diagnosis of cancer) had positive margins 55% of the time. Additionally, the use of the stereotactic biopsy resulted in a $1000 cost savings per patient.

In the cases of indeterminate mammographic findings, a MIBI scan may be helpful in assessing the relative risk of the lesion. As outlined in other chapters in this text, the use of Tc-99m sestamibi in breast tumor imaging may enhance the detection of breast cancer [28–30]. In a recent study, 157 women with 164 lesions appearing suspicious on mammography underwent scintimammography and biopsy [31]. The authors report a sensitivity of 92.3% for detecting breast cancer and a specificity of 87.5%. However, this study was done to determine correlation/reliability of suspicious mammographic findings with MIBI. The application of MIBI to help stratify indeterminate mammographic lesions or uninterpretable mammograms is still under investigation.

III. THERAPY: MASTECTOMY VERSUS BREAST CONSERVATION

Once the diagnosis of infiltrating breast cancer is made, the patient has several surgical options. Small lesions are often amenable to lumpectomy and axillary node dissection (AND) if the patient desires breast conservation. NSABP B-6 showed that lumpectomy and AND followed by radiation therapy to the breast have comparable survival and recurrence rates to mastectomy [32]. From this and other clinical trials, the 1990 NIH consensus conference on breast cancer recommended lumpectomy and AND as the preferred treatment for women with stage I and II cancers [33–35]. Early Breast Cancer Trialists' Collaborative Group and another recent meta-analysis similarly found no significant difference in survival between women undergoing breast conservation and mastectomy at 10 years [36,37].

In spite of legislation requiring physicians to disclose the options of BCT, only 30% to 35% of patients undergo breast conserving treatment [38]. While stage I and II breast cancer is amenable to BCT, breast-conserving surgery has been extended to patients with larger tumors. In a study of 68 patients with tumors 4 cm or larger undergoing lumpectomy and AND, the 5-year recurrence was reported as 8.5% and the overall survival as 76% [39]. Thus, in select patients whose breast size will accommodate lumpectomy with adequate margins, acceptable survival and recurrence rates can be obtained with BCT.

We advocate modified radical mastectomy (MRM) for those patients who:

1. Request it
2. Have large ulcerating tumors
3. Have large bulky tumors unresponsive to neoadjuvant chemotherapy or unwilling to undergo neoadjuvant chemotherapy
4. Have multiple sites of cancer on mammography
5. Have had prior irradiation to the breast
6. Are in the first or second trimester of pregnancy
7. Do not want radiation therapy

A small study by Leopold et al. found that two or more separate primary tumors in the breast may be associated with a higher incidence of local recurrence after

BCT [40]. Prior irradiation to the breast is considered a contraindication to breast-conserving treatment. Usually this is the case in patients who develop a recurrence after previous lumpectomy and AND. Thus, patients with recurrent breast carcinoma should undergo modified radical mastectomy.

Diffuse microcalcifications or more than two suspicious areas on mammography are indications for mastectomy. However, if those suspicious areas are confined to a quadrant, the patient may still undergo quadrantectomy.

Breast cancers diagnosed during the first or second trimesters of pregnancy are best treated with mastectomy. Although the fetus can be shielded from radiation, the standard breast treatment dose of 5000 cGy will potentially deliver 10 cGy to 200 cGy to the developing fetus. In mice, there is a 20% incidence of severe malformations with exposures to the fetus of as little as 18 cGy [41,42]. Retroareolar cancer and large tumor relative to breast size are other relative contraindications to breast conserving treatment.

A. Axillary Node Dissection

In the standard axillary node dissection, three levels of axillary nodes are identified (Fig. 1). Axillary dissection is viewed as a therapeutic modality as well as a prognostic one [43]. Since more patients are being treated with adjuvant therapy regardless of nodal status [44], the issue of need for axillary node dissection is controversial and under study. NSABP B-04 randomized patients with clinically negative axillary lymph nodes to modified radical mastectomy, total mastectomy with delayed axillary dissection if positive nodes developed, or total mastectomy with radiation therapy to the axilla [45]. Forty percent of patients undergoing axillary node dissection in clinically negative axillae had positive nodes. They found no difference in survival at 10 years, however. Thus, AND has not been shown to provide any survival benefit.

Generally, metastases occur in progression from levels I to III. The occurrence of "skip" metastases in level III (with no lesions in levels I or II) is unusual, occurring only 0.5% to 3% of the time [46–48]. Most surgeons perform a level II dissection to achieve at least 10 lymph nodes for sampling. Level III dissection is performed if there are large bulky nodes in level II or III.

As tumor size increases, the likelihood of axillary nodal involvement increases such that patients with tumors >5 cm have a 60% chance of axillary metastases. Silverstein et al. found the incidence of axillary metastases to be 3% in T1a tumors, 17% in T1b, 32% in T1c, 44% in T2, and 60% in T3 tumors [49]. Given the low incidence of positive axillary nodes in T1a tumors (T < 0.5 cm), some surgeons favor avoidance of AND [50]. Of note, a recent prospective study of 147 patients undergoing AND notes that of 29 patients with cancers <10 mm, five (17.2%) had axillary metastases [51]. All of these cancers were located in the upper outer quadrant. The authors argue that cancers located inferiorly or medially have an extremely low incidence of axillary metastases, such that AND can

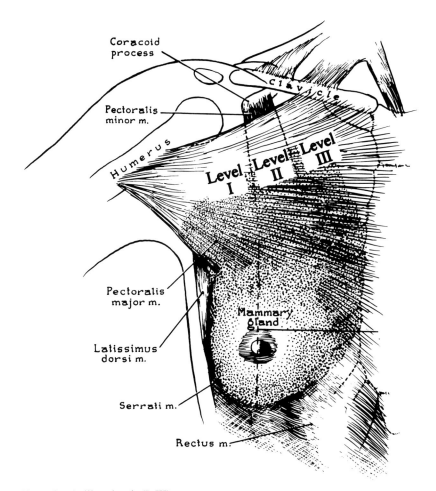

FIGURE 1   Axillary levels (I–III).

be omitted in this patient group. Thus, a more selective approach to AND for T1 tumors, relying on position of the cancer within the breast, may save some patients the potential morbidity of an AND. The side effects of AND can be arm swelling, seroma formation, and pain syndromes.

Whereas the patient with the clinically positive axilla may have the most to gain with AND, the prognostic significance of determining the involvement of the axilla is important. The presence of positive axillary lymph nodes has been shown to decrease 5-year survival by 28% to 40% [52,53]. Thus, there has been an evolution to more minimally invasive ways to assessing axillary involvement without

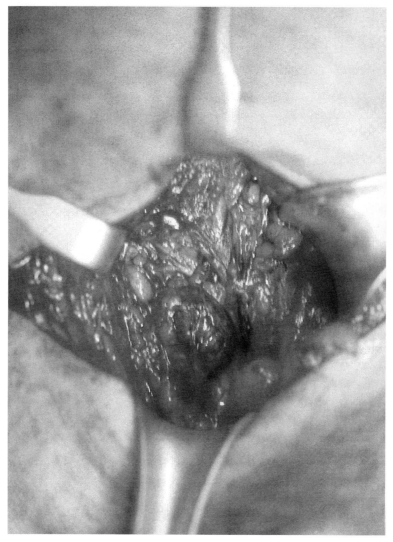

FIGURE 2   SLN dissection.

the morbidity of an AND. Sentinel node mapping has recently been applied to breast cancer. (Fig. 2).

Giuliano et al. report 95.6% accuracy in predicting axillary nodal status in 114 cases in which a sentinel node was identified (65% of the time) [54]. They noted a significant learning curve and subsequently found 100% predictability in the latter part of the study. Albertini et al. report the ability to locate the sentinel lymph node 92% of the time using Isosulfan Blue in combination with technetium-labeled sulfur colloid [55]. They found that all patients with positive axillary lymph nodes had positive sentinel nodes. The technique of sentinel lymph node mapping involves injecting the breast at the tumor site with Isosulfan Blue dye (and radiolabeled colloid). The radioactive colloid allows gamma probe assistance in locating the sentinel lymph node and enhances detection of the first nodal basin [56].

The first studies relied upon H&E staining in combination with cytokeratin immunohistochemistry to detect axillary metastases [54]. Other groups have recently advocated the use of reverse transcription PCR (RT-PCR) to detect micrometastases [57]. The micrometastases are thought to correlate with other prognostic factors such as tumor size and vascular invasion [58,59]. Patients with micrometastases when compared to node-negative patients have significant differences in recurrence and survival [60]. Thus, the debate as to the role of AND continues. Most node-negative patients are receiving adjuvant therapy, so is the difference between the micrometastatic patients and the node negative patients of clinical relevance?

Current practice would suggest a formal AND in those patients with clinically positive axillae because of the potential local therapeutic benefit. In patients with clinically negative axilla and small tumors, the sentinel lymph node sampling may allow maximal information with minimal risks. Patients with large primary tumors are likely to benefit from AND even though the axilla is clinically negative [61]. Ultimately, if the detection of axillary lymph node metastases can be done nonsurgically in a reliable fashion, the role of AND will be only to remove bulky disease.

A recent study of mammolymphoscintigraphy showed improved ability to detect sentinel lymph nodes [62]. Thirty-one of 34 patients had lymphatic drainage patterns identified. Of note, the authors identified drainage to supraclavicular or infraclavicular nodes in 20%. They also found unexpected drainage patterns of outer lesions to internal mammary nodes and inner lesions draining to axillary nodes in 32% of patients. If these methods of detecting drainage patterns can be reliably coupled with detection of metastases nonsurgically (i.e., with tracers such as MIBI), then surgery on the negative axilla can be avoided. In contrast to this viewpoint, others feel that patients should be offered chemotherapy regardless of the nodal status. The absolute role of AND remains under evolution.

B.   Locally Advanced Breast Cancers

Large tumors diagnosed by FNA or core needle biopsy may be treated initially with chemotherapy. This allows potential for breast conservation as well as improved resectability with MRM. Approximately 10% to 15% of breast cancers diagnosed each year are considered locally advanced [63]. Locally advanced cancers are those >5 cm in size with matted axillary nodes or skin/or chest wall involvement. Several studies summarizing the results of mastectomy alone for locally advanced breast cancer show 5-year survival rates of 5.7% to 53% [64–68] with 5-year recurrence rates of 6% to 50%. These studies illustrate the high rate of recurrence and death in patients undergoing radical surgery for advanced disease and confirm that surgery alone is inadequate treatment. Radiation therapy to the breast with and without surgery has been tried as well, with no survival benefit [69]. The combination of surgery with chemotherapy and radiation therapy has been shown to result in the greatest survival [70,71].

Induction or neoadjuvant chemotherapy was initially used for unresectable tumors or inflammatory cancers in an attempt to downstage these tumors to facilitate resection. From this application, the question arose as to whether patients treated initially with chemotherapy had improved survival. Results of NSABP B-18 were recently presented in abstract form. No improvement in survival was found [71]. Multiple clinical trials of neoadjuvant chemotherapy for locally advanced breast cancer show response rates of 51% to 92%. The results have been variable and interpretation of the data has been difficult secondary to widely varying drug regimens.

Nonetheless, the NSABP B-18 results show a >50% reduction in tumor size in 80% of patients [72]. Thus, induction chemotherapy may not improve survival, but it can allow improved resectability and even allow for breast conservation treatment. Bonadonna et al. in 1990 reported the use of induction chemotherapy to allow patients with large breast cancers to undergo BCT [73]. One hundred twenty-seven of the 157 patients were able to have lumpectomy with AND after three to four cycles of chemotherapy. Sixty percent of the women had a partial response, and 27 of 157 had a complete response. M.D. Anderson reported partial response in 70.7% and complete response in 16.7% in patients treated with adriamycin/cytoxan based chemotherapy [74], with a 27% rate of breast conservation [75]. More long-term follow-up data are needed, yet the locoregional control appears to be good.

C. Margins

In patients who have received lumpectomy with AND, there has been concern over the potential increased rate of recurrence when the lumpectomy specimen has positive margins. As defined by investigators from NSABP, a margin is positive if cancer cells are present directly at an inked surface. Patients with negative lumpectomy margins have recurrence rates of 1% to 7% at 5 years [76,77]. In NSABP B-6, patients treated with lumpectomy and AND with negative lumpectomy margins had a local recurrence rate comparable to mastectomy.

A recent study stratified patients treated with breast conserving treatment into groups with negative margins (>1 mm), close margins (≤1 mm), and positive margins [78]. The rates of recurrent disease were studied and compared among the groups with particular reference to extensive intraductal component (EIC). They found that patients with negative margins have a low rate of recurrence at 5 years regardless of whether the margin was close (<1 mm) or not and whether the cancer had EIC or not (2% to 3%). The recurrence rate increased to 9% for focally positive margins and 28% for more than focally positive margins (EIC-negative 19%, EIC-positive 42%). Their recommendations were for reexcision if >3 low-power microscopic fields (>focally positive margins) containing cancer are obtained. Some patients with focally positive margins can be candidates for breast conservation without reexcision if the tumor is EIC-negative [78,79].

D. Ductal Carcinoma In Situ (DCIS)

Ductal carcinoma in situ (DCIS) is defined as the transformation of ductal epithelial cells into malignant cells that are contained within the basement membrane [80]. DCIS is strictly contained within the breast and cannot, by definition, metastasize. DCIS should be treated with this concept in mind. High-grade or comedo-DCIS is characterized histologically by necrosis and cytologic atypia. Calcification is frequently present and accounts for 20% to 40% of all mammographically guided biopsies. Comedo-DCIS is frequently associated with microinvasive carcinoma and should be treated as an infiltrating carcinoma [81–83]. Unifocal comedo-DCIS can be treated by lumpectomy followed by radiation therapy to the breast. Other types of DCIS include lesions characterized as intermediate or low-grade.

DCIS can present as a mass (rarely), a mammographic abnormality, nipple discharge, or Paget's disease of the nipple. Breast conservation treatment without radiation therapy produces a high local recurrence rate (19% to 43%), of which half may be invasive cancer [84]. This recurrence rate drops to 9% if the breast is irradiated after lumpectomy. NSABP B-17 reported recurrence rates of 16.4% without radiation therapy (8.2% being invasive cancer), as compared to 7% recurrence after radiation to the breast (2.9% being invasive cancer) [85]. NSABP B-17 data confirm that DCIS treated with excision alone has an unacceptably high recurrence rate.

Patients with multiple areas of high-grade DCIS should be considered for mastectomy. However, focal areas of high-grade DCIS are best treated by lumpectomy with clear margins and radiation to the breast [86]. Currently, some intermediate grade lesions are treated like comedo DCIS. Work by Lagios et al. and Silverstein suggests that in intermediate- or low-grade lesions radiation may be unnecessary [87,88] Silverstein reports disease-free survivals of 93% in low-grade DCIS without necrosis. Lagios found that 0 of 33 low-grade lesions treated by excision alone recurred. Low-grade lesions can be treated with excision alone.

Paget's disease of the nipple appears as an eczematous-type lesion often causing an exudative, scaly area on the nipple-areolar skin. This finding has been found to correlate with underlying carcinoma. If no mass is palpable, a mammogram may reveal positive findings 24% to 97% of the time [89]. Confirmation of Paget's disease is made by skin biopsy. Research has substantiated the theory of Paget's arising from an underlying glandular neoplasm. Paget's cells express antigens characteristic of glandular cells and have similar immunoreactivity profiles as carcinomas [90]. Although BCT has been considered for Paget's disease, most surgeons treat Paget's with mastectomy. While reports show carcinoma in 97% of mastectomy specimens with Paget's, the type is usually in situ. Eusebio et al. report a 19% incidence of infiltrating carcinoma in mastectomy specimens with no palpable masses and a 90% incidence when a mass was palpable [91]. NSABP B-24 trial is under study to assess the utility of tamoxifen in the prevention of invasive cancer in patients with DCIS. Results of this study may elucidate the role of adjuvant therapy in DCIS.

E.   Lobular Carcinoma In Situ (LCIS)

LCIS should be viewed as a marker for increased risk of breast cancer and not as an indication for surgical intervention. LCIS is a proliferative breast lesion that can be present in both breasts diffusely. The finding of LCIS carries an increased risk for subsequent development of infiltrating breast cancer in both breasts of seven to nine times the general population risk [92]. LCIS is viewed as a marker of increased risk and warrants close patient surveillance (biannual clinical exam and annual mammography), rather than prophylactic mastectomy [93].

IV.   PROPHYLACTIC MASTECTOMY

The role of prophylactic mastectomy has changed as our perceptions of breast cancer biology/behavior have evolved. Since mastectomy itself does not completely eliminate the risk of breast cancer and we cannot currently predict with certainty those who will develop breast cancer, prophylactic mastectomy is rarely indicated.

Patients with hereditary breast cancer syndromes are the biggest risk group where prophylactic surgery may play a role. Members of these families typically have autosomal-dominant penetration whereby breast cancer affects multiple generations. This genetic cause accounts for only 5% to 10% of breast cancers [94,95]. These syndromes include hereditary early-onset breast cancer syndrome, breast-ovarian cancer syndrome, Li-Fraumeni syndrome, Muir-Torre syndrome, Peutz-Jegher's syndrome, ataxia telangectasia, and Cowden's disease.

The BRCA-1 gene was identified on chromosome 17q21 (96) and is found to be mutated in 45% of genetically linked breast cancer. This mostly involves the breast-ovarian cancer syndrome [97]. The BRCA-2 gene was also recently cloned and has been linked to early-onset breast cancer not associated with BRCA-1 [98]. The position statement of the Society of Surgical Oncology for prophylactic mastectomies does not incorporate genetic testing into its paradigm [99]. Since there have been many alleles of the BRCA-1 gene found and each may confer different relative risks for breast (or ovarian) cancer, further research is needed to characterize this breast cancer susceptibility gene. At this time, routine genetic testing should not be performed given the large degree of uncertainty and variance in interpretation of the results. Genetic counseling should be offered to those being tested in research centers. The National Advisory Council for Human Genome Research cautions against the use of testing for BRCA-1 gene mutations until further research has characterized the genetic risks [100].

Without the use of genetic testing, the SSO position statement suggests that patients with a pedigree of first-degree relatives with premenopausal bilateral cancer should be offered prophylactic mastectomy. However, genetic testing should not be used as a criterion for recommendation of prophylactic mastectomy.

Certainly the identification of the BRCA 1 and BRCA 2 genes has heightened the clinician's awareness to genetic risks. Prophylactic oopherectomy should be considered in premenopausal women with breast cancer found to have the BRCA-1 gene defect because of the high association of ovarian cancer.

Atypical hyperplasia, when multicentric or when associated with familial breast cancer, places the patient at high risk for the development of breast cancer. Thought should be given to the need for prophylactic mastectomy in these cases. Ultimately the decision for prophylactic mastectomy should be made only after the patient has been informed of the alternatives, has been told of the limits of genetic testing, has been presented at the hospital Ethics Committee, and has received a second opinion. The patient should not be scheduled for surgery without the passage of several weeks to months.

REFERENCES

1. EJ Feuer, LM Wun, CC Boring, et al. The lifetime risk of developing breast cancer. J Natl Cancer Inst 85:848–849, 1993.
2. BA Miller, LAG Ries, BF Hankey, et al., eds: Cancer Statistics Review: 1973–1989. Bethesda, MD: National Cancer Institute. NIH Publ. No. 92-2789, 1992.
3. American Cancer Society, Inc. Cancer Facts & Figures—1993, 1993.
4. BF Hankey, B Miller, R Curtis, C Kosary. Trends in breast cancer in younger women in contrast to older women. JNCI Monogr 16:7–14, 1994.
5. EJ Sondik, LG Kessler, LAG Ries, eds. Cancer Statistics Review: 1973–1986, including a report on the status of cancer control. Bethesda, MD: National Cancer Institute. NIH Publ. No. 89-2789, 1989, pp II.20–II.22.

6. U Veronesi, R Saccozi, M Del Vecchio, et al. Comparing radical mastectomy with quadrantectomy, axillary dissection, and radiotherapy in patients with small cancers of the breast. N Engl J Med 305:6–11, 1981.
7. B Fisher, M Bauer, R Margolese, et al. Five-year results of a randomized clinical trial comparing total mastectomy and segmental mastectomy with or without radiation in the treatment of breast cancer. N Engl J Med 312:665–673, 1985.
8. D Sarrazin, MG Le, J Rouesse, et al. Conservative treatment versus mastectomy in breast cancer tumors with macroscopic diameter of 20 millimeters or less: the experience of the Institut Gustave-Roussy. Cancer 53:1209–1213, 1984.
9. L Tabor, G Fagerberg, HH Chen, et al. Efficacy of breast cancer screening by age. New results from the Swedish two-county trial. Cancer 75:2507–2517, 1995.
10. WL Donnegan. Evaluation of a palpable breast mass. N Engl J Med 327:937–942, 1992.
11. HJ Wanebo, PS Feldman, MC Wilhelm, JL Covell, RL Binns. Fine needle aspiration cytology in lieu of open biopsy in management of primary breast cancer. Ann Surg 199:569–579, 1984.
12. SV Nicosia, SA Horowitz, JA Williams, NN Ku, DS Reintgen, C Cox. Fine needle aspiration biopsy of palpable breast lesions: review and statistical analysis of 1,311 cases. Acta Cytol 35:609–610, 1991.
13. MS Ballo, N Sneige. Can core needle biopsy replace fine-needle aspiration cytology in the diagnosis of palpable breast carcinoma. Cancer 78:773–777, 1996.
14. MM Shabot, IM Goldberg, P Schick, R Nieberg, YH Pilch. Aspiration cytology is superior to Tru-cut needle biopsy in establishing the diagnosis of clinically suspicious breast masses. Ann Surg 196:122–126, 1982.
15. WH Hindle, PA Payne, EY Pan. The use of fine-needle aspiration in the evaluation of persistent palpable dominant breast masses. Am J Obstet Gynecol 168:1814–1819, 1993.
16. EJ Wilkinson, JB Hendricks. Fine needle aspiration of the breast for diagnosis of preinvasive neoplasia. J Cell Biochem Suppl 17G:81–88, 1993.
17. JA Butler, HI Vargas, N Worthen, SE Wilson. Accuracy of combined clinical–mammographic–cytologic diagnosis of dominant breast masses. A prospective study. Arch Surg 125:893–895, 1990.
18. PA Cheung, KW Yan, TT Alagaratnam. The complementary role of fine needle aspiration cytology and Tru-cut needle biopsy in the management of breast masses. Aust NZ J Surg 57:615–620, 1987.
19. SH Parker, F Burbank, RJ Jackman, et al. Percutaneous large-core breast biopsy: a multi-institutional study. Radiology 193:359–364, 1994.
20. RJ Jackman, KW Nowels, MJ Shepard, SI Finkelstein, FA Marzoni Jr. Stereotactic large-core needle biopsy of 450 nonpalpable breast lesions with surgical correlation in lesions with cancer or atypical hyperplasia. Radiology 193:91–95, 1994.
21. LM Ellis, KI Bland. Techniques for obtaining the diagnosis of malignant breast lesions. Surg Clin North Am 70:815–830, 1990.
22. LW Norton. The cost effectiveness of breast biopsy techniques. Prob Gen Surg 8:267–275, 1991.
23. ML Palmer, TN Tsangaris. Breast biopsy in women 30 years old or less. Am J Surg 165:708–712, 1993.

24. J Zitarelli, LL Burkhart, SM Weiss. False negative breast biopsy for palpable mass. J Surg Oncol 52:61–63, 1993.

25. FM Hall, JM Storella, DZ Silverstone, G Wyshak. Nonpalpable breast lesions: recommendations for biopsy based on suspicion of carcinoma at mammography. Radiology 167:353–358, 1988.

26. MC Chan, HS Lam, E Gwi, TY Leung, Y Lau, WC Yip. Stereotactic fine needle aspiration in the management of mammographic abnormalities detected in breast screening. Aust NZJ Surg 66:595–597, 1996.

27. JH Yim, P Barton, B Weber, et al. Mammographically detected breast cancer. Ann Surg 223:688–700, 1996.

28. ME Stuntz, I Khalkhali, JF Moss, SR Klein. Breast imaging techniques and their application in breast disease. Breast J 1:284–294, 1995.

29. I Khalkhali, I Mena, E Jouanne E, et al. Prone scintimammography in patients with suspicion of carcinoma of the breast. J Am Coll Surg 178:491–497, 1994.

30. I Khalkhali, JA Cutrone, IG Mena, et al. Scintimammography: the complementary role of Tc-99m sestamibi prone breast imaging for the diagnosis of breast carcinoma. Radiology 196:421–426, 1995.

31. S Iraniha, I Khalkhali, JA Cutrone, LE Diggles, SR Klein. Breast cancer imaging: can Tc-99m sestamibi scintimammography fit in? Medscape Women's Health 2, 1997.

32. B Fisher, DL Wickerham, M Deutsch, S Anderson, C. Redmond, ER Fisher. Breast tumor recurrence following lumpectomy with and without breast irradiation: an overview of recent NSABP findings. Sem Surg Onc 8:153–160, 1992.

33. B Fisher, S Anderson, C. Redmond, N Wolmark, DL Wickerham, WM Cronin. Reanalysis and results after 12 years of follow-up in a randomized clinical trial comparing total mastectomy with lumpectomy with or without irradiation in the treatment of breast cancer. N Engl J Med 333:1456–1461, 1995.

34. U Veronesi, A Banti, B Salvaderi, et al. Breast conservation is the treatment of choice in small breast cancer: long-term results of a randomized trial. Eur J Cancer 26:668–670, 1990.

35. NIH Consensus Conference. Treatment of early stage breast cancer. JAMA 265:391–395, 1991.

36. Early Breast Cancer Trialists' Collaborative Group. Effects of radiotherapy and surgery in early breast cancer. An overview of the randomized trials. N Engl J Med 1995; 333:1444–1455.

37. AD Morris, RD Morris, JF Wilson, et al. Breast-conserving therapy vs. mastectomy in early-stage breast cancer: a meta-analysis of 10-year survival. Cancer J Sci Am 3:6–12, 1997.

38. AB Nattinger, RG Hoffmann, R Shapiro, MS Gottlieb, JS Goodwin. The effect of legislative requirements on the use of breast-conserving surgery. N Engl J Med 335:1035–1040, 1996.

39. MM Khanna, RJ Mark, MJ Silverstein, G Juillard, B Lewinsky, AE Giuliano. Breast conservation management of breast tumors 4 cm or larger. Arch Surg 127:1038–1043, 1992.

40. KA Leopold, A Recht, SJ Schnitt, et al. Results of conservative surgery and radiation therapy for multiple synchronous cancers of one breast. Int J Radiat Oncol Biol Phys 16:11–16, 1989.

41. EJ Hall. Effects of radiation on the developing embryo. In: EJ Hall, ed. Radiobiology for the Radiologist. New York: Harper and Row, 1973, pp 231–239.

42. JA Petrek. Breast cancer and pregnancy. Monogr Natl Cancer Inst 16:113–121, 1994.

43. WK Ruffin, A Stacey-Clear, J Younger, HC Hoover. Rationale for routine axillary dissection in carcinoma of the breast. J Am Coll Surg 180:245–251, 1995.

44. A Goldhirsch, WC Wood, H-J Senn, JH Glick, RD Gelber. Meeting highlights: International Consensus Panel on the Treatment of Primary Breast Cancer. J Natl Cancer Inst 87(19):1441–1445, 1995.

45. B Fisher, C Redmond, ER Fisher, et al. Ten-year results of a randomized clinical trial comparing radical mastectomy and total mastectomy with or without radiation. N Engl J Med 312:674–681, 1985.

46. RS Boova, B Roseann, F Rosato. Patterns of axillary metastasis: predictability of level one dissection. Ann Surg 196:642, 1982.

47. U Veronesi, A Luini, V Galimberti, et al. Extent of metastatic axillary involvement in 1446 cases of breast cancer. Eur J Surg Oncol 16:127, 1990.

48. RS Foster. The biologic and clinical significance of lymphatic metastases in breast cancer. Surg Onc Clin North Am 5:79–104, 1996.

49. MJ Silverstein, ED Gierson, JR Waisman, et al. Axillary lymph node dissection for T1a breast carcinoma: is it indicated? Cancer 73:664–667, 1994.

50. DM Dent. Axillary lymphadenectomy for breast cancer. Arch Surg (commentary) 131:1125–1127, 1996.

51. AA Kambouris. Axillary node metastases in relation to size and location of breast cancers: analysis of 147 patients. Am Surg 62:519–524, 1996.

52. CD Haagensen. Treatment of curable carcinoma of the breast. Int J Radiat Oncol Biol Phys 2:975–980, 1977.

53. G Bonadonna. Karnofsky Memorial Lecture. Conceptual and practical advances in the management of breast cancer. J Clin Oncol 7:1380–1397, 1989.

54. AE Giuliano, DM Kirgan, JM Guenther, DL Morton. Lymphatic mapping and sentinel lymphadenectomy for breast cancer. Ann Surg 220:391–401, 1994.

55. JJ Albertini, GH Lyman, C Cox, et al. Lymphatic mapping and sentinel node biopsy in the patient with breast cancer. JAMA 276:1818–1822, 1996.

56. JC Alex, DN Krag. The gamma-probe-guided resection of radiolabeled primary lymph nodes. Surg Onc Clin North Am 5:33–41, 1996.

57. A Schoenfeld, Y Luqmani, D Smith, et al. Detection of breast cancer micrometastases in axillary lymph nodes by using polymerase chain reaction. Cancer Res 54:2986–2990, 1994.

58. AG Huvos, RNP Hutter, JW Berg. Significance of axillary macrometastases and micrometastases in mammary cancer. Ann Surg 173:44–46, 1971.

59. International (Ludwig) Breast Cancer Study Group. Prognostic importance of occult axillary lymph node micrometastases from breast cancers. Lancet 335:1565–1568, 1990.

60. I De Mascarel, F Bonicham, JM Coindre, M Trojani. Prognostic significance of breast cancer axillary lymph node micrometastases assessed by two special techniques: reevaluation with longer follow up. Br J Cancer 66:523–527, 1992.

61. C Botti, P Vici, M Lopez, AF Scinto, F Cognetti, R Cavaliere. Prognostic value of

lymph node metastases after neoadjuvant chemotherapy for large-sized operable carcinoma of the breast. J Am Coll Surg 181:202–208, 1995.

62. RF Uren, RB Howman-Giles, JF Thompson, et al. Mammary Lymphoscintigraphy in breast cancer. J Nuc Med 36:1775–1782, 1995.

63. P Wingo, T Tong, S Bolden. Cancer Statistics: 1995. CA 45:8, 1995.

64. C Haagensen, A Stout. Carcinoma of the breast. II. Criteria of operability. Ann Surg 118:859, 1943.

65. D Arnold, G Lesnick. Survival following mastectomy for stage III breast cancer. Am J Surg 137:362, 1979.

66. A Fracchia, J Evans, B Eisenberg. Stage III carcinoma of the breast: a detailed analysis. Ann Surg 192:705, 1980.

67. D Schottenfeld, A Nash, G Robbins, et al. Ten-year results of the treatment of primary operable breast carcinoma: a summary of 304 patients evaluated by the TNM system. Cancer 38:1001, 1976.

68. KK Hunt, FC Ames, SE Singletary, AU Buzdar, GN Hortobagyi. Locally advanced noninflammatory breast cancer. Surg Clin North Am 76:393–410, 1996.

69. J Harris, J Sawicka, R Gelman, et al. Management of locally advanced carcinoma of the breast by primary radiation therapy. Int J Radiat Oncol Biol Phys 9:345, 1983.

70. G Bonadonna, P Valagussa, M Zambetti, et al. Locally advanced cancer: 10-year results after combined treatment. Proc Am Soc Clin Oncol 7:9, 1988.

71. M Lopez, D. Andriole, W. Kraybill, et al. Multimodal therapy in locally advanced breast carcinoma. Am J Surg 160:669, 1990.

72. B Fisher, A Brown, E Mamounas, et al. Effect of preoperative therapy for primary breast cancer (BC) on local-regional disease, disease-free survival (DFS) and survival (S). Proc ASCO 16:449, 1997.

73. G Bonadonna, U Veronesi, C Branbilla, et al. Primary chemotherapy to avoid mastectomy in tumors with diameters of 3 centimeters or more. J Natl Cancer Inst 82:1539, 1990.

74. G Hortobagyi, F Ames, A Buzdar, et al. Management of stage III primary breast cancer with primary chemotherapy, surgery and radiation therapy. Cancer 62:2507, 1988.

75. D Booser, D Frye, S Singletary, et al. Response to induction chemotherapy for breast cancer: a prospective multimodality treatment program. Proc Am Soc Clin Oncol 11:82, 1992.

76. SJ Schnitt, A Abner, R Gelman, et al. The relationship between microscopic margins of resection and the risk of local recurrence in patients treated with conserving surgery and radiation therapy. Cancer 74:1746–1751, 1994.

77. MC Smitt, JW Nowels, MJ Zdeblich, et al. The importance of the lumpectomy surgical margin status in long term results of breast conservation. Cancer 76:259–267, 1995.

78. I Gage, SJ Schnitt, AJ Nixon, et al. Pathologic margin involvement and the risk of recurrence in patients treated with breast-conserving therapy. Cancer 78:1921–1928, 1996.

79. R Heimann, C Powers, HJ Halpern, et al. Breast preservation in stage I and II carcinoma of the breast. Cancer 78(8):1722–1730, 1996.

80. AC Broders. Carcinoma in situ contrasted with benign penetrating epithelium. JAMA 99:1670, 1932.

81. P Borgen, C Swallow, K Van Zee, V Sacchini. Ductal carcinoma in situ. Curr Probl Surg Monogr 557–591, 1996.

82. J Warneke, D Grossklaus, J Davis, et al. Influence of local treatment on the recurrence rate of ductal carcinoma in situ. J Am Coll Surg 180:683–688, 1995.

83. K Kerlikowske, J Barclay, D Grady, E Sickles, V Ernster. Comparison of risk factors for ductal carcinoma in situ and invasive breast cancer. J Natl Cancer Inst 89:76–82, 1997.

84. ER Fisher, R Sass, B Fisher, et al. Pathologic findings from the National Surgical Adjuvant Breast Project (protocol 6). I. Intraductal carcinoma (DCIS). Cancer 57:197–208, 1986.

85. ER Fisher, J Costantino, B Fisher, et al. Pathologic findings from the National Surgical Adjuvant Breast Project (NSABP) Protocol B-17. Cancer 75:1310–1319, 1995.

86. MJ Silverstein, A Barth, DN Poller, et al. Ten-year results comparing mastectomy to excision and radiation therapy for ductal carcinoma in situ of the breast. Eur J Cancer 31A:1425–1427, 1995.

87. MJ Silverstein, DN Poller, JR Waisman, et al. Prognostic classification of breast ductal carcinoma-in-situ. Lancet 345:1154–1157, 1995.

88. MD Lagios, FR Margolin, PR Westdahl, et al. Mammographically detected duct carcinoma in situ: frequency and local recurrence following tylectomy and prognostic effect of nuclear grade on local recurrence. Cancer 63:618, 1989.

89. RH Sawyer, DL Asbury. Mammographic appearances in Paget's disease of the breast. Clin Radiol 49:185, 1993.

90. C Cohen, J Guarner, P De Rose. Mammary Paget's disease and associated carcinoma: an immunohistochemical study. Arch Pathol Lab Med 117:291, 1993.

91. RB Eusebio, PJ Deckers. Paget's disease of the nipple-areola complex: a plea for conservatism. Contemp Surg 40:13, 1992.

92. RG Margolese. Symposium: Breast Cancer 1984, precancerous and high-risk lesions. Can J Surg 28:242, 1985.

93. WC Wood. Management of lobular carcinoma in situ and ductal carcinoma in situ of the breast. Sem Oncol 23:446–452, 1996.

94. D Easton, D Ford, J Petro. Ingerited susceptibility to breast cancer. Cancer Surv 18:95–113, 1993.

95. DM Radford, BA Zehnbauer. Inherited breast cancer. Surg Clin North Am 76:205–220, 1996.

96. Y Miki, J Swensen, D Shattuck-Eidens, et al. A strong candidate for the breast and ovarian cancer susceptibility gene BRCA 1. Science 226:66, 1994.

97. SA Smith, DF Easton, DG Evans, et al. Allele losses in the region 17q12-21 in familial breast cancer and ovarian cancer involve the wild-type chromosome. Nat Genet 2:128, 1992.

98. R Wooster, G Bignell, J Lancaster, et al. Identification of the breast cancer susceptibility gene BRCA 1. Nature 378:789–791, 1995.

99. MJ Lopez, KA Porter. The current role of prophylactic mastectomy. Surg Clin North Am 76:231–242, 1996.

100. National Advisory Council for Human Genome Research. Statement on use of DNA testing for presymptomatic identification of cancer risk. JAMA 271:785.

3
Mammography and Interventional Breast Procedures

Saeed Iraniha and Iraj Khalkhali
Harbor-UCLA Medical Center, Torrance, California

I. INTRODUCTION

In 1913, Albert Salomon, a surgeon, was the first person who described the application of radiography in the diagnosis of breast cancer. He studied over 3000 mastectomy specimens and compared the radiographic and pathologic results and found that radiography is effective in differentiating the highly infiltrating carcinoma from circumscribed carcinoma, as well as in diagnosing of axillary lymph node metastasis [1]. Fourteen years later in Germany, Otto Kleinschmidt published the use of mammogram as a diagnostic tool for breast diseases [2]. In 1930, Stafford Warren reported the use of a stereoscopic technique for breast radiography. His studies of 119 patients indicated a high diagnostic accuracy of mammography for diagnosis of breast cancer [3]. Goyanes et al., in 1931, described the mammographic signs of normal breast and explained how to differentiate the mammographic signs of inflammatory lesions from cancer [4]. Paul Seabold, in 1931, reported the mammographic appearance of normal breasts in various physiologic states ranging from the puberty to menopause. He even described the mammographic changes during the menstrual cycle [5]. In 1932, Walter Vogel published the mammographic differentiation of benign and malignant breast lesions [6]. Ira Lockwood, in 1933, published a review of mammographic diagnostic criteria [7]. Once again, in 1938, Jacob Gershon-Cohen and Albert Strickler reported the range of normal mammographic appearance of the breast at different ages and physiologic status [8]. In 1951 in France, Gros and Sigrist published many articles regarding mammography and mammographic criteria of benign and malignant lesions. Gros developed a dedicated mammography unit with a device to compress the breast [9]. In 1952, Gershon-Cohen and Helen Ingleby (pathologists) studied the correlation of the mammography and pathology results and established the mammographic criteria for the diagnosis of benign and malignant lesions. Gershon-Cohen also emphasized the use of high-contrast images and breast compression [10]. In Uruguay, Raul Leborgne described the typical mammographic appearance of breast cancer. He emphasized the use of breast compression to immobilize the breast and decrease its thickness and enhance image quality. He was also the first person to report the significant association of microcalcifications to subclinical breast carcinoma [11].

In 1960, Robert Egan modified the routine x-ray equipment to optimize soft-tissue imaging. By using this new technique, Egan reported excellent imaging results of his first 1000 mammographies under study [12]. In 1962, he reported the diagnosis of 53 cases of occult breast carcinoma by mammography which were undetectable by usual diagnostic methods [13]. His success led to the widespread use of mammography for diagnosis of breast cancer. In 1963, the Cancer Control Program of the United States Public Health Service, the National Cancer Institute, and the M.D. Anderson Hospital conducted a multicenter trial involving 24 centers to verify Egan's results and to determine the possible clinical applications of mammography. The results of this study, published in 1965, demonstrated that (1) the Egan technique of mammography could be learned by other radiologists; (2) mammography could enable differentiation between benign and malignant lesions; (3) mammograms of acceptable quality could be reliably produced; and (4) mammography could be used as a screening tool for the breast cancer in asymptomatic women [14]. Following these results, the American College of Radiology established a mammography committee which initiated a nationwide training program for radiologists and technologists to perform and interpret mammograms [15].

It is important to note that technological advances that took place during the second half of 20th century led to better and improved imaging technique, increasing the diagnostic value of mammography and its widespread usage.

II. TECHNICAL ASPECTS OF MAMMOGRAPHY

The ultimate goal of x-ray mammography is to produce images with high spatial resolution and good contrast separation. Producing such images requires a complex interaction of many linked factors. The quality of mammographic images depends on the mammographic equipment, the image receptor system, and the film processing. By law, all mammography should be done on dedicated mammographic equipment which is an x-ray system designed specifically for breast radiography [16]. First dedicated mammography unit was developed by Charles Gros

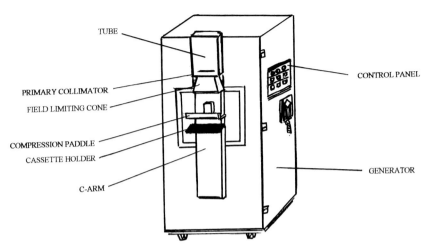

FIGURE 1   Dedicated mammography unit and its components.

in France in 1967 [17]. A dedicated mammography unit is expected to have the following components (Fig. 1): (1) breast compression device; (2) special target material and filter for soft-tissue imaging; (3) small focal spot (0.3 to 0.4 mm); (4) C-arm; (5) moving grid; (6) low x-ray attenuating cassette holder; and (7) automatic exposure control device [18]. Each component of dedicated mammographic unit significantly affects the overall clinical image quality.

Mammographic image quality is a combination of contrast, resolution, sharpness, and noise [19]. Image contrast is the difference in optical density between different regions of the mammogram and depends on subject contrast and image receptor contrast. Subject contrast is related to the attenuation of the x-ray beam as it passes through the breast. Image resolution is the ability to record small objects that are close together as separate objects. Image sharpness is the distinctness of the boundary or edges of a structure. Radiographic noise or mottle includes quantum mottle, screen mottle, and film grain. The major cause of this radiographic mottle is quantum mottle, which is caused by the statistical fluctuation in the number of x-ray photons absorbed at individual locations in the intensifying screen. The fewer x-ray photons that are used to make the image, the greater the amount of quantum mottle that results.

A.   Generator and X-Ray Source Assembly (Fig. 1)

Generator: A generator is a device that supplies electric power to the x-ray tube and regulates the length of the radiographic exposure [19].

Anode/Filter Combinations: The most commonly used anode/filter combination for mammography is a molybdenum (Mo) anode and molybdenum filter (25 to 30 μm thick). The Mo/Mo combination is preferred when imaging breasts with a compressed thickness of 2 to 5 cm, because this combination will provide the greatest sharpness and contrast. This combination is less effective in mammography of denser breasts. Dense breasts can be imaged with either an Mo/Rh (rhodium), Rh/Rh, or W(tungsten)/Rh combination [20].

Focal Spot: The focal spot size is a projection of the area of the target or anode on a film plane after an x-ray exposure [19]. X-ray mammography demands the highest resolution possible in order to image the fine structures and small calcifications (as small as 150 μm). Resolution is determined by the size of the focal spot and its distance from the structure within the breast to be imaged, by the distance from the structure to the detector, and ultimately by the ability of the detector to produce the image. Experimental findings correlated well with the theoretical prediction that the resolution of a system is inversely related to the size of the focal spot and the distance of the structure from the detector, and directly related to the distance from the focal spot to the lesion. Therefore, resolution can be increased by moving the small focal spot close to the object being imaged and moving the object away from the detector [19].

C-Arm: The C-arm rigidly supports the x-ray tube and cassette at opposite ends and is able to rotate to allow imaging in all projections [21].

Collimator: Collimators regulate the size and the shape of the x-ray beam. Beam collimation is intended to decrease scatter radiation and unnecessary patient exposure. In mammography, rectangular collimation is used to match the shape of the image receptor [19].

Compression Device: The compression device, consisting of a compression plate and mechanical components, is designed to help hold the breast stationary, to reduce the thickness of breast tissue, and to provide uniform taut breast compression so that the differences in attenuation of breast tissues can be appreciated [21]. In addition to making the breast thickness more uniform, compression has other advantages. It decreases the geometric unsharpness and improves the resolution by compressing the tissue against the detector. It also decreases the motion-related unsharpness because compression maintains the breast in the appropriate position. It reduces the image degradation from scatter, shortens the radiation exposure time, and decreases the radiation dosage. Finally, it spreads the tissues apart, separating often confusing overlapping structures on the mammogram.

Image Receptor System: Image receptor system includes the image receptor support, the antiscatter grid, the cassette, and the automatic exposure control detector. The image receptor support holds the cassette tightly to prevent its movement during C-arm motion [21]. Antiscatter grid is a set of thin, uniformly spaced lead strips, interspersed by low-attenuating material. The grid is located between the breast and the image receptor to reduce scatter radiation reaching the image receptor [21]. Automatic exposure control system, or phototimer, automatically determines and provides the exposure needed to produce an adequate film optical density. The AEC determines the appropriate exposure by sampling the x-ray intensity after it passes through the breast and image receptor [19].

B.   Magnification Mammography

Microfocus magnification mammography enhances image quality by improving apparent resolution, diminishing the effect of screen unsharpness, and decreasing image noise. Magnification is obtained by moving the object further away from the film and closer to the focal spot (Fig. 2). Currently, the recommended magnification is 1.5 to 2.0 times. Magnification more than two times leads to motion blur from long exposure times, increased geometric blur, and excessive radiation dose. For magnification mammography, the focal spot should be small and the SID (source-to-image distance) should be >60 cm [21].

C.   Positioning

The breast is a difficult organ to image. Not only does it contain tissue elements of very similar x-ray attenuation and low relative contrast, but also the geometry of the breast on the chest wall is complex. This geometry makes it extremely difficult to project all of the breast tissue onto a two-dimensional recording system. Careful attention to positioning is required to view as much of the tissue at risk as possible. Positioning is the maneuvers that the radiologic technologist uses to place the breast in the desired position on the film for a specific mammographic view. The art of mammographic positioning significantly enhances the detectability of subtle alterations of radiographic architecture, which may provide the earliest detectable signs of developing carcinoma.

Mammographic projections: A verity of positioning maneuvers and projections has been developed to better define the breast tissue and the lesions and/or to better localize the lesions. The remainder of this section addresses each of the standard projections and positions commonly used, as well as additional views, for mammography.

1.   Standard Views

The standard images for two-view screening mammography should include the mediolateral oblique (MLO) and craniocaudal (CC) views [22].

Mediolateral Oblique (MLO) (Fig. 3): The mediolateral oblique view is one of the standard views for the screening examination of an asymptomatic woman and, if it is performed properly, offers the best opportunity to image all of the

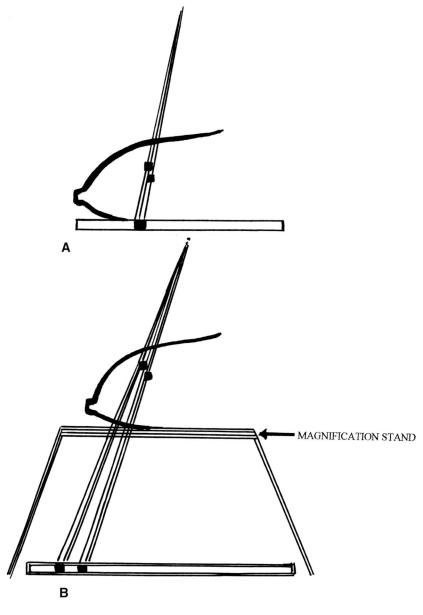

A

B

MAGNIFICATION STAND

FIGURE 2   Magnification, in order to improve resolution, is obtained by moving the object further away from the film and closer to focal spot. (A) On the contact image, the two small lesions are too close together to be identified in the film. (B) On the magnification image, the two objects are separated enough to be identified on the film.

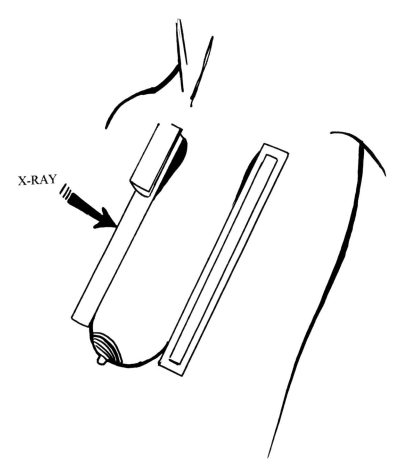

X-RAY

Figure 3   Mediolateral oblique view (MLO). The plane of cassette holder is angled 30° to 60° from the horizontal parallel to the plane of pectoralis muscle. The x-ray beam is directed from the superomedial to inferolateral aspect of the breast.

breast tissue in a single view [22]. For this view the plane of cassette holder is angled 30° to 60° from the horizontal, so that the cassette holder is parallel to the plane of the pectoralis muscle. The x-ray beam is directed from the superomedial to inferolateral aspect of the breast. It is important that the angle utilized be adjusted to the body habitus of patient to image the maximum amount of tissue. The properly positioned MLO projection should follow these criteria on the mammogram: (1) the pectoralis muscle is well visualized, with convex anterior shape, and extends to or below the nipple line; (2) the deep and superficial breast tissues are well separated; (3) the breast is not sagging; (4) close inspection shows no evidence of motion blur; (5) the inframammary fold is open; and (6) no posterior tissue is excluded [23].

Craniocaudal (CC) (Fig. 4): The craniocaudal view is the second standard projection, which is used for the screening of an asymptomatic woman. If any breast tissue is excluded from the MLO view, it is likely to be the medial tissue [22]. Therefore, it is necessary to show all of the medial tissue on the CC projection. This projection provides sagittal orientation of the breast tissue and, when properly performed, will include most of the breast with the exception of the far lateral portion [23]. For this view the plane of cassette holder is parallel to the floor and the x-ray beam is directed perpendicular to the floor. The properly positioned CC should follow these criteria: (1) all medial tissue visualized; (2) nipple centered; (3) visualization of pectoralis muscle or posterior nipple line measuring within one cm of the measurement on the MLO [23].

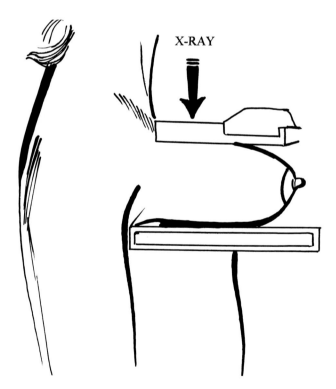

X-RAY

FIGURE 4   Craniocaudal view (CC). The plane of cassette holder is horizontal and x-ray beam is directed perpendicular to it.

2. Additional Views

In addition to standard views, many additional views can be useful to further evaluate a patient with a palpable mass or complete an abnormal screening mammogram. Additional views can help resolve questions relating to reality, location, or finite features of a perceived lesion.

Exaggerated craniocaudal: The XCC view is the most commonly performed additional view. This view depicts lesions deep in the outer aspect of the breast, including most of the axillary tail. The position is similar to the CC, but patient rotates until the lateral aspect of the breast is in contact with the cassette holder [23].

Spot Compression: Spot or coned compression views are especially helpful with obscure or equivocal findings in areas of dense tissue. In this view, by using a small compression plate, pressure can be applied to a smaller volume of breast. Compared with whole-breast compression, spot compression allows for greater reduction in thickness of the localized area of interest, improves separation of breast tissues, and results in greater contrast and more precise evaluation of findings. Spot compression is often combined with microfocus magnification to improve resolution [23].

Magnification: A magnification view allows more precise evaluation of margins and other architectural characteristics of a focal density or mass. It is also most effective in the delineation of the number, distribution, and morphology of calcifications [24]. Magnification is performed by moving the focal spot closer to the breast and moving the breast farther away from the detector. Optimal magnification mammography requires a tube with a microfocal spot of 0.1 mm or less [23].

Tangential: Tangential views can be used to image the palpable lesions that are obscured by surrounding dense glandular tissue in the mammogram. In this view superficial lesions are brought close to the skin surface for optimal visualization with least amount of overlapping parenchyma. This view can also be used to verify if calcifications seen on a mammogram are located within the skin. The x-ray tube is angled to any degree that will project areas of focal interest nearest to the skin.

90° Lateral (Mediolateral or Lateromedial) (Fig. 5): This view is one of the most commonly used additional view and is usually used in conjunction with the CC view to triangulate the exact location of the lesions in the breast. The most appropriate 90° lateral view, medial to lateral versus lateral to medial, is the one that provides the shortest object-to-film receptor distance, to reduce geometric unsharpness. For instance, if a questionable area is located medially, a lateromedial projection is obtained and vice versa. For either view, the tube arm is rotated to 90° [23].

Cleavage (Fig. 6): The cleavage view, or valley view, or double breast compression view, is performed to visualize deep lesions in the posteromedial aspect of the breast. The cleavage view is a CC view obtained with both breasts on the film holder and with the x-ray beam centered between the breasts or slightly off center, focusing on the medial aspect of one of the breasts [23].

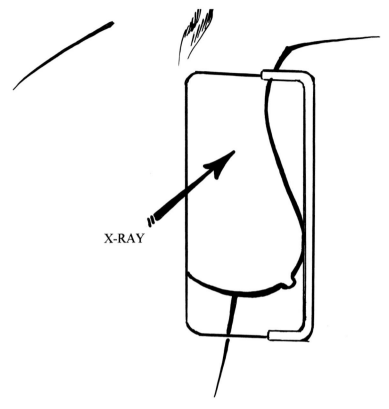

X-RAY

Figure 5   90° lateral. The plane of cassette holder is 90° from the horizontal, and the x-ray beam is directed perpendicular to it (from medial to lateral or lateral to medial sides).

Axillary Tail View (*Fig. 7*): The axillary tail view, or Cleopatra view, may be utilized to show the entire axillary tail as well as most of the lateral aspect of the breast. By reclining the patient's back (Cleopatra style), a slightly angled view of the lateral breast could be obtained [23].

Roll View (*Fig. 8*): Roll view, or change-of-angle view, offers a mechanism for uncovering lesions masked by overlapping structures. The purpose of this view is to confirm the presence of an abnormality, to better define a lesion, or to determine the location of a finding seen on only one of the standard views [23]. The patient is repositioned using the same projection that showed the abnormality, and breast tissue is rolled in opposite directions.

Caudocranial View: The caudocranial view or reverse CC improves the visualization of lesions in the uppermost aspect of the breast by providing a reduced object-to-film distance. This view can also be used during needle local-

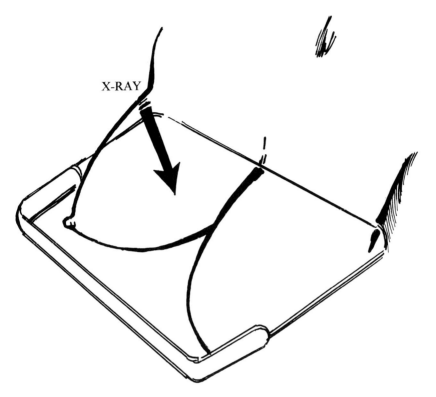

X-RAY

FIGURE 6   Cleavage view (valley view). This view is a craniocaudal view obtained with both breasts on the film holder and x-ray beam centered between the breasts or slightly off center.

ization to provide a shorter route to an inferior lesion or can be used to maximize the amount of tissue visualized on the breast of male patient or in women with kyphosis [23].

Lateromedial Oblique: This view improves the visualization of the medial breast tissue by providing a reduced object-to-film distance. The x-ray beam directed from the lower outer to the upper-inner aspect of the breast.

Implant-Displaced Views (*Fig. 9*): These views are CC and MLO or 90° lateral projections used in patients with breast implant. In these views, the prosthesis is displaced posteriorly and superiorly against the chest wall, and breast tissue is pulled anteriorly and held in place with compression device. With this technique the breast tissue can be well compressed and visualized free of the implant [25]. It is important to stress inclusion of the standard views with the implant in the field together with the modified compression views as part of the complete

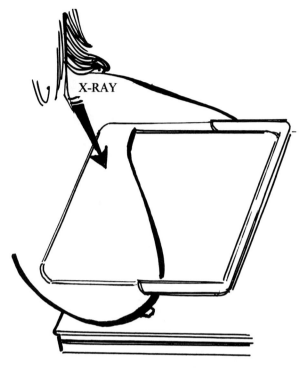

FIGURE 7   Cleopatra view. The plane of cassette holder is horizontal. By reclining the patient's back, axillary tail is placed in contact with cassette holder and x-ray beam is directed perpendicular to it.

mammographic evaluation of the breast that has implants [25]. The standard views permit visualization of breast tissue surrounding the implant posteriorly that may not be seen on the modified views.

D.   Quality Control

Quality assurance (QA) is defined as all of the policies and systematic procedures that provide confidence that a valid mammography was performed, including everything from recruitment and monitoring of patients to assessment of outcome data. Quality control (QC) refers only to those QA activities that specifically involve the technical aspects of performing the mammographic examination.

Equipment and positioning are the two most important factors in obtaining high-quality mammograms. Good technique requires constant attention to detail. Quality control throughout the imaging sequence must be maintained. The x-ray system should be routinely monitored for tube output and beam quality as well as

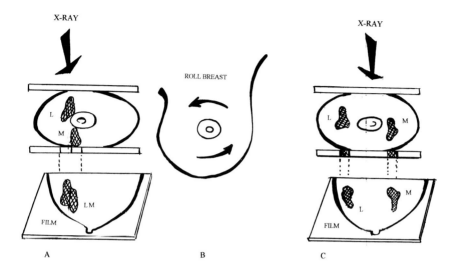

FIGURE 8   Roll view. This view is used to separate superimposed breast lesions (A). Breast tissue is rolled to lateral or medial directions (B) and while the breast is in new position the same view is obtained (C).

for patient dose. Automatic exposure control will reduce the number of underpenetrated and overpenetrated studies. Processor system requires routine maintenance, and the screens should be routinely cleaned to eliminate dust particles which compromise the images. The importance of proper positioning cannot be overemphasized. Failure to image the deep tissue of the breast will lead to false-negative results and missed early cancers. Symmetrical positioning with firm compression will help minimize interpretive error. In general, constant attention to quality control, with every image evaluated for adherence to strict technical standards, is essential for maintaining image quality.

E.   Analyzing the Mammogram

A systematic approach to image analysis is important to appreciate subtle changes and reduce false-negative interpretations due to observer error. While individuals will develop their own routine, as long as the basic conventions are maintained there is no one "correct" sequence. Radiologists should adhere to one system to avoid mistakes in interpretation. The observer should compare the current study with all previous studies because a subtle abnormality may only be apparent as a progressive change over a long period of time and difficult to appreciate over the short interval. The breasts should always be viewed as symmetrical organs. It is preferred to position the mammograms as mirror images with the chest wall side of the breasts

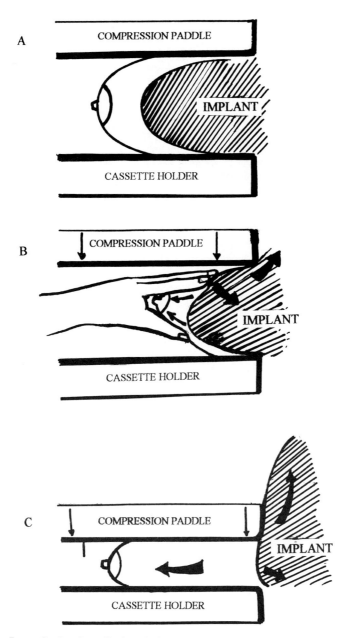

FIGURE 9   Implant-displaced views. These views are the standard projections used in patients with breast implants. (A) Standard view without displacing the implant. (B and C) Implant is displaced posteriorly and superiorly against the chest wall and breast tissue is pulled anteriorly and held in place with compression device.

against one another. Viewing the breasts as mirror images aids the appreciation of asymmetry. Since the breasts are remarkably symmetrical and the finding lesions is based on observing disruption of normal patterns, the reader should assess asymmetric density and architectural differences in mammograms. The overall breast composition should be described. This overall assessment of the attenuating tissues in the breast indicates the relative possibility that a lesion could be hidden by normal tissues in mammogram. This description has been classified into four patterns, including entirely fat, scattered fibroglandular densities, heterogeneously dense, and extremely dense breast in mammogram (Figs. 10–13) [29]. This global evaluation is followed by a close-up individual review of each image looking for abnormal densities, areas of architectural distortion, and microcalcification. Magnifying lenses are used to further search for microcalcifications.

After reading the mammogram, the radiologist should be able to report the finding in an organized manner. The American College of Radiology Reporting and Data System (BIRADS) has been designed to provide a dictionary of terminology and a report organization that leads to a decision-oriented final assessment of a mammogram [26,29]. The BIRADS categorizes the mammographic findings into five groups:

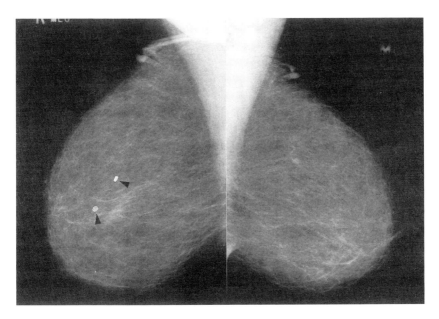

FIGURE 10   A 74-year-old woman with no breast mass on physical examination. Standard mammogram (MLO view) was consistent with predominantly fatty breast (pattern 1 in ACR classification). Note: This mammogram also showed two calcified densities with central lucency in right breast, characteristics of fat necrosis (arrowhead).

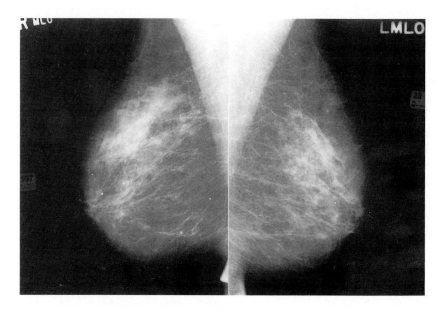

FIGURE 11   A 60-year-old woman with no breast mass on physical examination. Standard mammogram (MLO view) showed scattered fibroglandular densities in both breasts (pattern 2 in ACR classification). These densities could obscure a breast lesion on mammogram.

1. A negative mammogram meaning no abnormality
2. A benign finding indicating the presence of a benign lesion such as calcifying fibroadenoma, but no evidence of a cancer
3. A probably benign finding indicating the presence of an abnormality that is probably benign (prevalence of cancer <2%) but short interval follow-up is recommended to confirm its regression or stability
4. An indeterminate finding indicating the probability of malignancy between 2% and 50%; biopsy should be considered
5. A malignant finding indicating the presence of a lesion likely to be a cancerous (80% or more); biopsy is a must [26,29].

Each mammogram should be assessed for the presence of asymmetry; architectural distortion; masses; calcifications; skin, nipple, and trabecular changes; and axillary nodal abnormalities.

1. Asymmetry

a. Asymmetrically Dense Breast Tissue

Asymmetrically dense breast tissue is a broad area of radiographically dense tissue that does not form masses but is distinctly different from the corresponding

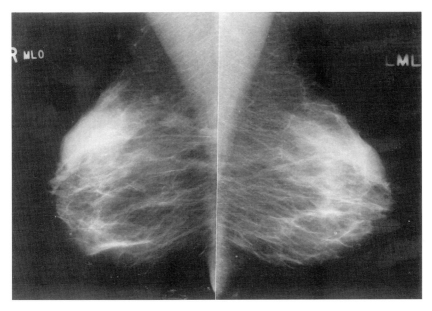

FIGURE 12   A 45-year-old woman with no breast mass on physical examination. Standard mammogram (MLO view) showed heterogeneously dense breasts (pattern 3 in ACR classification). This pattern may lower the sensitivity of mammogram for detecting the breast lesions.

contralateral volume of tissue. It refers to a relative increase in the volume of fibroglandular tissue compared with the corresponding area in the contralateral breast. The architecture of the breast is maintained, the underlying trabecular pattern is preserved, and fat can be frequently seen distributed through the area. Simple benign asymmetrically dense tissue should not have definable margins, and it does not have an easily defined center. If calcifications are present, the entity is no longer a simple asymmetry and may require biopsy. Nonspecific dense areas are evident in about 3% of mammograms. Virtually all are normal variations which occur due to either developmental asymmetry or different end-organ response to hormonal stimuli. The upper outer quadrant is the most common site. Asymmetrically dense breast tissue, if cancerous, is virtually always clinically evident (palpable). Therefore, biopsy of simple asymmetric breast tissue is recommended only when a corresponding palpable mass is present (Fig. 14) [26].

b.   Focal Asymmetric Density

A focal asymmetric density is a three-dimensional structure with definable margins that either fade into the surrounding tissue or are obscured by it. This suspi-

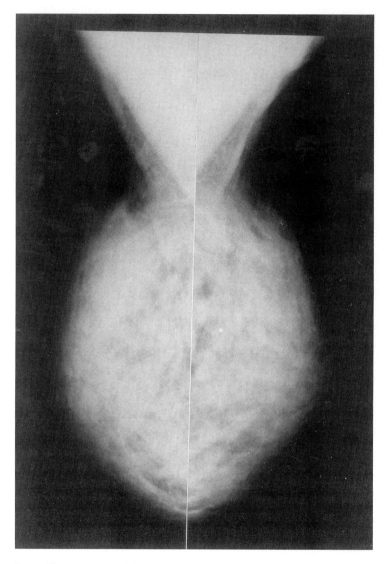

FIGURE 13   A 39-year-old woman with no breast mass on physical examination. Standard mammogram (MLO view) showed extremely dense breasts (pattern 4 in ACR classification). This pattern significantly lowers the sensitivity of mammogram in detecting the breast lesions.

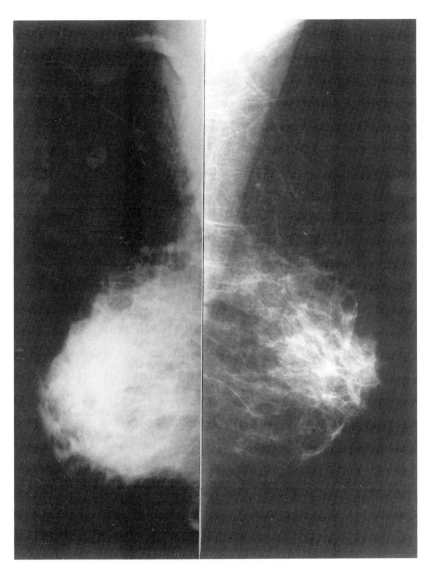

FIGURE 14   A 44-year-old woman with right breast palpable mass. Standard mammogram (MLO view) showed diffuse asymmetrical density and skin thickening of right breast. Result of excisional biopsy indicated infiltrative ductal carcinoma. Note: Mammogram showed no abnormality in left breast.

cious asymmetric density has a dense central zone with density tapering toward the periphery. Focal asymmetric density should be considered suspicious and warrants biopsy (Fig. 15).

c. Asymmetric Prominent Ducts

Asymmetric prominent ducts have been described as a secondary sign of malignancy [28] only if a mass or microcalcifications are present. Cancerous tissue detected is very likely to be palpable on physical examination and warrants biopsy [28]. Asymmetric prominent ducts in the absence of a mass or calcifications represent a normal variation or duct ectasia.

d. Asymmetric Vasculature

The vessels of the breast are generally symmetrical in size and distribution. They may become engorged because of either distal obstruction or increased flow due to hyperemia. A dilated vessel can accompany inflammation as well as neoplasia; however, it is generally either a normal variation or secondary to differences in mammographic compression.

2. Architectural Distortion

The structures of the breast are loosely arranged along duct lines, and the normal flow is toward the nipple. This pattern is superimposed on the crescentic planes of Cooper's ligaments, which form acinar curvilinear densities that criss-cross the breast to insert on the undersurface of skin, producing concave scalloped surfaces at the edge of the mammary parenchyma. Disturbances in this normally symmetrical flow, especially the pulling in of structures toward a point eccentric to the nipple, is called architectural distortion. In other words, an architectural distortion is a focal abnormal arrangement of the parenchymal tissues (the ducts and ligaments) with no definite mass including spiculation radiating from a point and focal retraction or distortion of the edge of the parenchyma (Fig. 15) [29]. In the absence of previous surgery, cancer is the major cause of architectural distortion. Postsurgical scarring, as well as benign lesions such as radial scars, can produce areas of architectural distortion. If a three-dimensional architectural abnormality is present, biopsy is indicated unless the disruption clearly relates to prior surgery.

3. Masses

The most common mammographic sign of a breast cancer is a mass. A mass can be defined as a three-dimensional area of density with margins distinguishing it

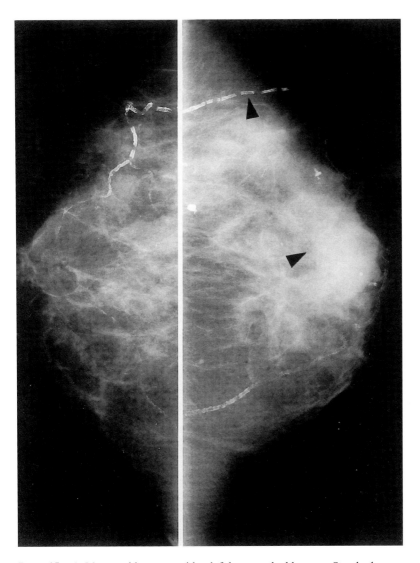

FIGURE 15   A 56-year-old woman with a left breast palpable mass. Standard mammogram (CC view) showed asymmetrical density and architectural distortion, involving 2/3 of left breast (lower arrowhead). Result of excisional biopsy indicated infiltrative ductal carcinoma. Note: This mammogram also demonstrated benign arterial calcifications or rail-road calcifications (upper arrowhead).

from the surrounding parenchyma [29]. Such lesions should be evaluated for location, density, size, shape, margins, and the presence of associated calcifications.

a. Location

The mammographer must first determine that a lesion is in fact within the breast and not on the skin. These can easily be differentiated by placing a marker on the skin lesion and repeating the mammogram or obtaining a tangential view. Although statistically the most common location for breast cancer is the upper outer quadrant, cancer may be found anywhere in the breast where there are epithelial elements.

b. Density

In general, malignant lesions have greater radiographic density than an equal volume of fibroglandular breast tissue, probably due to the dense fibrosis associated with these lesions. Lucent lesions are always benign. Lucent lesions have a capsule whose inner wall is visible in contrast to the high-fat material making up the lesion. These encapsulated lesions containing fat such as lipoma and galactoceles are not malignant and can be detected directly from the mammogram as benign processes.

c. Size

Although benign lesions such as cysts and fibroadenomas can reach very large sizes, in general, the larger a lesion, the more suspicious. The size of a cancer is directly related to the probability of involvement of the axillary nodes and thus to prognosis [30].

d. Shape

The shape of the lesion is an important indicator of malignancy. Lesions may be round, ovoid, lobulated, irregular, or a combination. The more irregular the shape, the more likely a lesion is to be cancer.

e. Margins

The interface between a lesion and the surrounding tissue is one of the most important factors in determining the significance of a mass. The margins of a lesion may be sharply defined, producing circumscribed densities; ill-defined; stellate; or spiculated. Analysis of the margins of lesions is complicated by the superimposition of normal structures that occur in any two-dimensional view of a three dimensional organ. Coned-down spot compression with magnification can help by spreading overlying structures and by improving the resolution. Infiltrative margins should prompt a biopsy.

4.   Masses with Circumscribed Margins

Statistically, a lesion with sharply defined borders that abruptly separate it from the surrounding tissues has a very high likelihood of being benign. However, lymphoma, papillary carcinoma, and infiltrating carcinoma can all on occasion appear as round, smoothly marginated lesions. Isolated, small (<8 mm), round, smoothly marginated densities require follow-up at 4- to 6-month intervals if close evaluation reveals no suspicious morphology. This is particularly true when there are many similar densities scattered throughout the breast. An isolated density, however, particularly one >1 cm in size, is more suspicious and should be investigated further, by aspiration or ultrasound—in general, any circumscribed lesion that has any irregular contour, distorts the architecture, or has suspicious calcifications requires biopsy.

a.   Fibroadenoma

Fibroadenoma is the most common benign breast tumor encountered in women <35 years and the most common solid masses found in women of all ages. They rarely develop or grow after menopause [31]. On mammograms, it is seen as well-circumscribed mass with round, oval, or nodular borders which does not distort the architecture. They are frequently multiple and bilateral. Calcification, which is coarse or primarily distributed at the periphery of the mass, is characteristic [31]. When the typical large, "popcorn" calcification is present within the fibroadenoma, the diagnosis can be made without biopsy (Fig. 16). Fibroadenoma with diffusely distributed calcification need to be biopsied because the intraductal carcinoma may have the same appearance [32].

b.   Cysts

Beginning in the fourth decade of life, cysts become more common. They are more common than fibroadenoma among women in their 40s and 50s [31]. They most likely represent dilatation of the terminal ducts within the lobules, as a result of duct obstruction and/or an imbalance between secretions and resorption. Cysts are usually round or oval and have well-circumscribed margins. They are usually multiple and bilateral and do not distort the architecture of the breast (Fig. 17). Calcification is infrequent, but may be seen as a thin peripheral eggshell, which may extend along part or all of the circumference [31]. Intracystic cancer is extremely rare but if aspiration reveals old blood, or they recur after multiple aspiration, biopsy is warranted.

c.   Intramammary Lymph Node

Benign intramammary lymph nodes are usually well-circumscribed oval or reniform noncalcified masses. They also have a fairly classic appearance of a lucent

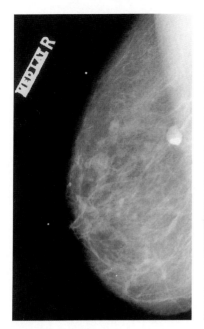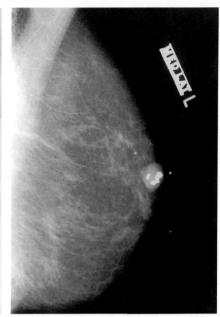

Figure 16   A 65-year-old woman with left breast palpable mass. Standard mammogram (MLO view) showed a 2-cm well-circumscribed mass with internal, coarse calcification (popcorn calcifications) in left breast, corresponding to the palpable mass. This finding is consistent with classic calcified fibroadenoma. Note: This mammogram also demonstrated a nonpalpable calcified fibroadenoma in the right breast. Metallic skin markers were placed on the nipple and palpable mass in the left breast and on the nipple and a skin mole in the right breast.

center with an invaginated hilum or notch (Fig. 18). On mammography, they are mostly seen at the periphery of upper outer quadrant, usually as far as three-quarters of the way toward the nipple. Typically, intramammary nodes are <1 cm in size. Enlargement of intramammary lymph nodes is uncommon but may result from inflammation dermatitis, hyperplasia, breast cancer, or metastasis [31]. If an intramammary lymph node is enlarged, it loses its hilar notch and becomes rounded. In this condition biopsy should be strongly considered.

d. Fibrosis

Fibrosis is a benign proliferation of fibrous connective tissue of the breast. Occasionally, these focal areas of fibrosis may appear as isolated islands of density with well-circumscribed margins [34]. They usually do not disrupt the architec-

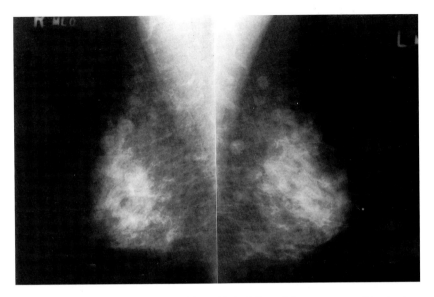

FIGURE 17   A 39-year-old woman with multiple, bilateral breast masses. Standard mammogram (MLO view) showed multiple, bilateral, well-circumscribed masses with no architectural distortion. Result of fine-needle aspiration was consistent with cystic lesions.

ture of the breast. They might also appear as ill-defined or spiculated masses with architectural distortion which warrant the biopsy.

e. Hematoma

A contusion may appear as very subtle, diffuse infiltration of tissues by blood or edema. It produces mild architectural changes with some thickening of the breast trabeculations. If trauma results in a true hematoma, a fairly circumscribed lesion may usually develop in the mammogram (Fig. 19). They usually resolve spontaneously, and permanent architectural distortion is fairly unusual [31]. On rare occasions, architectural distortion and scarring may persist, forming a worrisome spiculated density.

f. Hamartoma

Hamartoma, or lipofibroadenoma, is a breast mass with multiple areas of fatty and fibroglandular densities surrounded by a fibrotic psudocapsule (due to dis-

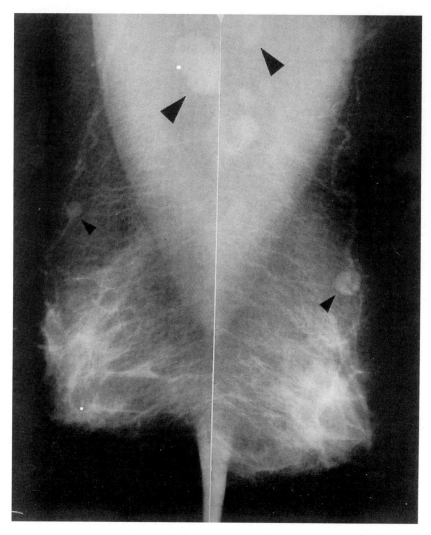

FIGURE 18   A 52-year-old woman with no palpable mass and incidental finding in screening mammogram. Standard mammogram (MLO view) showed a well-circumscribed mass with central lucency in the upper outer quadrant of each breast, consistent with intramammary lymph nodes (small arrowheads). Note: There are multiple bilateral lymph nodes in the axillary area, which are common findings on screening mammogram (large arrowheads).

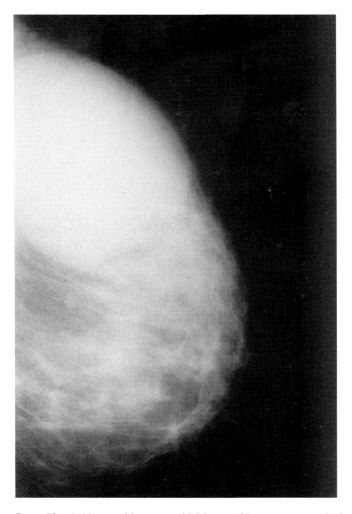

FIGURE 19   A 44-year-old woman with history of breast trauma and a breast mass 24 hours after trauma. Standard mammogram 3 months after trauma (on presentation) showed a 10 cm × 11 cm dense mass in upper outer quadrant of left breast. Result of excisional biopsy indicated hematoma.

placement of breast trabeculae). They usually appear in women >35 years. These lesions are usually circumscribed, containing fat and soft tissue density with a thin radiopaque capsule [33]. When they have the typical mammographic appearance (47%), no further follow-up or intervention is required [33]. On the other hand, the atypical lesions would require close-interval follow-up mammography or biopsy, depending on the lesion's size, imaging features, and clinical findings.

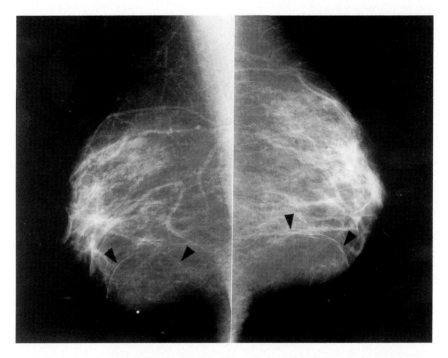

FIGURE 20   A 55-year-old woman with right breast soft, palpable mass. Standard mammo-gram (MLO and CC views) showed a 5-cm fatty mass with a thin capsule around it, corre-sponding to the palpable mass (arrowhead). This is a classic mammographic finding of lipoma. Note: Metallic skin marker was placed over the palpable mass.

g. Lipoma

Lipoma is a circumscribed fat-containing, completely radiolucent lesion sur-rounded by a thin radiopaque capsule (Fig. 20). This appearance is diagnostic of a benign lesion, and further workup or intervention is not required.

h. Papilloma

An intraductal benign papilloma usually occurs in the retroareolar region and may cause a serous or sanguinous nipple discharge. These lesion are usually small and are mammographically occult [35]. However, they may appear as a small circum-scribed mass with or without mulberry-like calcification along the periphery [31].

i. Galactocele

A galactocele is a milk-containing cyst that develops during or within a few months after lactation. The mammographic appearance depends on the amount of fat and proteinaceous material within the milk. If the fat content is very high, the mass may be completely radiolucent, mimicking a lipoma. However, the mammographic finding of a circumscribed mass with a fat-fluid level on upright horizontal beam films (ML or LM views) is diagnostic [36]. In some patients, the fat and water densities may be mixed, producing a mottled pattern similar to hamartoma [36].

j.   Phyllodes Tumor

Phyllodes tumor is an uncommon benign tumor with both epithelial and mesenchymal elements similar to fibroadenoma, with more cellular elements in the stroma. The most common clinical presentation is a large, rapidly growing mass. Although usually benign, the tumor can recur if not completely excised. Malignant degeneration can occur in 5% to 10% of cases. On mammography, most phyllodes are smooth-bordered, round, oval, or multilobulated circumscribed noncalcified masses (Fig. 21) [37]. When they are small, the appearance is identical to fibroadenoma.

k.   Lymphoma

Primary breast lymphoma is a relatively rare phenomenon. Secondary involvement of breast with lymphoma is more frequent. Malignant lymphoma of the breast can have varying morphologic characteristics, from diffuse increased density to sharply marginated lesion. The most common form of involvement is a circumscribed mass that is well defined or shows minimal irregularity [38]. Moderate to marked spiculation, however, is not infrequent. The mammographic findings are nonspecific, but bilateral axillary lymphadenopathy suggests the possibility of lymphoma [31].

l.   Sarcoma

Fewer than 1% of primary breast cancers are of mesenchymal origin such as lymphosarcoma or fibrosarcoma. They usually have a round or lobular shape with circumscribed margins and no spiculations or calcifications [31]. They cannot be distinguished mammographically from benign phyllodes tumor.

m.   Metastases to the Breast

Metastatic disease to the breast from extramammary primary lesions is unusual. Melanoma, lymphoma, and other hemotologic malignancies and lung cancer are the three most common bloodborne sources, followed by ovarian cancer, soft-tissue sarcomas, and other gastrointestinal and genitourinary cancers [39]. On mammograms, these metastases will be seen as discrete, round nodules with circumscribed to ill-defined margins with no spiculation. They are often solitary (85%)

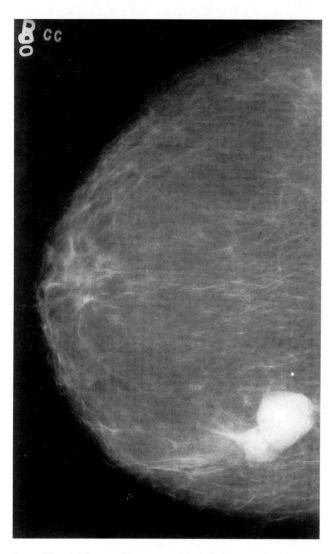

FIGURE 21   A 37-year-old woman with right breast palpable mass. Standard mammogram showed 4-cm lobulated mass with internal microcalcifications in right breast, suspicious for malignancy. Result of excisional biopsy indicated phylloides tumor. Note: Metallic skin marker was placed over the palpable mass.

and sometimes multiple (15%). On initial presentation, metastatic nodules will be unilateral in 75% and bilateral in 25% of cases. The majority will be found in the upper outer quadrant [40]. The presence of one or more discrete nodules in a patient with known extramammary cancer should alert one of the possibility of bloodborne metastases. With the exception of psammomatous calcification in metastatic ovarian carcinoma, metastases to the breast do not calcify [39].

n. Circumscribed Breast Cancer

Circumscribed carcinoma is a descriptive term referring to any ductal carcinoma that appears as a circumscribed mass with well-defined margin and no spiculation [31]. Circumscribed carcinoma includes all medullary [41], papillary [42], and mucinous carcinoma as well as some invasive ductal carcinoma [43] and some in situ ductal carcinoma [44]. Uncommonly, invasive lobular carcinoma can present as a circumscribed mass [31]. The likelihood of malignancy for a completely well-defined circumscribed mass of 1 cm or less is extremely low [31]. If these well-defined circumscribed masses are >1 cm, palpable or nonpalpable, the chance of cancer is 2% [45,46].

o. Masses with Ill-Defined Margins

Most breast cancers have ill-defined margins as a result of tumor infiltration into the surrounding tissue and the fibrosis that frequently accompanies it (Fig. 22) [47]. However, virtually every benign lesion of the breast can also be found with radiographically ill-defined margins. Benign lesions such as cysts with pericystic inflammation or fibrosis, fibroadenoma, contusion, or hematoma, or infection including true abscess may have ill-defined margins (Fig. 23) [47]. Many benign lesions may appear as an ill-defined mass secondary to the superimposition of normal breast tissue. Spot compression and magnification views may aid in spreading overlapping structures and improve the visualization of the lesion's margins, respectively. In general, solitary lesions with ill-defined margins that are not cysts (ultrasound can be useful) require biopsy [47].

p. Lesions with Spiculated or Stellate Margins

The presence of spiculations or a more diffuse stellate appearance is probably the most significant mammographic feature of breast cancer (Fig. 24). These are radially oriented filamentous structures that represent fibrosis interspersed with tumor extending into the tissue surrounding the breast cancer and distorting the surrounding tissue. The spicules can be as small as a few millimeters in size, producing "brush border," or extended over several centimeters. There are rare benign lesions, such as extra-abdominal desmid tumors, granular cell tumors, adenosis, fat necrosis, and radial scars that can mimic the classic appearance of breast can-

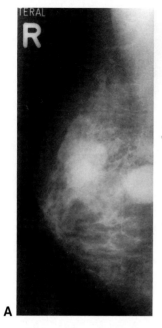
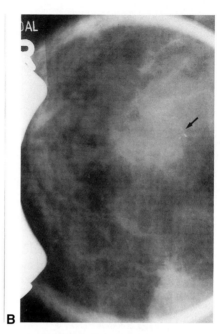

FIGURE 22   A 61-year-old woman with right breast palpable mass. (A) Standard mammogram (MLO view) showed multiple ill-defined masses with microcalcifications (not seen clearly). (B) Cone compression magnification view of the lesion demonstrated a large ill-defined mass with heterogeneous microcalcifications, suggestive of malignancy (arrow). Result of excisional biopsy of right breast mass indicated infiltrative ductal carcinoma.

cer (spiculated mass) and cannot be safely diagnosed without a biopsy [47–49]. Postoperative architectural distortion and increased density in the breast may persist for many months after surgery; however, the breast usually heals without radiographically visible scarring.

It is not unusual for the biopsy site to appear spiculated soon after the biopsy (Fig. 25) [50]. This appearance may persist for as long as 6 months to a year after surgery, and postoperative radiation therapy may delay its resolution. Many women have no residual mammographic or sonographic changes 1 year or more after biopsy [47]. However, some women have visible sequela for life. This sequela may present itself as an ill-defined or spiculated mass or area of architectural distortion [50]. It is also not unusual to see these mammographic changes after reduction mammoplasty [51]. In order to make the diagnosis of a scar, it is important to review prebiopsy mammograms to determine if the changes are truly in the area of the previous lesion. If there is any question, biopsy may be required.

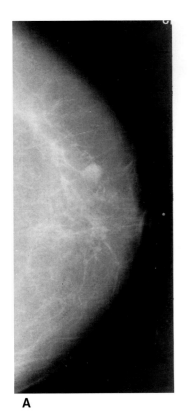

A

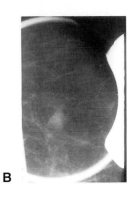

B

FIGURE 23   A 63-year-old woman with left breast palpable mass. (A) Standard mammogram (CC view) showed a 9-mm, ill-defined mass in the outer portion of left breast. (B) Cone compression magnification view of the lesion demonstrated the indistinctive border of the mass, suspicious for malignancy. Result of excisional biopsy indicated fibroadenoma with focal epithelial hyperplasia.

III. MASSES WITH ASSOCIATED CALCIFICATIONS

A. Calcified Involuting Fibroadenomas

Dense, large calcifications of a benign involuting fibroadenoma when seen within a lobulated mass are diagnostic of a benign lesion [47]. When these calcifications begin they may be very small, irregular, worrisome in appearance, and indistinguishable from malignant deposits. In such cases, biopsy is required. However, in later phases the calcification has a typical appearance that has been described as popcorn shape (Fig. 16). Generally fibroadenomas calcify from the center, and are so characteristic that they do not need to be biopsied [47]. Some fibroadenomas,

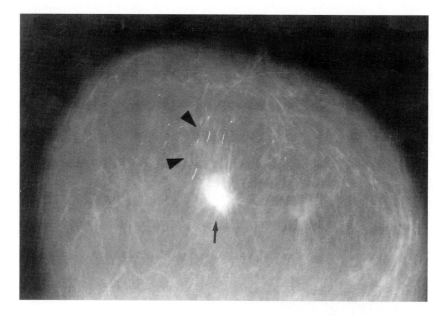

FIGURE 24   A 63-year-old woman with right breast palpable mass. Standard mammogram (CC view) showed a 2.3-cm spiculated mass in the central portion of right breast, suggestive of malignancy (arrow). Note: Mammogram also demonstrated multiple coarse, thick ductal calcifications adjacent to the cancer, which seems to be benign secretary calcifications (arrowhead). Result of excisional biopsy of right breast mass indicated infiltrative ductal carcinoma.

however, calcify from the periphery [52] and are indistinguishable from cancer and warrant a biopsy.

B.   Calcified Fat Necrosis and Cysts

Fat necrosis may appear as a radiolucent circumscribed mass with peripheral calcification ("eggshell") rim. This appearance is characteristic and known as "oil cyst" [48]. Similar deposits can occur within cysts walls. Very rarely, circumscribed malignant lesions can have such peripheral calcification; however, the calcification rim usually appears as thicker, more continuous deposits (Fig. 10).

C.   Calcifications in Cancer

Punctate, pointed, irregularly surfaced calcifications within a mass that are heterogeneous in size and morphology, as well as fine, linear, branching calcifications filling the duct with narrowed lumen are strong indications of cancer (Fig. 26) [52]. Up to 50% of malignant masses have calcifications [47].

1. Calcifications Without an Associated Mass

Calcification is the deposition of calcium salts (calcium hydroxyapatite or trical-cium phosphate) in the breast tissue [53]. Calcium deposits are extremely common in the breast tissue. Pathogenesis of calcification in the breast is variable. Some are the result of active secretion, while others form in necrotic cellular debris [53]. They may be a response to inflammation, trauma, radiation, foreign bodies, or cancer [47]. Calcifications are found within the ducts, alongside the ducts, in the lobular acini, in the vascular structures, in the interlobular stroma, in fat, and in the skin. Depending on their etiology and location they may be punctate, branching, linear, spherical, fine, coarse, cylindrical, smooth, jagged, regular in size and shape, or heterogeneous. When calcifications are lobular, they are virtually always benign and usually within dilated acini. Intraductal cancers may narrow the duct, and calcium deposits may fill the narrowed lumen, producing a characteristic fine linear pattern that branches with the duct. Most calcifications have characteristically benign morphology, but certain shapes and patterns require biopsy. A careful search for the clustered microcalcifications that may herald an early stage breast cancer should be done on all mammograms.

The visibility of calcifications is enhanced by obtaining a high-contrast image. Microfocus magnification mammography and spot compression will improve the clarity of these particles [52]. Unfortunately, benign and malignant processes can produce similar patterns of calcium deposition and frequently cannot be differentiated. Biopsy is often required for diagnosis. Analysis of the morphology, distribution, size, and number of the calcifications, however, eliminates many of these calcifications from suspicion.

D. Morphology

Morphology is the most important element in the analysis of calcifications. Typically, benign calcifications include those with vascular, lucent-centered, coarse (popcorn), or sedimenting appearance. These calcifications often do not require any follow-up other than mammography. Calcifications that are amorphous (hazy and irregular) in appearance are of intermediate concern and usually require further investigation. Pleomorphic calcifications are of greatest concern for presence of malignancy and require biopsy.

Calcifications associated with breast cancer are usually extremely variable in shape as well as in size. These calcifications appear as either comma-shaped deposits with pointed projections and irregular surfaces, or small, fine linear deposits within narrowed lumen that may be branching or appear as punctate calcifications in a "dot-dash" pattern [47].

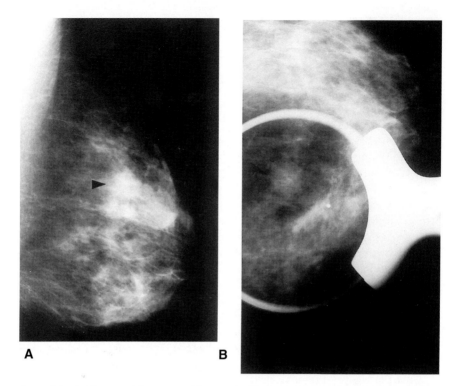

A   B

FIGURE 25   A 50-year-old woman with no palpable breast mass. Standard mammogram (MLO view) (A), and cone compression magnification view (B) showed a 1.8-cm mass with ill-defined border in the left breast, suspicious for malignancy (arrowhead). Result of needle localization excisional breast biopsy indicated fibrocystic changes with apocrine metaplasia and sclerosis adenosis. Three months later, her follow-up mammogram (C: CC view; D: cone compression magnification view) demonstrated a large spiculated mass consistent with post operative scar tissue (arrow). Metallic markers in left breast were placed on the skin scar. Note: Surgical scar can mimic mammographic findings of invasive carcinoma.

Some shapes are typically benign and do not require biopsy. Isolated shell-like or spherical calcifications with radiolucent center are always benign. These may occur in areas of fat necrosis [48]. The extrusion of cellular debris into the tissues around the ducts can result in an inflammatory reaction and produce extensive thick, rod-shape calcification seen in "plasma cell mastitis" [47]. Solid rod-shaped calcifications, which may form within the duct, are benign mammographic findings. Since the benign process does not narrow the lumen and may in fact lead to duct ectasia, these calcifications are generally larger than the fine, irregular

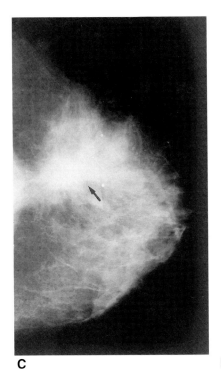
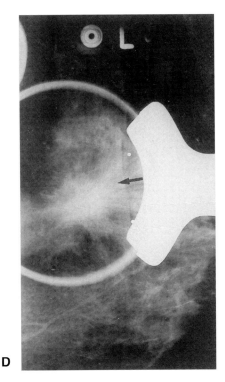

C   **D**

FIGURE 25   Continued

intraductal deposits found in malignancy [54]. Tubular (lucent-centered rods) calcifications that are oriented along duct lines, rarely branched, and thicker than 0.5 mm are virtually always a form of benign secretory deposit within the normal or dilated ducts or the periductal stroma [52,54].

Skin calcifications are usually lucent-centered calcifications that are round, dumbbell-shaped, or polygonal and appear near the periphery of the breast and are almost always benign [52].

Vascular calcifications are intimal calcium deposits in the arterial wall which are characterized by linear, parallel calcifications in a "railroad track" configuration on mammography (Fig. 15) [52]. Arterial calcifications are virtually always a consequence of age. They have also been reported in younger women with diabetes [55]. Vascular calcifications rarely confused with significant calcifications, and their presence has no clinical significance [55].

Milk of calcium is the term associated with the benign process in which free-floating calcium precipitates in the small, cystically dilated acini of the lob-

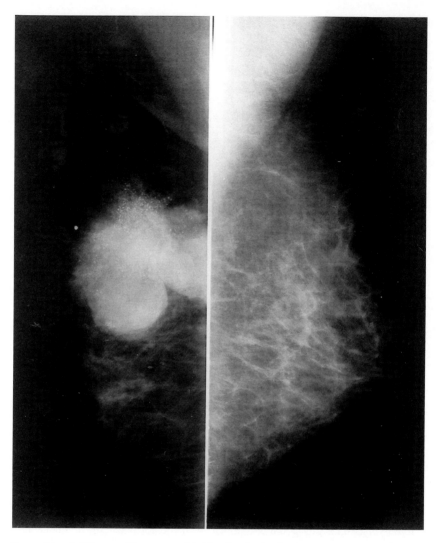

FIGURE 26   A 62-year-old woman with bloody nipple discharge from right breast for 6 years' duration. Standard mammogram (MLO view) showed a 6-cm × 6.5-cm lobulated mass in upper portion of right breast with multiple heterogeneous calcifications, suspicious for malignancy. Metallic marker in right breast was placed on palpable mass. Result of excisional biopsy indicated invasive ductal carcinoma. Note: Mammogram showed no abnormality of left breast.

ules, similar to the sediment at the bottom of a cup of tea (teacup calcifications) [56]. On the craniocaudal view with the x-ray beam perpendicular to the floor passing down through the fluidic calcium pooled in the bottom of the cyst, the precipitated calcium appears as amorphous, small, round, or oval smudged dots. When a lateral view is obtained with the beam parallel to the floor, the calcium projects as small linear to crescent-shaped calcification as the beam passes from the side through the concave meniscus of the material (Fig. 27) [52].

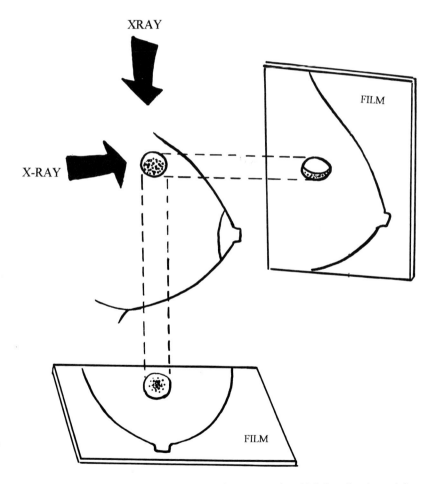

FIGURE 27   Cyst calcification. This is a benign process in which free-floating calcium precipitates in a cyst, and on the craniocaudal view (bottom), calcium appears as amorphous, small, round, or oval smudged dots; on lateral view (right), it appears as crescent-shaped calcification.

Large, coarse, solid, and sharply marginated calcifications usually represent completely involuted calcified fibroadenomas [52]. Other large calcifications may form in breast after surgery or irradiation. Many of these postirradiation calcifications are probably related to calcified suture material [47].

Foreign body in the breast can elicit calcification. Some forms of suture material appear to produce parallel, tubular-appearing calcifications with a radiating pattern from a central area in the immediate vicinity of previous surgery. This pattern is most common after radiation therapy [47].

Deodorant sprays, talc powders, and ointment (electrocardiogram paste) can cause the artifact and appear as calcifications. Tattoos also may look like calcification on mammogram. Scratches on the film, hair superimposed on the film, dust, dirt particles, and fingerprints on the screen and deposits of processing chemicals on the film also may simulate calcification on mammogram [52].

E.   Distribution

Distribution is the second most important element in analysis of calcifications. Calcifications may appear as cluster, linear, segmental, regional, or diffuse arrangement. Many cancer calcifications form in nonspecific patterns. However, cluster or linear arrangements of calcifications are usually worrisome and require biopsy. Calcifications whose distribution represents the presence of calcium deposits within a single duct network are of concern and also require biopsy. Diffusely scattered, lucent-centered calcifications generally represent skin deposits and are almost always benign. In general, diffuse calcifications randomly distributed across large volumes of breast tissue are caused by benign processes [52]. This is especially true when they are bilateral and fairly uniform in shape although varying in size.

F.   Size

Calcifications may occur in the tumor when it has infiltrated beyond the duct, or occur inside the involved ducts and form template of its lumen [52]. The diameter of these involved ducts is often diminished by the heaped-up layers of the tumor cells, which leads to appearance of intraductal calcifications with different sizes and densities on mammography. Although calcifications up to 2 mm in diameter may still be considered suspicious, those associated with cancer are usually <0.5 mm in diameter [47]. Calcifications as small as 0.2 and 0.3 mm are visible on mammography [47]. The smaller the calcification particles, the greater the suspicion for malignancy.

G.   Number of Calcifications

The use of threshold number of calcification to categorize suspicious calcifications has caused much discussion. It is reported that the probability of cancer increases with the number of calcifications in the tissue volume. Eagan et al. found that in 115 patients biopsied for microcalcifications alone, all lesions diagnosed as cancer had at least five visible flecks of calcium in a 0.5-by-0.5-cm field [57]. No absolute minimum threshold exists, because some cancers contain fewer than five calcifications. However, the risk seems to increase significantly when there are five or more calcifications visible in a square cm of the mammogram in a volume of approximately 1 cc [52].

IV.   SKIN, NIPPLE, AND TRABECULAR CHANGES

The skin generally forms a smooth convex surface, surrounding the breast parenchyma with a layer of subcutaneous fat in between. Normal skin is approximately 0.5 to 2 mm in thickness, except at the inframammary fold, near the cleavage, and in the periareolar region, where the skin is normally thicker.

A.   Thickening

Cooper's ligament produces a fine trabecular pattern of curvilinear septations coursing through the breast. Fibrous extensions of Cooper's ligaments extend through the subcutaneous fat and insert in the skin as the retinacula cutis, giving a scalloped, concave appearance to the edge of the parenchymal cone. Mammographic appearance of skin or trabecular thickening is nonspecific. Both benign and malignant process can result in thickening of these structures. Skin thickening may have a focal or a diffuse pattern. Infection or postsurgical scarring is the most likely cause of focal thickening. Invasive carcinoma also may appear as focal thickening on mammography, which suggests direct infiltration of the skin by the tumor (Fig. 14). Diffuse skin thickening is more common than focal. In the case of malignancy, diffuse skin thickening may be due to diffuse involvement of dermal lymphatics by tumor cells (inflammatory carcinoma), distal lymphatic obstruction secondary to underlying carcinoma, or metastasis to the axillary lymph nodes. Diffuse skin thickening may also be associated with mastitis, abscess, progressive systemic sclerosis, obstruction of superior vena cava, pemphigus, nephrotic syndrome, congestive heart failure, Milroy's syndrome, lymphoma, lymphatic extension from contralateral breast carcinoma, or changes secondary to radiotherapy [58].

B.   Retraction

Although malignant lesions may produce alterations in the nipple and skin, these are usually late changes and a palpable lesion is frequently evident. Cancers tend to elicit a contractile fibrotic response, and this can result in traction on the skin or nipple through direct extension or through Cooper's ligaments. Even deep lesions may cause retraction of the skin as a result of the tethering effect of Cooper's ligaments through the skin insertions of the retinacula cutis [58]. Skin or nipple retraction may result from benign scarring, usually in a postsurgical setting along the skin incision. Fat necrosis and inflammation from bacterial infection have also been reported as benign causes of skin retraction [48]. Nipple inversion is usually the result of benign idiopathic process and is often bilateral. Benign changes invariably occur over a long period of time. If nipple inversion happens over a short interval, a malignant etiology should be sought.

C.   Calcifications

Calcifications of the nipple occur infrequently. On occasion, the clinically evident extension of intraductal carcinoma onto the surface of the nipple known as Paget's disease can produce microcalcifications extending along the duct network in a single-file pattern. Calcification in the skin, however, is extremely common. They usually have typical appearance of spherical or polygonal shapes with central lucency and are widely scattered over the breast [47].

D.   Axillary Lymph Nodes

Lymphatic drainage of the breast is primarily through the axillary lymph nodes. Attempts to stage the axilla by mammography have been unsuccessful. Mammography with dedicated units generally provides a limited view of the axilla. The lower axillary lymph nodes can be seen on mediolateral oblique views, but mammography is relatively inaccurate in determining their status [59]. Normal axillary lymph nodes are <2 cm in size and have a fairly typical hilar notch or lucent center. When replaced by fat, axillary lymph nodes may become extremely large, but the lucent fat is obvious. Lymph nodes without central lucency that are >1.5 to 2 cm in size should be considered abnormal (Fig. 28) [47]. These are nonspecific and may be secondary to reactive hyperplasia. Furthermore, axillary lymph nodes may appear normal by mammography and still contain tumor. Surgical sampling is the most accurate method of assessing the involvement of axillary lymph nodes.

On very rare occasions, calcifications appear in axillary nodes. When calcifications are present in axillary nodes, metastasis should be suspected, especially if tumor in the breast contains similar calcifications.

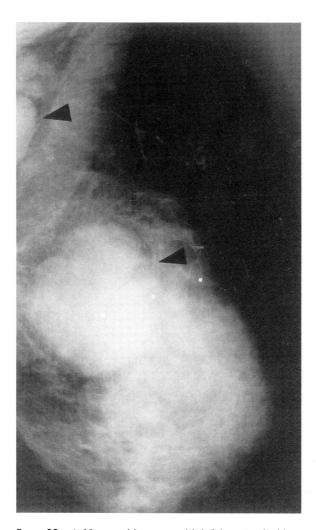

FIGURE 28   A 33-year-old woman with left breast palpable mass. Standard mammogram (MLO view) showed a 6-cm × 6.5-cm ill-defined mass in upper portion of the left breast, highly suspicious for malignancy (lower arrowhead). This mammogram also demonstrated several enlarged, dense lymphadenopathy in the left axillary area (upper arrowhead). Result of lumpectomy and axillary lymph node dissection indicated invasive ductal carcinoma with involvement of axillary lymph nodes. Note: Metallic skin marker was placed on the area of previous biopsy in Mexico.

V. SCREENING MAMMOGRAPHY

Breast cancer is the most common cancer and the second leading cause of cancer-related death in women living in the United States [60]. In the United States in 1995, 183,400 new breast cancer patients were reported and 46,000 women died from the disease [61]. The incidence of breast cancer is increasing by about 3% per year in the United States [61]. Recent statistics show that one in eight women in the United States has the lifetime risk of developing breast cancer [61]. The risk of developing breast cancer increases markedly with age; >75% of breast cancers occur in women who are >50 [62]. Methods to prevent breast cancer have not yet been established, and most of the scientific efforts have concentrated on developing the new and improved ways to detect the breast cancer at early stages and to treat the cancer once it occurs.

Early detection of breast cancer is a potentially important means for reducing the mortality of breast cancer and increasing life expectancy of the patients [63–65]. It leads to earlier treatment of breast cancer before spreading of the tumor. The main screening methods for early detection of breast cancer are physical examination of breast by a trained health professional and mammography [66].

Other potential methods of screening, such as self-examination of the breasts, have not demonstrated to be of great value [67], and some methods, such as thermography and CT scanning, have been shown to be of no value [66]. In this section, various studies on the screening mammography will be reviewed.

A. Screening Mammography

The purpose of screening for breast cancer is to decrease the mortality by detecting the breast cancer at earlier, more curable stages. Recently the usefulness of mammography has been enhanced by technical advances that provide increased visualization of the breast parenchyma, reduced exposure to radiation, improvements in film quality and processing, refined technique of imaging, better guidelines for the diagnosis of the cancer, and wider availability of well-trained mammography technicians [66]. These newer techniques detect a large percentage of cancers that are 2 cm or less in diameter [66]. Randomized trials are the only way to accurately evaluate the effect of screening mammography on breast cancer mortality. Since around 30 years ago, in addition to several case control and cohort studies, eight major randomized controlled trials of breast cancer screening have been conducted. Table 1 summarizes eight major randomized clinical trials. This section includes summary of these randomized clinical trials and a discussion of the data from randomized trials for women in three age groups: 40 to 49, 50 to 69, and 70 or older.

TABLE 1   Randomized Clinical Trials of Mammography

Study (dates)	Age range	Sample size		Screening modality (periodicity, mo)	Breast cancer mortality relative risk (Follow-up, yr)
		Study	Control		
HIP, New York (1963–1969)	40–64	30,239	30,756	2-view MM + CEB (12 mo, 3 times)	0.71 (10 yr)
Two-County, Sweden (1977–1985)	40–74	78,085	56,782	1-view MM <50y, 24 mo, 4 times >50y, 33 mo, 3 times	0.70 (11 yr)
Malmo, Sweden (1976–1986)	40–69	21,088	21,195	2-view MM (18–24 mo, 5 times)	0.81 (12 yr)
Stockholm, Sweden (1981–1985)	40–64	39,164	19,943	1-view MM (28 mo, 2 times)	0.80 (8 yr)
Gothenborg, Sweden (1982–1988)	40–59	20,724	28,809	2-view MM (18 mo)	0.86 (7 yr)
Edinburg, Scotland (1979–1988)	45–64	23,226	21,904	2-view MM + CBE (12–24 mo)	0.84 (10 yr)
NBSS 1, Canada (1980–1985)	40–49	25,214	25,216	2-view MM + CBE (12 mo)	1.36 (7 yr)
NBSS 2, Canada (1980–1985)	50–59	19,711	19,694	2-view MM + CBE (12 mo)	0.97 (7 yr)

Source: From Ref. 68.
MM: Mammogram; CBE: Clinical Breast Examination.

B.   Randomized Clinical Trials

In order to understand the purpose, design, and major limitations of randomized clinical trials, each of these trials will be summarized in this section. Together, these trials include more than 500,000 women, with 180,000 women aged 40 to 49 years. There is a wide variation in design among these trials [68]. The design varied based on the age of the participants, whether one-view or two-view screening mammography was being used, and screening interval.

C.   Health Insurance Plan of New York

The first randomized clinical trial of breast cancer screening was conducted by the Health Insurance Plan of Greater New York (HIP) from 1963 to 1970 [69]. HIP trial included women aged 40 to 64 years at entry. Nearly 62,000 women were randomly assigned to either the study group or the control group. Women in study group underwent two-view mammography and clinical breast examination every 12 months in 4-year study period; those in control group offered no screening. Follow-up was continued for 18 years. This trial demonstrated the reduction of breast cancer mortality in the study group 4 years after entry for women aged

50 and older and 7 years after entry for women between 40 and 49 years. By 18-year follow-up, this reduction was almost similar in both groups (23% and 21%, respectively) [69].

D.   Swedish Two-County Study

This trial, in Kopparberg and Ostergotland, began in 1977 with enrollment of almost 135,000 women. Women 40 years of age and older were randomly assigned to either a single-view mammogram (study group) or their usual care (control group). Screening examination were conducted at 2-year intervals for those aged 40 to 49 and at 33-month intervals for those aged 50 to 74. Screening continued for four rounds for the younger group and three rounds for the older group. A 31% reduction in mortality from breast cancer was found among women 40 to 74 years old after 8 years of follow-up [70,71].

1.   Malmo Trial

This trial was started in Malmo, Sweden, in 1976 and randomized 42,284 women aged 45 to 69 years old to have a two-view mammogram every 18 to 24 months for five rounds or to have usual care [72]. The result of this study demonstrated a nonsignificant reduction of 4% in breast cancer mortality in women having two-view mammogram after a mean follow-up of 8.8 years. However, this reduction was 20% in women age 55 years or older [72].

2.   Stockholm Trial

This trial was started in Stockholm, Sweden, in 1981 and randomized about 60,000 women age 40 to 64 years old to have a single-view mammogram every 28 months for two rounds or to have usual care [68]. The result of this trial showed a non-significant reduction of 29% in breast cancer mortality after 7 years follow-up in the screened group.

E.   Gothenborg Trial and Combined Swedish Trials

This study was started in Gothenborg, Sweden, in 1982 and randomized 52,000 women age 40 to 59 years old to have a two-view screening mammography every 18 months. Although the result of this study has not been published, it was included in an overview of the five Swedish trials since 1976 [73,74]. The overview of Swedish trials included nearly 2.5 million women age 40 to 74 years old. The results of these combined trials showed a significant reduction of 24% for breast cancer mortality in screened group. This reduction was even higher (29%) and appeared earlier (4 to 5 years) for women age 50 to 69 years old but nonsignificant (13%) and appeared later (8 years) for women age 40 to 49 years old [73,74].

F. Edinburgh Trial

This trial was started in Edinburgh in 1978 and randomized 23,226 women age 45 to 64 years old to have a yearly physical examination and a two-view mammogram every 12 or every 24 months. The result of this study showed a nonsignificant reduction of 17% in breast cancer mortality in screened patients after 7 years' follow-up [75].

G. Canadian Trials

Two trials were started in Canada in 1980 in two different age groups. National Breast Screening Study 1 (NBSS 1) randomized 50,430 women age 40 to 49 years old to have annual physical examination and two-view mammogram or to have only an initial physical examination [76]. Unexpectedly, at the initial examination more node-positive cancers were found in the screened group than in the control group. Therefore, the result of this study showed a higher rate of death in the screened population. Survival rates were similar in the two groups. This study has failed to show any benefit from screening mammography in women age 40 to 49 years old.

The second Canadian study (NBSS 2), also started in 1980, randomized nearly 43,000 women age 50 to 59 years old to have annual breast examination and two-view mammogram or to have only clinical breast examination [77]. The results of this study indicated that the number of cancers discovered by mammography was doubled, but there was no significant difference of overall survival or death rates from breast cancer between the study group and the control group [77].

Canadian trials have been criticized on several study flaws, including randomization and quality control of mammograms [78]. Unlike the other trials, Canadian trials recruited volunteers who were different from the general population in several ways [79]. Furthermore, having had participants undergoing physical examination prior to randomization may have been responsible for assignment of an excess number of women with advanced incurable breast cancer to the study group [79,80] Lack of optimal mammographic technique was another major problem of the NBSS [79,81]. Over 50% of the mammograms obtained during the first 4 years of the trial were found to be technically inadequate due to poor quality equipment, technique, and film processing [82,83].

VI. FINAL SUMMARY OF RESULTS OF RANDOMIZED TRIALS IN DIFFERENT AGE GROUPS

A. Randomized Trials in Women Aged 40 to 49 Years

Table 2 summarizes the subgroup data from each randomized clinical trial in women aged 40 to 49 years. Of these eight trials, only the NBSS-1 trial was specif-

TABLE 2   Randomized Controlled Trial Results for Women Ages 40 to 49 Years

Study (dates)	Sample size		Follow-up (yr)	Breast cancer mortality relative risk
	Study	Control		
HIP, New York (1963–1969)	14,432	14,701	18	0.77
Kopparberg, Sweden (1977–1985)	9582	5031	12	0.73
Ostergotland, Sweden (1977–1985)	10,262	10,573	12	1.02
Malmo, Sweden (1976–1986)	3658	3679	12	0.51
Stockholm, Sweden (1981–1985)	14,375	7103	8	1.04
Gothenburg, Sweden (1982–1988)	10,600	12,800	7	0.73
Edinburg, Scotland (1979–1988)	5913	5810	11	0.78
NBSS 1, Canada (1980–1985)	25,214	25,216	7	1.36

Source: From Ref. 84.

ically designed to study women ages 40 to 49 years [76]. Meta-analysis of these randomized clinical trials data for women ages 40 to 49 years was performed by Smart et al. in 1995 [84]. This analysis of all currently available results of these clinical randomized trials on women ages 40 to 49 years after 7 to 18 years of follow-up suggests a nonsignificant 16% reduction in mortality in the group invited to screening compared with women assigned to an unscreened control group [84]. As mentioned before, the NBSS-1 trial has been criticized for several important points, including randomization design and quality of mammography [79–83]. With the exclusion of the NBSS-1 trial from the randomized clinical trial meta-analysis of current data, a statistically significant 23% reduction in mortality from breast cancer exists in women ages 40 to 49 years (95% confidence level) [84]. The rationale for excluding the Canadian trial data in the second meta-analysis was the belief that design flaws in the Canadian study significantly s kewed the results. It is important to mention that the potential benefit of screening mammography takes longer to manifest in women ages 40 to 49 years than in older women [73]. This benefit begins to appear only after 8 to 10 years of follow-up.

B.   Randomized Trials in Women Aged 50 to 69 Years

The most convincing evidence for the benefit of screening mammography has been shown for women aged 50 to 69 years [Table 3]. Five randomized studies of screening mammography have been done in Sweden. These trials demonstrate the largest reduction of breast cancer mortality (29%) among women aged 50 to 69 who underwent the screening mammography in comparison with the similar patients with no screening mammography [73]. A meta-analysis of data from

TABLE 3   Relative Risk for Breast Cancer Mortality; Results of
Randomized Clinical Trials in Women Aged 50 and Older

Trial age at entry	Follow-up (yr)	Breast cancer mortality relative risk
HIP		
50–64	10	0.68
Swedish centers combined		
50–59		0.71
60–69	12	0.71
70–74		0.94
Edinburgh		
50–64	10	0.85

Source: From Ref. 68.

seven clinical randomized trials (excluded data from the Canadian NBSS-1 and NBSS-2 trials because of study design differences compared with the seven other trials) conducted by Wald et al. for women age 50 years and older showed a statistically significant benefit from mammography [85]. Another meta-analysis of data of the five randomized trials on women age 50 to 69 years old after 7 years of follow-up by Elwood et al. showed a 34% reduction in mortality among patients in the study group compared with those in the control group [86]. In summary, the evidence from the randomized trials consistently points out the substantial benefit attainable from screening mammography and the mortality reduction of about 30% to 35% for women aged 50 to 69 years old after 10 to 12 years follow-up [68].

C.   Effectiveness of Screening in Women Aged 70 Years or Older

Advancing age is the most significant single risk factor for breast cancer. In other words, the incidence of this disease is increased as women age [87,88]. None of the randomized trials has included a sufficient number of women over age 70 to determine the benefits of screening in this group [68]. Unfortunately, older women who are most likely to develop breast cancer are least likely to be compliant to mammography compared to younger women [89]. The reasons cited for poor compliance of older women to screening mammography include lack of physician recommendation or referral for mammography, lack of understanding of the benefit of screening in asymptomatic women, cost, lower income status and education level, and difficulty of access to mammography facilities [90–92].

Faulk et al. reviewed age-specific screening results from more than 65,000 mammographic examinations done over a 9-year period. In this survey, 21,226 women were 50 to 64 years of age and 10,914 were 65 or older. They concluded that mammographic screening is at least as effective in detecting early breast cancer in women 65 or older as it is in those of ages 50 to 64. Since screening is of proven efficacy in the relatively younger group, screening may also benefit women of 65 and older [93]. The National Institutes of Health Breast Screening Forum urged that decisions regarding screening for older women be based on the women's general health, be made jointly by the woman and her physician, and reflect a consideration of comorbid diseases or other medical conditions [94,95].

It is important to emphasize that the true benefit of mammography today is likely to exceed the benefit demonstrated in the randomized control trials for at least two reasons: (1) Randomized controlled trials test the efficacy of the offer of mammography to a predefined study group compared with a predefined control group. Compliance rates for obtaining the first screening mammogram among the women who were offered screening ranged from 61% to 89% in those randomized clinical trials. Assuming benefit exists, the true benefit to women who receive regular screening mammography in the general population will be higher than the benefit demonstrated among women who were offered mammography in the randomized controlled trials [84]. (2) The technology of mammography has improved significantly since the time of even the most recent randomized controlled clinical trials [96]. Women receiving regular, high-quality mammography today are more likely to have their cancers detected at smaller sizes and at earlier stages than women who participated in the eight randomized controlled trials [96,97].

D.   Screening Guidelines

In 1988, 12 medical organizations met to develop consensus recommendations for breast cancer screening. They agreed to the following breast screening guideline: (1) clinical breast examination and mammography are both essential for optimal screening; (2) mammography should be done at 1- to 2-year intervals for women 40 to 49 years old; (3) annual mammography should be done for women aged 50 and over; (4) the conference could not reach a consensus on the role of breast self-examination in breast cancer screening [66]. The National Cancer Institute and National Institute on Aging sponsored a forum on breast cancer screening in older women in 1990. The screening recommendations for older women derived from this Forum are summarized below:

1.   Women ages 65 to 74: clinical breast examination annually and mammography every 2 years
2.   Women 75 and over in good general health with good life expectancy: clinical breast examination annually and mammography every 2 years
3.   All women 65 and over: breast self-examination monthly [94]

VII.   ANALYSIS OF CANCER MISSED AT SCREENING MAMMOGRAPHY

The true sensitivity of screening mammography is uncertain because of many ways sensitivity has been calculated and reported in the literature [98,99]. Bird et al. demonstrated that the sensitivity of screening mammography without physical examination ranges from 85% to 90% [100]. In an attempt to increase the sensitivity of screening mammography, they also studied some common characteristics of the lesions that were missed in screening mammography [101]. They analyzed 320 breast cancers found in a screened population between 1985 to 1990 and revealed 77 breast cancers that were missed at the screening mammography. These lesions were found among approximately 50,000 screening mammographies done during that period. The missed lesions were compared with 121 cancers that were correctly diagnosed at their first screening mammography. Of these 77 missed breast cancers, 40 lesions were misinterpreted as benign appearance, present on previous mammogram, seen only on one view, and site of previous biopsy. Of the rest of the missed cancers, 33 lesions were overlooked, and four lesions were missed secondary to suboptimal technique of screening mammogram. Comparison of the 77 missed lesions in the study group with the 121 patients in the comparison group showed that the breasts in the study group were significantly denser than those in the comparison group. Microcalcifications were also found much less commonly among the study group than comparison group. Developing opacities were significantly more common among the missed cancer because small, irregular opacities are easy to overlook or to misinterpret as benign. In regard to the position of the missed lesions, Bird et al. found that the lesions in the retroglandular areas were particularly difficult to detect. In summary, they concluded that the increased sensitivity of screening mammography depends on properly interpreted radiographs of optimal technical quality [101].

Another case control study, by Ma et al., showed that the failure of mammography to detect some breast cancers is due to poor mammographic technique that excludes the tumor from the area examined, observer error, radiologic density of the breast, tumor growth pattern, lack of tumor calcification, and the histology of intraductal carcinoma [102]. In this study, Ma et al. found that three variables were independently and significantly associated with failure to detect breast cancer by mammography. The independent variables comprise the presence of extensive parenchyma densities within the breast, a tumor of lobular histology, and tumors of small size. They concluded that current mammography has limitations due to the biologic nature of the tissue examined [102]. Improvement of the imaging techniques and future developments in computerized digital analysis of mammograms may help detect tumors with a diffusely infiltrative growth pattern or help detect in situ carcinomas that rarely produce a localized density or that have no associated calcification [102].

VIII.   MANAGEMENT OF WOMEN WITH
ABNORMAL MAMMOGRAM

Screening mammography is usually limited to two views (craniocaudal and me-diolateral oblique) of each breast, done with the highest image quality at the low-est possible radiation exposure of the patient. Women with an abnormal mammo-gram may need additional views to classify the abnormality as suspicious or questionable. Most (80% to 85%) breast cancers can usually be seen in mammog-raphy as a mass, a cluster of calcification, or a combination of the two [103]. Mammography is a sensitive but often nonspecific examination, and its true-pos-itive rate ranges from 10% to 30% of all mammographic abnormalities. The false-negative rate of mammography is 10% to 15% when breast cancer is palpable. Therefore, a negative mammogram in the presence of a palpable mass does not relieve the clinician of the obligation to biopsy the mass. Most mammographi-cally detected nonpalpable breast lesions do not have pathognomonic appear-ances; therefore, morphologic features are used to guide the decision to recom-mend biopsy. In general, malignant lesions on mammography have a greater radiographic density than an equal volume of normal fibroglandular breast tissue.

Radiolucent lesions on mammography are always benign. Therefore, iso-lated solitary noncystic densities >8 mm in diameter need to be biopsied. Irregu-lar or spiculated margin is the most important feature indicating a malignant mass. Benign lesions such as fibroadenomas or cysts usually have sharply defined mar-gin on mammography. A mass with this appearance may be malignant in about 7% of cases. Less infiltrating cancers such as papillary, medullary, and colloid breast carcinoma may have only slightly irregular or even well-circumscribed margins. Lesions with ill-defined margins on mammography should be biopsied. Lesions with spiculated or stellate margins must also be biopsied. Most nonspe-cific circumscribed masses on mammography have <7% chance of being cancer and should be followed up with clinical breast examination and/or mammogra-phy.

Asymmetrical breast tissue is nearly always distinguishable from a true mass by mammography. The differentiation of a small stellate mass from an early invasive breast cancer is often extremely subtle. Thus, optimal technique and meticulous interpretation of the mammogram, with biopsy if there is any ques-tion, are essential. Only mammography can depict malignant breast calcifications, and this is one of the major reasons that no other diagnostic tests, including sonog-raphy, thermography, light scanning, or MRI, can replace mammography for the early detection of breast cancer. When calcifications are identified on routine mammographic views, microfocus magnification mammography combined with spot compression should improve the clarity of the calcifications [52]. The calci-fications of malignancy are typically grouped or clustered, pleomorphic, fine and branching, and numerous. The greater the number of calcifications of a cluster, the greater the likelihood of malignancy. A group containing fewer than five calcifications is unlikely to represent malignancy [104]. Up to 50% of malignant breast masses contain calcifications visible on mammography, and about 20% to 35% of radiographically detected clustered calcifications without a mass on mammography are malignant (mostly noninvasive carcinoma). Mammography is highly sensitive in detecting breast calcifications, but the specificity in distinguishing benign from malignant calcifications is only 50% to 60%. Large, dense calcifications of a benign, involutional fibroadenoma, when associated with a lobulated mass, are diagnostic of a benign process. However, when an involutional process is developing (early stage), it may be indistinguishable from a malignant process and must be biopsied.

IX.   MAMMOGRAPHY-GUIDED NEEDLE LOCALIZATION AND BIOPSY OF NONPALPABLE BREAST LESIONS

During the late 1960s and early 1970s, developments in the fight against breast cancer focused on refining the diagnostic biopsy of nonpalpable breast lesions. Since the vast majority of these biopsies were blind surgical procedures, accurate prebiopsy localization of these nonpalpable breast lesions needed to be developed. In 1963, Gerald Dodd was probably the first radiologist to perform prebiopsy needle localization of nonpalpable, mammographically detected breast lesions [105]. He reported that prebiopsy needle localization allows for more precise resection and less chance of resultant breast deformity. Prebiopsy localization using standard needle was rapidly replaced with another technique using special needle-hook wire system for better fixation in the lesion.

In 1976 Howard Frank, Ferris Hall, and Michael Steer described a needle-hook wire assembly for preoperative localization of mammographically detected, nonpalpable breast lesions [106]. Once the needle was inserted in the breast, it could be withdrawn over the wire, allowing the hook to stabilize the wire in the lesion. A significant drawback was that the wire was preloaded into the needle with the hook protruding beyond the bevel of the needle, and the needle-hook wire assembly was then inserted into the breast through a small skin incision.

In 1980, Daniel Kopans and Salvatore Deluca reported their experience with preoperative localization using a new wire with an overbent hook that remained retracted while the wire was entirely within the needle and sprang open when the needle was withdrawn over the wire [107]. Therefore, the needle could be repositioned before the hook was engaged. Once the hook was open, however, it anchored the wire so firmly that it could not be withdrawn. In 1985, Marc Homer reported his study with a curved end retractable wire for preoperative localization [108]. The J-shape end of the wire was manufactured from a pseudoelastic metal alloy with a "memory" allowing it to slide in and out of the distal end of the needle for easy repositioning. One of the problems of this J-wire was inadvertent repositioning or dislodgment of hook wire prior to or during the biopsy. In 1988, Hawkins et al. presented another hook wire assembly that not only can be easily repositioned but also is able to anchor firmly in the breast lesion and prevent dislodgment [109,110].

Currently, excisional biopsy after needle localization has been the gold standard for the diagnosis of mammographically detected, nonpalpable lesions because it is the most accurate method of separating benign from malignant lesions and is the only method that permits pathologists to fully characterize malignant lesions. This procedure requires the coordinated efforts of the radiologist, surgeon, and pathologist. This combined procedure should be planned with the goal of minimizing the trauma for the patient while providing her with accurate and complete characterization of the mammographic lesion. Guide placement for most mammographically detected, nonpalpable lesions can be easily accomplished by using mammography, ultrasound [111], computed tomography [112], MRI [113], and sestamibi scintimammography [114].

Many guides have been developed to assist the surgeon in resecting the nonpalpable breast lesions. The principle of guide placement is similar, positioning of a needle under imaging observation and guidance. There are several choices of needle localizer system that basically differ in the configuration of the anchoring end. Among the more commonly used needle hook wire system are Kopans [107], Homer [108], and Hawkins II [109] needle hook wire systems (Fig. 29) All of these needle localizer systems involve a wire with a hook at the end. The hook wire is passed through a needle and hook reforms when the needle is withdrawn over the wire, anchoring the wire in the breast tissue. The needle is first positioned to achieve a satisfactory relation to the lesion, and the wire is then engaged in the appropriate tissue volume.

The length of wire is important. Wire must be of sufficient length to ensure that, when the breast is in its natural position the wire will not be drawn beneath the skin. Surgical dissection is made easier if the surgeon has a palpable guide to follow. Some systems have addressed this need by thickening the distal end of the wire, using a stiffening needle or allowing both the wire and needle to be left in the tissue [115]. The combination of needle and hook wire allows a three-dimensionally accurate, surgically palpable guide. These wires must be placed in the breast lesion or in close proximity to the lesion (<5 mm) [116] and maintained in that position. Dislodgment or inadvertent repositioning of the hook wire prior to or during the biopsy might happen and may be one of the reasons for failed biopsies. The most stable needle-hook wire system is the one in which the hook protrudes from the side of the needle [109,110]. This needle hook wire system introduced in 1988 by Howkins et al. [109]. They reported 60 needle localization

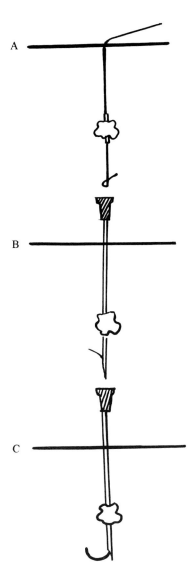

FIGURE 29   Needle hook wire systems. (A) Hook wire placed into the lesion, leaving a flexible wire for the surgeon to follow. (B) Homer's Needle Hook Wire System with a curved wire protruding from the end of the needle. (C) Hawkins' Needle Hook Wire System with the hook protruding from the side of the needle.

biopsies with no failure by using this system. This system consists mainly of a 20-gauge, outer cannula (which has a fenestration approximately 1.5 cm from its tip), an inner, 23-gauge cannula with a sharp tip, and a 0.012-inch spring wire barb which protrudes from a slot in the inner cannula. This needle hook wire system not only can be easily repositioned but also appears to anchor firmer in the breast tissue than the other systems, preventing dislodgment or migration [109,110].

The injection of vital dyes to stain the tissue and provide a track from the lesion to the skin has been used for guiding the biopsy [117]. Success with dye injection requires avoidance of overinjection and minimization of the time between injection and biopsy to lessen the possibility of dye diffusion into a large volume of tissue. In a recent study the success rate of using the metylen blue, one of the more commonly used vital dyes, alone for spot localization biopsy of the breast lesions was 91% [118]. This report also demonstrated that combining hook wire system with dye does not improve the success rate [118]. Another study suggested that methylen blue may interfere with estrogen receptor analysis [119].

A. Needle Localization Technique

Before the needle localization (Fig. 30), the radiologist must have an accurate idea of the three-dimensional location of a lesion and be confident of ability to place the tip of the needle at the lesion. An additional straight lateral projection should be obtained before needle placement to provide true perpendicular coordinates to the craniocaudal view. If the location is uncertain, methods have been described to assist in confirmation and triangulation [120,121]. Procedure should be explained to the patient in details. Premedication is not recommended because it reduces the patient's ability to be fully cooperative for the localization procedure. Local anesthesia can be used, but it is not needed for most women and may be more painful than the localization itself. The development of dedicated mammography equipment has led to the ability to accurately position needles into or alongside the smallest mammographically detected abnormalities. This is most accurately and safely accomplished by introducing the needle while the breast is held in the mammographic compression system and the needle usually introduced parallel to the chest wall. This approach uses compression plates with a series of holes permitting access to the breast and the lesion while the breast is held compressed. To reduce the amount of tissue that must be traversed by the surgeon, the shortest distance to the lesion from the skin should be chosen for the introduction of the needle. Using the appropriate technique, the needle shaft should be placed >5 mm from the lesion [116].

Precise wire placement permits less tissue to be removed. It also leads to reduce the failure of excision of a breast cancer to <1%. Mammograms should be sent to the operating room to allow the surgeon to determine the three-dimensional location of the lesion in the breast when the patient is supine, as well as the

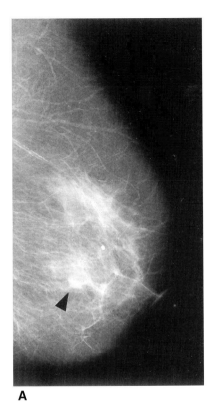

A

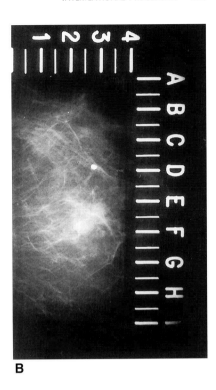

B

FIGURE 30 A 64-year-old woman with no palpable breast mass. (A) Lateral view of the left breast showed a cluster of microcalcifications, suspicious for malignancy (arrowhead). (B) Localizer grid was placed in craniocaudal position in order to determine the coordinates of the lesion in X and Y axes. (C) Needle hook wire system was placed adjacent to the lesion, according to predetermined coordinates. After confirming the depth of the tip of the needle (Z coordinate), blue methylen was injected and guidewire was engaged. (D) Postbiopsy, specimen magnified radiograph confirmed the presence of microcalcifications in the specimen (arrow). Result of excisional biopsy indicated ductal carcinoma insitu. Note: Mammogram also showed a large coarse calcification (short arrow) which is a benign finding.

position of the lesion to the wire. The position of the hook relative to the nipple remains fairly constant, despite movement of the breast into the supine position, and can be used to estimate the location of the lesion within the breast. Jones et al. [122] reported a modified technique of localization biopsy of the breast in order to identify the position of the wire tip after placement and before biopsy. In this technique, after wire placement, two metallic skin markers are placed on the nip-

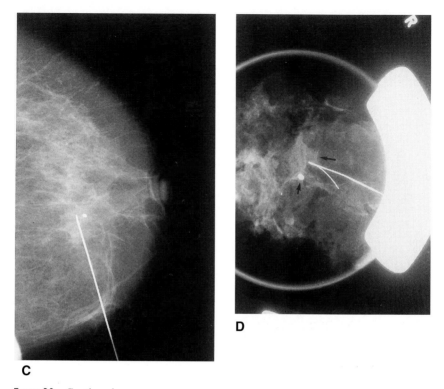

C

D

FIGURE 30 Continued

ple and wire entry site. Patient is then positioned on an x-ray table in the same position to be used during biopsy, and a supine x-ray of the breast is obtained. They reported 53 biopsies of nonpalpable breast lesions with this technique. In all instances, the biopsy incision was independent of the wire insertion site, the lesion was excised in a single specimen, and the amount of tissue dissection was reduced without decreasing the accuracy [122].

B. Surgical Principle

Although the excision of a nonpalpable, needle-localized breast lesion is technically more difficult than excision of a palpable lesion, the same principle apply. Each lesion should be treated as if it were a malignancy and excised through an incision that could be contained within a future mastectomy incision or converted into a cosmetically acceptable partial mastectomy incision. Effort should be made to excise the lesion completely, with a rim of surrounding normal tissue. However, given that most needle-localized breast biopsies ultimately prove to be benign, the volume of tissue excised should be as small as possible with wide excision reserved for highly suspicious lesions malignancy. After the localization is completed, the surgeon reviews the postlocalization films with the radiologist to gain precise understanding of the spatial relationship between the localizer and lesion. Patient is then transferred to the operating room and placed in a supine position with her arms at her side. Excisional biopsy is usually performed under local anesthesia with lidocaine 1% with or without intravenous sedation. After preparation of the skin with betadine and draping the breast, local anesthetic is injected. The incision is placed so that it is closed to the lesion to be biopsied as determined by the mammogram and the skin lines in the breast. After the skin incision, the surgeon dissects downward to identify the wire within the breast tissue and follows it to the thickened segment of wire. The tissue is then removed around the thick segment to encompass the lesion and a small amount of surrounding normal tissue. For a lesion shown to be malignant by previous fine or core needle biopsy, an appropriately wide margin should be taken. The amount of tissue taken around the wire depends on the actual distant of the lesion from the wire, as indicated on the postlocalizing images.

Immediately after the surgical excision the specimen should undergo radiography with some compression and magnification to confirm that the lesion has been removed [123,124]. If the lesion is not seen at the first image of the specimen, an additional excisional attempt is worthwhile [123]. If the lesion in question is not contained within the second biopsy, it is generally best to close the skin and obtain a repeat follow-up mammographic views, usually 2 to 3 weeks later [123], to evaluate whether the lesion has been removed; if not, another localization and biopsy should be done later. The specimen needs to be marked with suture or ink for orientation and identification of margins.

C.   In the Pathology

After obtaining the radiography of the specimen, the pathologist measures the specimen and paint the tissue with India ink (if it has not been previously done in the operating room), which serves to facilitate subsequent evaluation of margins [125]. The specimen is then sliced at 2 to 3 mm intervals and fixed in 10% neutral buffered formaldehyde solution for a minimum of 5 to 6 hours and processed for permanent slides. If the biopsy was done for calcifications, it is important for the pathologist to be sure that the calcifications are seen in histologic tissue sections to ensure that the area containing the lesion has been examined. If the calcifications are not found on routine examination of tissue, roentgenographic images of the paraffin-embedded tissue blocks can be obtained to identify

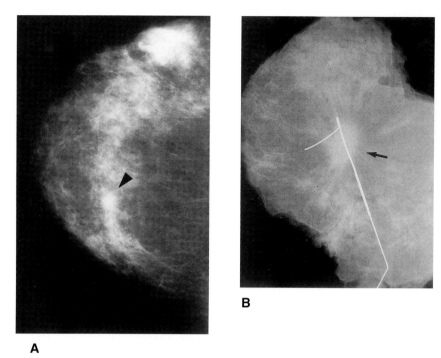

A

B

Figure 31   A 64-year-old woman with no palpable breast mass. (A) Standard mammogram (CC view) showed a 1-cm spiculated mass in right breast, suspicious for malignancy (arrowhead). (B) Specimen magnified radiograph of the right breast lesion after excisional biopsy demonstrated the total removal of the mass (arrow). Result of excisional biopsy indicated infiltrative ductal carcinoma. Subsequently, patient underwent modified radical mastectomy of right breast. One year later, she presented with a palpable chest wall mass at the site of mastectomy. (C) Standard mammogram (CC view) of the skin flap demonstrated a large posterior dense mass (small arrowhead) with diffuse skin thickening (large arrowhead). Result of excisional biopsy of the chest wall mass indicated recurrent carcinoma.

the sections containing the calcifications, and those blocks containing calcifications can be recut [126].

D.   Specimen Radiography and Missed Lesions

One of the important complications seen after needle localization biopsy of non-palpable lesions is a surgically missed lesion. The incidence of missed lesion varies from 0% to 17% in different reports [127–129,104]. Specimen radiographs are important to evaluate the adequate excision of the breast lesion and reduce the missed lesions (Fig. 31) [123,124]. The accuracy of the specimen x-ray is of great importance because a false-negative specimen x-ray may lead to unnecessary

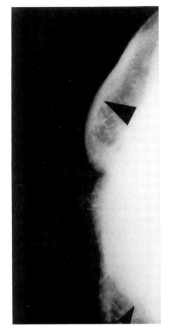

C

FIGURE 31   Continued

reexcision of tissue with resultant breast deformity and waste of expensive operating time; on the other hand, a false-positive specimen x-ray may give both surgeon and patient an unjustified feeling of security and delay the recognition of a
missed lesion. Studies show that specimen x-ray can be false-negative or false-
positive even when calcified lesions are removed [130,131].

The reasons for false-negative specimen x-ray may include distortion of
architecture of the lesion during operation or specimen roentgenography, or disappearance of the lesion such as rupturing of a cyst. The reasons of a false-positive specimen x-ray may be removal of calcification adjacent to but other than the
target calcification or distortion of specimen during roentgenography, giving rise
to a radiographic picture similar the lesion of which biopsy was performed. In one
study, Hasselgren et al. showed that the sensitivity, specificity, and accuracy of
specimen x-ray in this series were 96%, 28%, and 89%, respectively [130]. The
incidence of the missed lesions was 3.2%, which was similar to other reports
[129–131]. On the basis of this study, Hasselgren et al. concluded that postoperative mammography should always be done after needle localization breast biopsy
regardless of the result of the specimen x-ray in order to make certain the lesion
was not missed. The follow-up mammogram is best obtained about 3 months post-

biopsy to confirm the absence of the lesion and to reestablish the baseline mammogram.

E.   Pathologic Analysis of Nonpalpable Breast Lesions

Needle localization breast biopsy is an important and effective method in the early detection of breast carcinoma. It is a safe procedure and easily performed in an outpatient setting under local anesthesia.

Needle localization biopsy of nonpalpable breast masses or calcifications leads to a diagnosis of malignancy in 9% to 38% of biopsies, and 19% to 60% of these malignancies are noninvasive or in situ [132–137]. In contrast, only about 3% of cancers detected by excisional biopsy of palpable masses are noninvasive [132,138]. Invasive carcinomas detected by needle localization biopsy in patients with nonpalpable lesions are more likely to be stage 1 than are invasive carcinomas detected by excisional biopsy of palpable lesions [139]. While approximately 50% of women with clinically detected invasive carcinoma have axillary lymph node metastasis, most series report only 7% to 33% involvement with nonpalpable, mammographically detected breast carcinoma [140–149]. Therefore, the apparent increase in survival with mammographic screening may be due to detection of invasive carcinoma at an earlier stage or detection of in situ carcinoma that might later develop into or mark an increased risk of invasive cancer [139].

F.   Positive Predictive Value

The sensitivity of mammography in detection of nonpalpable, clinically occult breast lesions needs to be high, but it is also important to achieve a high diagnostic specificity to avoid the morbidity associated with unnecessary surgical biopsy. The overall positive predictive value of nonpalpable mammographic lesions in most series is 22% to 35% [140,150–155]. Therefore, for every 10 lesions undergoing localization biopsy, only two to three lesions prove to be malignant, and seven to eight benign. Burrell et al. reviewed the mammographic features of nonpalpable breast lesions to identify features which may improve the specificity of mammographic interpretation [156]. They studied mammographic abnormalities of 425 nonpalpable breast lesions which were biopsied with needle localization technique. This study showed the high positive predictive value of 94% for spiculated masses, which is similar to other series [151,154,157], and 4% for well-defined masses. Positive predictive value of all calcifications was 45%. They concluded that all spiculated masses, parenchymal deformities, and high-risk microcalcifications require surgical biopsy. Ill-defined masses and indeterminate microcalcification may be managed according to the core and/or fine needle biopsy. Masses which are entirely well-defined are regarded as benign and are not recalled for assessment unless they are new or enlarging [156].

X.   STEREOTACTIC CORE BREAST BIOPSY

Screening mammography is a valuable technique for detecting small nonpalpable breast cancers. Currently the average size of nonpalpable invasive breast cancer detected by mammography is about 10 mm [158]. In addition, a large proportion (25% to 50%) of cancers detected by mammography are noninvasive [159]. By early detection of breast cancer, screening mammography has been shown to be effective to reduce the mortality and increase the survival of breast cancer patients in several randomized trials [68]. With acceptance of the effectiveness of screening mammography, the number of mammograms performed in the United States has been increased, from which 2% to 4% are referred for a breast biopsy [159]. Approximately 500,000 breast biopsies, initiated by mammographic finding, are performed in the United States each year. Of these biopsies, 60% to 90% are benign [157]. Although the surgical biopsy has been considered the gold standard technique of evaluation of these lesions, it has several disadvantages. One of the most significant disadvantages is cost. The surgical biopsy accounts for the largest fraction of induced costs of screening [160]. Other significant disadvantages include physical and psychological trauma, anesthetic risks, a failure rate of 0.2% to 22% [123,129,161,162], removal of more tissue than necessary (in case of benign lesions), and the creation of mammographic pseudolesions by postsurgical scarring.

Recently, stereotactic core needle biopsy of mammographically detected lesions offers an attractive alternative to surgical biopsy. In addition to being potentially more cost-effective, stereotactic core needle breast biopsy results in a shorter procedure time, less patient discomfort, less complication and cosmetic deformity, and fewer artifacts on postbiopsy mammogram.

A.   Historical Aspect of Stereotactic Core Biopsy

Stereotactic localization for percutaneous needle biopsy of mammographic lesions was originated in Sweden. In 1977, Bolmgren et al. became the first to develop and report the stereotactic instrumentation for fine needle aspiration of mammographic lesions [163]. The same year, Nordastrom et al. reported the first series of patients who underwent breast biopsy with screw needle by using stereotactic technique [164]. In 1987, Dolatshahi et al. introduced the stereotactic fine needle breast biopsy technique in the United States [165]. There have been a number of reports over the past decade on the efficacy of stereotactic fine needle breast biopsy that demonstrated an unsatisfactory results because the tissue sample obtained with fine needle was often inadequate or nondiagnostic and the reading was highly dependent on cytopathologist experience and slide preparation [165–168]. Subsequently, Parker et al. adapted the concept of core needle biopsy for stereotactic breast biopsy [169]. They established the safety and increased efficacy of utilizing a larger needle (14-gauge) with greater excursion (23 mm) [167,169,170]. Unlike fine needle breast biopsy, core needle breast biopsy provides a histologic diagnosis and does not require a skilled cytopathologist for interpretation. Parker et al. showed that the results obtained with stereotactic core needle biopsy were equivalent to surgical biopsy with high accuracy and low morbidity [167,169,170]. The introduction of automated core biopsy gun has escalated interest in this technique due to increased confidence in histologic samples obtained and the ability to make specific benign diagnosis more frequently [158].

Based on current estimates, there are now over 1000 centers either investigating or using stereotactic core needle biopsy for nonpalpable breast lesion in the United States [158].

B.   Core Biopsy Needles and Automated Biopsy Gun

Currently, many needles are available for percutaneous needle breast biopsy. These needles are divided into two categories, fine needle (20 to 23 gauge) and core needle (14 to 18 gauge). Both fine and core needle can be used either manually or in an automated biopsy gun. Unlike the fine needle aspiration biopsy, which collects some cellular material for cytologic evaluation, core needle biopsy is able to provide tissue that can be analyzed histologically in the same manner as surgical specimens. Most core needles consist of an inner trocar with a sample notch at its distal end and an outer cutting cannula (Fig. 32).

During the procedure, the trocar portion is pushed forward first, and tissue is collected within the sample notch. Then the outer cutting cannula is pushed forward, shearing off the sample from the surrounding tissue and enclosing it within the walls of the cannula. This procedure may be done manually but requires two hands and some level of experience. It is also possible for the needle to slide off of or away from very firm or fibrotic lesions. The introduction of the Bard Biopsy

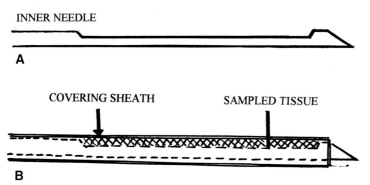

FIGURE 32   Core biopsy needle. (A) Inner trocar with a sample notch at its distal end. (B) Outer cutting canula or covering sheath.

Gun in the mid-1980s solved these problems [171]. The core needle fits into an automatic biopsy gun, and the outer needle covers the inner needle in prefire position. When firing mechanism is activated, the spring in the gun cause the inner needle to advance and a sample of tissue becomes lodged in the tissue slot. Then the outer needle slides over the inner needle, cutting the tissue and securing it in the slot.

This sequence of events occurs in a fraction of a second and is not visible except for the excursion of the entire needle. The distance the needle must travel to obtain a core of tissue called the "throw" of the biopsy gun is variable. The speed of penetration of needle in automated biopsy gun makes biopsy of very firm or fibrotic lesions as wall as mobile lesions very easy and accurate before they slip out of the way. In addition, the tissue sample obtained with automated biopsy gun has better quality and integrity than has manually obtained specimen [172,173]. The biopsy results by automated biopsy gun with fine needle and short throw (1.15 cm) were not entirely satisfactory [166,169]. Currently, the combination of 14-gauge needle biopsy gun with long throw (2.3 cm excursion) is being used. The results of breast biopsy with this equipment is as accurate as surgical biopsy [170,174].

C. Principles of Stereotactic Localization Mammography

All stereotactic mammographic devices use the principle of triangulation (Fig. 33). In this technique, two planar radiographic views are obtained at different x-ray source positions to determine the location of radiographically visible object in three spatial dimensions [171]. The two planar views differ only in horizontal position of the x-ray source with x-ray beam directed at $+15°$ and $-15°$ relation to a line perpendicular to the image receptor. In order to prevent overlapping of the two views, the screen-film cassette is shifted horizontally to the right and left for $+15°$ view and $-15°$ view, respectively. Since the horizontal shifts of the x-ray tube and the screen-film cassette are the only changes from one view to the other, the vertical location of the lesion does not change in these views. Therefore, if X is the amount of parallax shift of the lesion from the $+15°$ view to the $-15°$ view, by simple geometry the distance of the lesion from the image receptor (Z) is:

$$Z = X / 2 \tan(15°) = 1.866 \cdot X$$

Two types of stereotactic equipment are available—devices that add on to standard upright mammography units, and dedicated prone tables [158,171]. The add-on devices are relatively inexpensive, are small, and allow multipurpose use. Unfortunately, it is difficult for the patient to remain motionless while sitting or standing upright, and also the risk of vasovagal reaction is higher (7%) [175]. Dedicated prone stereotactic devices are expensive, take a large space, and are for single use. However, since the patient is lying prone and the breast is in a depen-

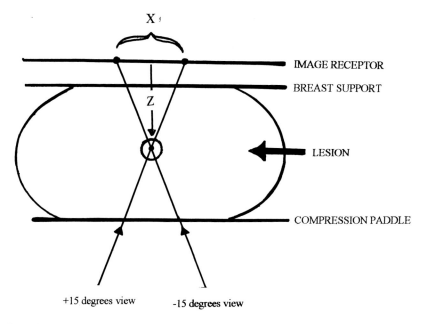

FIGURE 33 Principle of stereotactic localization. This diagram shows the horizontal shifts of the x-ray tube ($\pm$ 15°) with no change in the vertical location of the lesion and its geometric relationship to the distance of the lesion from the image receptor.

dent position, the patient's motion is minimal, patient is unable to see the needle during the procedure, vasovagal reaction is very rare, and the procedure is easier and more accurate [171].

D. Procedure

First the patient's mammogram is reviewed to determine the best way to approach the breast lesion. In most cases, the best approach is the skin surface closest to the lesion. Patient is then placed in prone position on the table while the breast is in a dependent position. Then the breast is compressed with the lesion positioned within the window of the compression paddle and a 0° scout film is obtained to verify the location of lesion. The skin is then prepared with povidone-iodine. Stereo images are obtained with the x-ray source shifted first 15° to the right and then 15° to the left on the same cassette. The computer calculates the horizontal, vertical, and depth coordinates of the center of the lesion. Then a sterile needle is placed in the biopsy gun and attached to the punction arm. The punction arm is positioned with respect to the horizontal and vertical coordinates and biopsy gun is advanced so that the needle is at the surface of the breast.

The patient is given local anesthetic (1% lidocaine), and a small skin puncture is made at the point of entry of the biopsy needle. Then the needle is inserted to the specified depth coordinate to locate the tip of the biopsy needle at the center of the lesion. Once again, stereo images at +15° and –15° are obtained on a single cassette to confirm the placement of the needle within the lesion on both views. The needle is then withdrawn 5 mm and the biopsy gun is fired. After the first firing, stereo images at +15° and –15° are obtained to document the needle passing the lesion. Additional samples (at least four) are acquired by retargeting various areas within the lesion at different horizontal and vertical locations without making a separate skin puncture for each passes. After each biopsy the needle is removed, the specimen is placed in formalin, and firm pressure is applied on biopsy site to reduce the bleeding and chance of hematoma [171].

E. Complications

Hematoma, infection, and possible tumor seeding are the possible complications of stereotactic core needle breast biopsy. In a multicenter experience, just six complications (0.2%) were reported among 3765 cases of stereotactic core needle biopsies for which follow-up was available [176]. Three complications were hematoma-required surgical drainage, and the other three were infection which required drainage, antibiotic treatment, or both. Minor bruising around the biopsy site is common but can be minimized by maintaining pressure on biopsy site or using an ice pack after the needle has been removed.

There has been one report of needle track seeding of malignant cells in a case of mucinous carcinoma diagnosed with core needle biopsy [177]. This report documents the presence of malignant cells along the course of the needle, but the viability of those cells is questionable. The theoretical possibility of the needle track tumor seeding exists with any types of needle procedures including the fine needle aspiration biopsy and needle localization, but the significance of this phenomenon is unknown. In a review of needle track tumor seeding, the incidence was reported <0.01% [178]. Parker et al. also reported no cases of needle track tumor seeding in a series of nearly 1000 cancers following core needle biopsy [176].

F. Efficacy of Stereotactic Core Needle Breast Biopsy

There have been a number of studies over the past decade on the efficacy of stereotactic core needle breast biopsy [162,166,169,170,179–181]. Schmidt reviewed these studies which compared the result of stereotactic core needle breast biopsies with mammographically needle localized open surgical biopsies [158]. Table 4 summarizes these studies as well as the sensitivity of core needle breast biopsy relative to surgery in each group. In this review, Schmidt pointed out that with stereotactic core needle breast biopsy, an experienced operator can produce a sufficient sample nearly 100% of the time with a sensitivity of 95% or more. Mammographically needle localized surgical breast biopsy has a reported failure rate

TABLE 4   Stereotactic Core Needle Breast Biopsy Compared with Surgery

Study	No. of cases	No. of cancers (percent)	Needle size (gauge)	Sensitivity of core biopsy[a] relative to surgery (percent)	Insufficient samples (percent)
Parker et al., 1990 [169]	102	16 (16)	14–20	94	1
Dowlatshahi et al., 1991 [166]	250	76 (30)	20	71	17 (11/43=CA)
Parker et al., 1991 [170]	102	23 (23)	14	96	0
Dronkers, 1992 [179]	53	45 (85)	18	95	6 (2/3=CA)
Elvecrog et al., 1993 [180]	100	35 (35)	14	100[b]	0
Gisvold et al., 1994 [181]	160	65 (41)	14	92[c]	<1
Parker et al., 1994 [176]	1363	910 (67)[d]	14	98	(None reported)

Source: From Ref. 158.
[a]Excluding insufficient samples.
[b]Core biopsy and surgery each missed one cancer.
[c]Counting three cases of atypical ductal hyperplasia on stereotactic biopsy as positive and three cases of lobular carcinoma in situ at surgery as negative.
[d]25 percent of the cancers were diagnosed by ultrasound guidance.

of 0.2% to 22% [129,162,189], with up to a 5% failure rate even at a major center with experienced personnel [123]. It appears that the reported results of stereotactic core needle biopsy are at the very least equivalent to those of open surgical biopsies [188]. Stereotactic core needle breast biopsy also offers the advantages of increased efficacy of preoperative diagnosis, lower cost, minimal complications and cosmetic deformity, and lower psychological trauma to the patient while maintaining an accuracy of diagnosis equivalent to open surgical biopsy. It also seems to be a method to facilitate the planning of single-step definitive surgical procedure in breast cancer therapy [158].

G.   Detection of Invasive and Noninvasive Carcinoma

One of the advantages of the core needle breast biopsy is the ability to obtain a sufficient tissue for histological analysis similar to surgical specimen. Unfortunately, the potential for misdiagnosis of borderline atypia or missing areas of microinvasion remains a serious problem for core needle breast biopsy. Jackman et al. found that stereotactic core needle breast biopsy was able to diagnose ductal carcinoma in situ but failed to show the microinvasion in eight out of 43 core biopsies (19%) [182]. In a similar comparison of 15 cases read as atypical ductal hyperplasia on core biopsy, 10 cases were found to be cancerous at surgical biopsy (73% discordance for core needle biopsy diagnosed atypical ductal hyperplasia) [183].

Therefore, stereotactic core needle biopsy of breast carcinoma can help confirm invasion with high accuracy but cannot reliably indicate the absence of tumor invasion when only ductal carcinoma in situ is found. Parker et al. also, in a multicenter study, reported that a complete agreement occurred between core needle and surgical biopsy with 741 out of 752 (98.5%) invasive lesions, 140 out of 158 (89%) intermediate to high-grade ductal carcinoma in situ lesions, and 116 out of 173 (67%) lesions classified as low-grade ductal carcinoma in situ, atypical ductal hyperplasia, lobular carcinoma in situ, or atypical lobular hyperplasia [176]. Therefore, when core needle breast biopsy result is ductal carcinoma in situ, lobular carcinoma in situ, atypical ductal hyperplasia, or atypical lobular hyperplasia, surgical biopsy is usually recommended.

H. Indications

In today's medical and economic environment, surgical treatment of breast cancer is usually a two-step procedure. Surgical biopsy is followed by a definitive procedure either lumpectomy with or without axillary dissection or mastectomy with or without reconstruction. However, because of core needle biopsy, this pattern is changing. Before biopsy, radiologist and referring physician should consider whether a specific tissue diagnosis by needle biopsy will improve patient care. If the procedure shortens the diagnostic process and potentially replaces the surgical biopsy, it is valuable and should be done. There has been some controversy regarding the indications of stereotactic core needle breast biopsy. Radiologists recommend biopsy based on the level of suspicion associated with a mammographic lesion [189]. American College of Radiology Breast Imaging Reporting and Data System (BI-RADS) suggests a standardized method of breast imaging reporting including five categories which correlate with level of suspicious of mammographic lesions [29] and indication of stereotactic core needle breast biopsy.

1. Probably Benign Lesions (Bi-Rads 2)

Since the likelihood of breast cancer in patients with probably benign lesions on mammography is <2%, the magnitude of a core needle breast biopsy benefit for these lesions over the mammographic surveillance is very small [185]. There are two occasions when early core biopsy may be of considerable help even though a lesion appears to be probably benign on mammography and can be followed-up with periodic mammography:

1. When it can be determined that periodic mammogram will not take place (e.g., when a patient plans to move, even temporarily, to a remote location where mammography is not available).
2. In patients who are overwhelmingly anxious over the inherent uncer-

tainty about the presumed benign nature of a mammographically identified abnormality despite appropriate counseling.

The sense of well-being resulting from a benign core biopsy can provide profound relief to women who otherwise might have severe anxiety during periodic follow-up [185].

2. Indeterminate Lesions (Bi-Rads 3–4)

Indeterminate mammographic lesions are generally considered to be the lesions most appropriately biopsied by stereotactic core needle breast biopsy [180,189]. Based on the accuracy of this procedure, definitive benign diagnosis by stereotactic core needle breast biopsy should eliminate the need for surgical biopsy if the result is consistent with initial mammographic finding. Since lesions diagnosed as benign will receive only clinical and mammographic follow-up without surgical confirmation, considering the high frequency of benign lesions among indeterminate mammographic lesions, stereotactic core needle breast biopsy in this group would provide the greatest overall cost advantage [190]. Stereotactic core needle breast biopsy also has the cost advantage for the lesion diagnosed malignant, because the result of this procedure eliminates positive margins and reexcision of tissue and allows for a single definitive operation [190].

3. Highly Suspicious Lesions (Bi-Rads 5)

The Indication of stereotactic core needle breast biopsy in this group is controversial. Since the chance of malignancy is about 80% in these lesions, some surgeons prefer the surgical excision as the first diagnostic and therapeutic maneuver [180,189]. Other surgeons recommend stereotactic core needle breast biopsy as the best initial approach in this group. Most studies demonstrated the positive margin or residual tumor in 45% to 83% of patients after needle localization excisional breast biopsy [191–195]. Yin et al. showed that a mammographic diagnosis of high-suspicion lesion did not significantly reduce the number of positive margins [190]. However, a histologic diagnosis of invasive cancer by stereotactic core needle breast biopsy almost completely eliminated positive margins and need for reexcision in women who chose breast conservation. Therefore presurgical malignant diagnosis in this group of patients by stereotactic core needle breast biopsy allows discussion of the treatment options before surgery, performance of a better lumpectomy, increased likelihood of adequate margins with a single procedure, and potential cost benefit. Another, less frequent but clear indication for stereotactic core needle breast biopsy is lesions characterized by multiple clusters of microcalcifications and/or multiple masses in different quadrants of the same breast. If two or more can be proven malignant by core biopsy, the patient is not a breast conservation candidate and can proceed with mastectomy with or without reconstruction [184].

Only a few instances exist in which core needle biopsy is not helpful:

1. The histologic diagnosis of the lesion by needle biopsy will not shorten the diagnostic process.
2. The removal of the entire lesion is necessary for diagnosis.
3. The lesion cannot be successfully targeted [184].

Some patients or lesions may not be technically suited for stereotactic biopsy. Women who cannot lie prone or undergo extended breast compression are not candidates for the procedure. In addition, some lesions located far posteriorly in the breast cannot be imaged satisfactorily with the stereotactic device [184].

I. Stereotactic Biopsy and Cost Factor

As mentioned before, surgical consults and biopsies represent the largest fraction of induced cost of screening [160]. On the other hand, the overall cost for stereotactic core needle biopsy in most institutions is one-third to one-fourth of cost of surgical biopsy [184]. Schmidt reported that the use of stereotactic core needle biopsy saved 86% of the patients a surgical biopsy or the anxiety of close follow-up, which translates into a cost savings of about 60% [155]. He also reported that the cost savings per biopsy is about $1500 to $2000. Considering the 500,000 breast biopsies initiated by mammographic findings annually in the United States, the use of stereotactic core needle breast biopsy could result in yearly savings of $750 million to $1 billion [186]. A theoretical model suggests that the use of stereotactic core needle biopsy in a mammographic screening program could lower the marginal cost per year of life saved by a maximum of 23%, from $20,770 to $15,934 [187]. Therefore, approximate use of stereotactic core needle biopsy rather than surgical biopsy could result in tremendous cost savings.

Acknowledgments

Special acknowledgments must be made to Ali Massoudi for his artwork and to Dr. Kathy Massoudi for helping us immeasurably with our editorial tasks.

REFERENCES

1. Salomon A. Beitrage zur pathologie und klinik der mammacarcinome. Arch Klin Chir 101:573–668, 1913.
2. Kleinschmidt O. Brustdruse. In: Zweife P, Payr E, eds. Die Klinik der Bosartigen Geschwulste. Leipzig: S. Hirzel, 1927, pp 5–90.
3. Warren SL. Roentgenologic study of the breast. AJR 24:113–124, 1930.
4. Goyanes J, Gentil F, Guedes B. Radiography of mammary gland and its diagnostic value. Arch Espano Oncol 111–142, 1931.

5. Seabold PS. Procedure in roentgen study of the breast. Am J Roentgenol Radium Ther 39:850–851, 1993.

6. Vogel W. Die roentgendarstellung der mammatumoren. Arch Klin Chir 171:618–626, 1932.

7. Lockwood IH. Roentgen-ray evaluation of breast symptoms. Am J Roentgenol Radium Ther 29:145–155, 1933.

8. Gershon-Cohen J, Strickler A. Roentgenologic examination of the normal breast: its evaluation in demonstrating early neoplastic changes. Am J Roentgenol Radium Ther 40:189–201, 1938.

9. Gros CM, Sigrist R. Radiography and transillumination of the breast. Strasbourg Med 2:451–456, 1951.

10. Gershon-Cohen J, Ingleby H. Roentgenology of cancer of the breast: a classified pathological basis for roentgenologic criteria. Am J Roentgenol Radium Ther Nucl Med 68:1–7, 1952.

11. Leborgne R. The Breast in Roentgen Diagnosis. Montevideo, Uruguay: Impresora, 1953.

12. Egan RL. Experience with mammography in a tumor institution: Evaluation of 1000 cases. Radiology 75:894–900, 1960.

13. Egan RL. Fifty-three cases of carcinoma of the breast, occult until mammography. Am J Roentgenol Radium Ther Nucl Med 88:1095–1111, 1962.

14. Clark RL, MM Copeland, RL Egan, et al. Reproducibility of the technique of mammography (Egan) for cancer of the breast. Am J Surg 109:127–133, 1965.

15. Scott WG. Mammography and the training program of the American College of Radiology. Am J Roentgenol Radium Ther Nucl Med 99(4):1002–1008, 1967.

16. Public Law (PL) 102–539. Mammography Quality Standards Act of 1992. 354.

17. Gros CM. Methodologie. Symposium sur le sein. J Radiol Electrol Med Nucl 48:638–655, 1967.

18. Gabbay E. Mammography x-ray source. In: AG Haus, MJ Yaffe, eds. Syllabus: A Categorical Course in Physics: Technical Aspects of Breast Imaging. Oak Brook, IL: Radiological Society of North America, 1994, pp 47–62.

19. Curry III TS, Dowdey JE, Murry RO Jr. Physics of Diagnostic Radiology. 4th ed. Philadelphia: Lea & Febiger, 1990.

20. Desponds L, Depeursinge C, Grescescu M, et al. Influence of anode and filter material on image quality and glandular dose for screen-film mammography. Phys Med Biol 36:1165–1182, 1991.

21. American College of Radiology and Centers for Disease Control and Prevention. Recommended Specifications for New Mammography Equipment. Reston, VA: ACR, April 1995.

22. ESickles A, Weber WN, Galvin HB, Ominsky SH. Baseline screening mammography: one vs two views. AJR 147:1149–1153, 1986.

23. Eklund GW, Cardenosa G . The art of mammographic positioning. Radiol Clin North Am 30:21, 1992.

24. Feig SA. Importance of supplementary mammographic views to diagnostic accuracy. AJR 151:40–41, 1988.

25. Eklund GW, Busby RC, Miller SH, et al. Improved imaging of the augmented breast. AJR 151:469, 1988.
26. D'Orsi CJ, Kopans DB. Mammographic feature analysis. Semin Roentgenol 28:204, 1993.
27. Kopans DB, Swann CA, White G, et al. Asymmetric breast tissue. Radiology 171:639–643, 1989.
28. Sickles EA. Mammographic feature of early breast cancer. AJR 143:461–464, 1984.
29. American College of Radiology. Breast Imaging Reporting and Data System. (BI-RADS). Reston, VA: American College of Radiology, 1995.
30. Carter CL, Allen C, Henson DE. Relation of tumor size, lymph node status, and survival in 24,740 breast cancer cases. Cancer 63:181, 1989.
31. Feig SA. Breast masses: mammographic and sonographic evaluation. Radiol Clin North Am 30(1):67–92, 1992.
32. Mitnick JS, Roses DF, Harris MN, et al. Circumscribed intraductal carcinoma of the breast. Radiology 170:423 425, 1989.
33. Helvie MA, Adler DD, Rebner M, et al. Breast hamartomas: variable mammographic appearances. Radiology 170:417–421, 1989.
34. Hermann G, Schwartz IS. Focal fibrous disease of the breast: mammographic detection of an unappreciated condition. AJR 140:1245–1246.
35. Woods ER, Helvie MA, Ikeda MD, et al. Solitary breast papilloma: comparison of mammographic, galactographic and pathologic findings. AJR 159:487–491, 1992.
36. Gomez A, Mata JM, Donoso L, et al. Galactocele: three distinctive radiographic appearances. Radiology 158:43–44, 1986.
37. Page JE, Williams JE. The radiological features of phylloides tumors of the breast with clinico-pathological correlation. Clin Radiol 44:8–12, 1991.
38. Paulus DD. Lymphoma of the breast. Radiol Clin North Am 28:833–840, 1990.
39. Paulus DD, HI Libshitz. Metastasis to the breast. Radiol Clin North Am 20:561–568, 1982.
40. Bohman LG, Bassett LW, Gold RH, et al. Breast metastases from extramammary malignancies. Radiology 144:309–312, 1982.
41. Meyer JE, Amin E, Lindfors KK. Medullary carcinoma of the breast: mammographic and ultrasound appearance. Radiology 170:79–82, 1989.
42. Mitnick JS, Vazquez MF, Harris MN, et al. Invasive papillary carcinoma of the breast: mammographic appearance. Radiology 177:803–806, 1990.
43. Stomper PC, Davis SP, Weidner N, et al. Clinically occult noncalcified breast cancer: serial radiologic-pathologic correlation in 27 cases. Radiology 169:621–626, 1988.
44. Ikeda DM, Andersson I. Ductal carcinoma in situ: atypical mammographic appearances. Radiology 172:661–666, 1989.
45. Moskowitz M. The predictive value of certain mammographic signs in screening for breast cancer. Cancer 51:1007–1011, 1983.
46. Sickles EA. Periodic mammographic follow-up of probably benign lesions: results in 3,184 consecutive cases. Radiology 179:463–468, 1991.
47. Kopans DB. Breast Imaging. 1st ed. Philadelphia: Lippincott, 1989.

48. Bassett LW, Gold RH, Cove HC. Mammographic spectrum of traumatic fat necrosis: the fallibility of "pathognomonic" signs of carcinoma. AJR 130:119–122, 1978.

49. Ciatto S, Morrone D, Catarzi S, et al. Radial scars of the breast: review of 38 consecutive mammographic diagnoses. Radiology 187:757–760, 1993.

50. Stigers KB, King JG, Davey DD, et al. Abnormalities of the breast caused by biopsy: spectrum of mammographic findings. AJR 156:287–291, 1991.

51. Swann CA, Kopans DB, White G, et al. Observations on the post-reduction mammoplasty mammogram. Breast Dis 1:261–267, 1989.

52. Bassett LW. Mammographic analysis of calcifications. Radiol Clin North Am 30(1):93–105, 1992.

53. Lanyi M. Pathogenesis, pathophysiology, and composition of breast calcifications. In: Diagnosis and Differential Diagnosis of Breast Calcifications. New York; Springer-Verlag, 1986, p 27.

54. Dixon JM, Anderson TJ, Lumsden AB, et al. Mammary duct ectasia. Br J Surg 70:601, 1983.

55. Sickles EA, Galvin HB. Breast arterial calcification in association with diabetes mellitis: too weak a correlation to have clinical utility. Radiology 155:577, 1985.

56. Linden SS, Sickles EA. Sedimented calcium in benign breast cysts. AJR 152:957, 1989.

57. Egan RL, McSweeney MB, Sewell CW. Intramammary calcifications without an associated mass in benign and malignant diseases. Radiology 137:1, 1980.

58. Bassett LW, Jackson VP, Jahan R, et al. Diagnosis of Diseases of the Breast. 1st ed. Philadelphia: Saunders, 1997, p 466.

59. Kalisher L, Peyster RG. Clinicopathological correlation of xerography in determining involvement of metastatic axillary nodes in female breast cancer. Radiology 121:333, 1976.

60. American Cancer Society. Cancer Facts and Figures. Atlanta, GA; American Cancer Society, 1992.

61. Wingo PA, Tong T, Bolden S. Cancer statistics, 1995. CA Cancer J Clin 45:8–30, 1995.

62. Surveillance, Epidemiology, and End Results: Incidence and Mortality Data, 1973–1977. DHEW Publ. No. (NIH)81-2330. Bethesda, MD: Public Health Service, 1981.

63. Rodes N, Lopez M, Peurson D. The impact of breast cancer screening on survival: a 5- to 10-year follow-up study. Cancer 57:581–585, 1986.

64. Tabar L, Feberberg C, Grad A. Reduction in mortality from breast cancer after mass screening with mammography: randomized trial from the breast cancer screening working group of the Swedish National Board of Health and Welfare. Lancet 1:829–832, 1985.

65. Habbema JDF, Van Cortmarssen GV, Van Putten DJ, et al. Age-specific reduction in breast cancer mortality by screening: an analysis of the results of Health Insurance Plan of Greater New York study. J Natl Cancer Inst 77:317–320, 1986.

66. Harris JR, Lippman ME, Veronesi U, Willett W. Breast cancer (review articles). N Engl J Med 327(5):319–328, 1992.

67. Morrison AS. Is self-examination effective in screening for breast cancer? J Natl Cancer Inst 83:226–227, 1991.

68. Fletcher S, Black W, Harris R, et al. Special article: Report of the international workshop on screening for breast cancer. J Natl Cancer Inst 85:1644–1656, 1993.
69. Shapiro S , Venet W, Strax P, Venet L. Periodic Screening for Breast Cancer. The Health Insurance Project and Its Sequelae, 1963–1986. Baltimore, MD: Johns Hopkins University Press, 1988.
70. Tabar L, Fagerberg G, Duffy S, et al. Breast imaging: current status and future directions. Update of the Swedish two-county program of mammographic screening for breast cancer. Radiol Clin North Am 30:187, 1992.
71. Tabar L, Duffy S, Burhenne L. New Swedish breast cancer detection results for women aged 40–49. Cancer 72:1437, 1993.
72. Andersson I, Aspegren K, Janzon L, et al. Mammographic screening and mortality from breast cancer: the Malmo mammographic screening trial. BMJ 297:943–948, 1988.
73. Nystrom L, Rutqvist LE, Wall S, et al. Breast cancer screening with mammography: overview of Swedish randomized trials. Lancet 341:973–978, 1993.
74. Chamberlain J. Firmer evidence on the value of breast screening: the Swedish overview. Eur J Cancer 29A(13):1804–1805, 1993.
75. Roberts MM, Alexander FE, Anderson TJ, et al. Edinburgh trial of screening for breast cancer: mortality at seven years. Lancet 335:241–246, 1990.
76. Miller AB, Baines CJ, To T, et al. Canadian national breast screening study: breast cancer detection and death rates among women aged 40 to 49 years. Can Med Assoc J 147:1459–1476, 1992.
77. Miller AB, Baines CJ, To T, et al. Canadian national breast screening study: breast cancer detection and death rates among women aged 50 to 59 years. Can Med Assoc J 147:1477–1488, 1992.
78. Mettlin CJ, Smart CR. The Canadian national breast screening study. Cancer 72:1461–1465, 1993.
79. Boyd NF, Jong RA, Yaffe MJ, et al. A critical appraisal of the Canadian National Breast Screening Study. Radiology 189:661–663, 1993.
80. Kopans DB, Feig SA. The Canadian National Breast Screening Study: a critical review. AJR 161:755–760, 1993.
81. Burhenne L, Burhenne H. The Canadian National Breast Screening Study: a Canadian critique. AJR 161:761, 1993.
82. Kopans DB. The Canadian Screening Program: a different perspective. AJR 155:748–749, 1990.
83. Baines CJ, Miller AB, Kopans DB. Canadian National Breast Screening Study: assessment of technical quality by external review. AJR 155:743–747, 1990.
84. Smart CR, Hendrick RE, Rutledge JH III, Smith RA. Benefit of mammography screening in women aged 40–49: current evidence from randomized trials. Cancer 75:1619–1626, 1995.
85. Wald N, Chamberlain F, Hackshaw A. Report of the European Society for Mastology: Breast Cancer Screening Evaluation Committee (1993). Breast 2:209–216, 1993.
86. Elwood JM, Cox B, Richardson AK. The effectiveness of breast cancer screening by mammography in younger women. Online J Curr Clin Trials, 1993, Feb. 25, Doc. No. 32.

87. Constanza ME. Breast cancer screening in older women: overview. J Gerontol 47:1–3, 1992.
88. Constanza ME, Annas GJ, Brown ML, et al. Supporting statements and rational. J Gerontol 47:7–16, 1992.
89. Smith RA, Haynes S. Barriers to screening for breast cancer. Cancer 69:1968–1978, 1992.
90. Breast Screening Consortium. Screening mammography: a missed clinical opportunity? Results of the NCI Breast Cancer Surveillance System, 1987. MMWR 38:137–140, 1989.
91. Dawson DA, Thompson GB. Breast cancer risk factors and screening: United States, 1987. Vital Health Stat 10(172):18–26, 1989.
92. Weinberger M. Physicians' knowledge, attitudes and behaviors with respect to breast cancer screening in older women. Presented at the Forum on Breast Cancer Screening in Older Women, Sturbridge, MA, Aug. 1, 1990.
93. Faulk RM, Sickles EA, Sollitto RA, et al. Clinical efficacy of mammographic screening in the elderly. Radiology 194:193–197, 1995.
94. Costanza ME . Breast cancer screening in older women: synopsis of a forum. Cancer 69:1925–1931, 1992.
95. Screening recommendations of the forum panel. J Gerontol 47:5, 1992.
96. Sickles EA, Kopans DB. Deficiencies in the analysis of breast cancer data. J Natl Cancer Inst 85:1621–1624, 1993.
97. Byrne C, Smart CR, Cherk C , Hartmann WH. Survival advantage differences by age: evaluation of the extended follow-up of the Breast Cancer Detection Demonstration Project. Cancer 74:301–310, 1994.
98. Moskowitz M. Breast cancer screening: all's well that ends well, or much ado about nothing? (Letter.) AJR 152:891–892, 1989.
99. Schmidt RA, Metz CE. Please be specific. (Letter.) AJR 154:1121–1122, 1990.
100. Bird RE. Professional quality assurance for mammography screening programs. (Letter.) Radiology 177:587, 1990.
101. Bird RE, Wallace TW, Yankaskas BC. Analysis of cancer missed at screening mammography. Radiology 184(3):613–617, 1992.
102. Ma L, Fishell E, Wright B, et al. Case-control study of factors associated with failure to detect breast cancer by mammography. J Natl Cancer Inst 84:781–785, 1992.
103. McKenna RJ. The abnormal mammogram radiographic findings, diagnostic options, pathology, and stage of cancer diagnosis. Cancer 74:244–255, 1994.
104. Powell RW, McSweeney MB, Wilson CE. X-ray calcifications as the only basis for breast biopsy. Ann Surg 197:555–559, 1983.
105. Dodd GD, Fry K, DelanyW. Pre-op localization of occult carcinoma of the breast. In: Nealon TF, ed. Management of Patient with Breast Cancer. Philadelphia; W.B. Saunders, 1965, pp 88–113.
106. Frank HA, Hall FM, Steer ML. Preoperative localization of nonpalpable breast lesions demonstrated by mammography. N Engl J Med 295:259–260, 1976.
107. Kopans DB, DeLuca S. A modified needle-hook wire technique to simplify preoperative localization of occult breast lesions. Radiology 134:781–782, 1980.

108. Homer MJ. Nonpalpable breast lesion localization using a curved-end retractable wire. Radiology 157:259–260, 1985.

109. Urrutia EJ, Hawkins MC, Steinbach BG, et al. Retractable-barb needle for breast lesion localization: use in 60 cases. Radiology 169:845–847, 1988.

110. Czarnecki DJ, Berridge DL, Splittgerber GF, Goell W. Comparison of the anchoring strengths of the Kopans and Hawkins II needle-hook wire systems. Radiology 183:573–574, 1992.

111. Kopans DB, Meyer JE, Lindfors KK, et al. Breast sonography to guide aspiration of cysts and preoperative localization of occult breast lesions. AJR 143:489, 1984.

112. Kopans DB, Meyer JE. Computed tomography guided localization of clinically occult breast carcinoma: the "N" skin guide. Radiology 145:211, 1982.

113. Greenstein Orel S, Schnall MD, Powell CM, et al. Staging of suspected breast cancer: effect of MR imaging and MR-guided biopsy. Radiology 196(1):115–122, 1995.

114. Khalkhali I, Mishkin FS, Diggles LE, Klein SR. Radionuclide-guided stereotactic prebiopsy localization of nonpalpable breast lesions with normal mammograms. J Nucl Med 1997 38(7):1019–1022, 1997.

115. Kopans DB, Meyer JE. The versatile spring-hook wire breast lesion localizer. AJR 138:586, 1982.

116. Gallagher WJ, Cardenosa G, Rubens JR, et al. Minimal-volume excision of nonpalpable breast lesions. AJR 153:957, 1989.

117. Horns JW, Arndt RD. Percutaneous spot localization of nonpalpable breast lesions. AJR 127:253, 1976.

118. Weyant M, Carroccio A, Tartter PI, et al. Determinants of success with spot localization biopsy of the breast. J Am Coll Surg 181(6):521–524, 1995.

119. Hirsch J, Banks WL, Sullivan JS, et al. Effect of methylene blue on estrogen receptor activity. Radiology 171:105, 1989.

120. Berkowitz JE, Gatewood OMB, Gayler BW. Equivocal mammographic findings: evaluation with spot compression. Radiology 171:369, 1989.

121. Swann CA, Kopans DB, McCarthy KA, et al. Practical solutions to problems of triangulation and preoperative localization of breast lesions. Radiology 163:577, 1987.

122. Jones MK, Vetto JT, Pommier RF, et al. An improved method of needle localized biopsy of nonpalpable lesions of the breast. J Am Coll Surg 178(6):548–552, 1994.

123. Homer MJ, Smith TJ, Safaii H. Prebiopsy needle localization: methods, problems, and expected results. Radiol Clin North Am 30(1):139–153, 1992.

124. Stomper PC, Davis SP, Sonnenfeld MR. Efficacy of specimen radiography of clinically occult noncalcified breast lesions. AJR 151:43, 1988.

125. Carter D. Margins of "lumpectomy" for breast cancer. Hum Pathol 17:330, 1986.

126. Rebner M, Helvie MA, Pennes DR, et al. Paraffin tissue block radiography: adjunct to breast specimen radiography. Radiology 173:695, 1989.

127. Pitzen RH, Urdancta LF, Al-Jurf AS, et al. Specimen xeroradiography after needle localization and biopsy of non-calcified, non-palpable breast lesions. Am Surg 51:50–57, 1985.

128. Proudfoot RW, Mattingly SS, Stelling CB, Fine JG. Non-palpable breast lesions. Wire localization and excisional biopsy. Am Surg 52:117–122, 1986.

129. Norton LW, Zeligman B, Pearlman NW. Accuracy and cost of needle localization breast biopsy. Arch Surg 123:947–950, 1988.
130. Hasselgren PO, Hummel RP, Smith DG, Fieler M. Breast biopsy with needle localization: accuracy of specimen x-ray and management of missed lesions. Surgery 114:836–842, 1993.
131. Reid SE, Scanlon EF, Bernstein JR, et al. An alternative approach to non-palpable breast biopsies. J Surg Oncol 44:93–96, 1990.
132. Molloy M, Azarow K, Garcia V, Daniel J. Enhanced detection of pre-invasive breast cancer: combined role of mammography and needle localization biopsy. J Surg Oncol 40:152–154, 1989.
133. Choucair R, Holcomb M, Matthews R. Biopsy of non-palpable breast lesions. Am J Surg 156:453–456, 1988.
134. Silverstein M, Gamagami P, Rosser R, et al. Hooked-wire-directed breast biopsy and over-penetrated mammography. Cancer 59:715–722, 1989.
135. Kapaln C, Matallana R, Wallack M. The use of state-of-the-art mammography in the detection of non-palpable breast carcinoma. Am Surg 56:40–42, 1990.
136. Knaus J, Dolan J, Isaacs J. Detection of localized breast cancer by prospective mammographic screening criteria. Am J Obstet Gynecol 158:147–149, 1988.
137. Meyer J, Eberlein T, Stomper P, Sonnenfield M. Biopsy of occult breast lesions. JAMA 263:2341–2343, 1990.
138. Rosner D, Bedwani R, Vana J, et al. Non-invasive breast carcinoma: results of a national survey. Ann Surg 192:139–147, 1990.
139. Perdue P, Page D, Nellestein M, et al. Early detection of breast carcinoma: a comparison of palpable and non-palpable lesions. Surgery 111:656–659, 1992.
140. Alexander HR, Candela FC, Dershaw DD, et al. Needle-localized mammographic lesions. Results and evolving treatment strategy. Arch Surg 125:1441–1444, 1990.
141. Marrujo G, Jolly P, Mall MH. Non-palpable breast cancer: needle localized biopsy for diagnosis and considerations for treatment. Am J Surg 151:599–602, 1986.
142. McCreery BR, Frankl G, Frost DB. An analysis of the results of mammographically guided biopsies of the breast. Surg Gynecol Obstet 172:223–226, 1991.
143. Jeter DD, Vest GR, Buday SJ. Mammographic guide-wire localization of non-palpable breast lesions. Am Surg 57:431–433, 1991.
144. Tinnemans JGM, Wobbes T, Holland R, et al. Treatment and survival of female patients with non-palpable breast carcinoma. Ann Surg 209:249–253, 1989.
145. Silverstein MJ, Gamagami P, Colburn WJ, et al. Non-palpable breast lesions: diagnosis with slightly over-penetrated screen-film mammography and hook wire-directed biopsy in 1014 cases. Radiology 171:633–638, 1989.
146. Schwartz GF, Feig SA, Patchefsky AS. Significance and staging of nonpalpable carcinomas of the breast. Surg Gynecol Obstet 166:6–10, 1988.
147. Hena MA, Warheit AC, Crowther JC. Occult breast cancer in two community hospitals in New York State. NY State J Med 89:612–613, 1989.
148. Thompson WR, Bowen JR, Dorman BA. Mammographic localization and biopsy of non-palpable breast lesions. Arch Surg 126:730–734, 1991.
149. Sickle-Santanello BJ, O'Dwyer PJ, McCabe DP, et al. Needle localization of mammographically detected lesions in perspective. Am J Surg 154:279–282, 1987.

150. Tresadern JC, Asbury D, Hartley G, et al. Fine wire localization and biopsy of non-palpable breast lesions. Br J Surg 77:320–322, 1990.
151. Gisvold JJ, Martin JK. Prebiopsy localization of non-palpable breast lesions. AJR 143:477–481, 1984.
152. Rissanen TJ, Makarainen HP, Mattila SI, et al. Wire localized biopsy of breast lesions: a review of 425 cases found in screening or clinical mammography. Clin Radiol 47:14–22, 1993.
153. Meyer JE, Kopans DB, Stomper P, et al. Occult breast abnormalities, percutaneous preoperative needle localization. Radiology 150:335–337, 1984.
154. Ciatto S, Cataliotti L, Distante V. Non-palpable lesions detected with mammography: review of 512 consecutive cases. Radiology 165:99–102, 1987.
155. Bassett LW, Liu TH, Giuliano AE, et al. The prevalence of carcinoma in palpable vs. impalpable mammographically detected lesions. AJR 157:21–24, 1991.
156. Burrell HC, Pinder S, Wilson ARM, et al. The positive predictive value of mammographic signs: a review of 425 non-palpable breast lesions. Clin Radiol 51:277–281, 1996.
157. Hall FM, Storella JM, Silverstone DZ, et al. Non-palpable breast lesions: recommendation for biopsy based on suspicion of carcinoma at mammography. Radiology 167:353–358, 1988.
158. Schmidt RA. Stereotactic breast biopsy. CA 44:172–191, 1994.
159. Sickles EA. Quality assurance: how to audit your own mammography practice. Radiol Clin North Am 30:265–275, 1992.
160. Cyrlak D. Induced costs of low-cost screening mammography. Radiology 168:661–663, 1988.
161. Yankaskas BC, Knelson MH, Abernethy ML, et al. Needle localization biopsy of occult lesions of the breast: experience in 199 cases. Invest Radiol 23:729, 1988.
162. Kopans DB. Review of stereotaxic large-core needle biopsy and surgical biopsy results in non-palpable breast lesions. Radiology 189:665, 1993.
163. Bolmgren J, Jacobson B, Nordenstrom B. Stereotaxic instrument for needle biopsy of the mammogram. AJR 129:121–125, 1977.
164. Nordenstrom B, Zajicek J. Stereotaxic needle biopsy and preoperative indication of non-palpable mammary lesions. Acta Cytol 21:350–351, 1977.
165. Dowlatshahi K, Jokich PM, Schmidt R, et al. Cytologic diagnosis of occult breast lesions using stereotaxic needle aspiration. Arch Surg 122:1343–1346, 1987.
166. Dowlatshahi K, Yaremko ML, Kluskens LF, Jokich PM. Non-palpable breast lesions: findings of stereotaxic needle-core biopsy and fine-needle aspiration cytology. Radiology 181:745–750, 1991.
167. Parker SH. When is core biopsy really core? Radiology 185:641–642, 1992.
168. Pettine S, Place R, Babu S, et al. Stereotactic breast biopsy is accurate, minimally invasive, and cost effective. Am J Surg 171:474–476, 1996.
169. Parker SH, Lovin JD, Jobe WE, et al. Stereotactic breast biopsy with a biopsy gun. Radiology 176:741–747, 1990.
170. Parker SH, Lovin JD, Jobe WE, et al. Non-palpable breast lesions: stereotactic automated large-core biopsies. Radiology 180:403–407, 1991.

171. Parker SH, Jobe WE. Percutaneous Breast Biopsy. 1st ed. New York: Raven Press, 1993.
172. Hopper KD, Baird D, Reddy VV, et al. Efficacy of automated biopsy guns versus conventional biopsy needles in the pygmy pig. Radiology 176:671–676, 1990.
173. Parker SH, Hopper KD, Yakes WF, et al. Image-directed percutaneous biopsies with a biopsy gun. Radiology 171:663–669, 1989.
174. Meyer JE. Value of large-core biopsy of occult breast lesions. AJR 158:991–992, 1992.
175. Helvie MA, Ikeda DM, Adler DD. Localization and needle aspiration of breast lesions: complications in 370 cases. AJR 157:711–714, 1991.
176. Parker S, Burbank F, Tabar L, et al. Percutaneous large core breast biopsy: a multi institutional experience. Radiology 193:359–364, 1994.
177. Harter LP, Curtis JS, Ponto G, et al. Malignant seeding of the needle track during stereotaxic core needle breast biopsy. Radiology 185:713, 1992.
178. Smith EH. Complications of percutaneous abdominal fine-needle biopsy. Review. Radiology 178:253–258, 1991.
179. Dronkers DJ. Stereotaxic core biopsy of breast lesions. Radiology 183:631–634, 1992.
180. Elvecrog EL, Lechner MC, Nelson MT. Non-palpable breast lesions: correlation of stereotaxic large-core needle biopsy and surgical biopsy results. Radiology 188:453–455, 1993.
181. GisvoldJJ, Goellner JR, Grant CS, et al. Breast biopsy: a comparative study of stereotaxically guided core and excisional techniques. AJR 162:815–820, 1994.
182. Jackman RJ, Nowels KW, Shepard MJ, et al. Stereotaxic large-core needle biopsy of 450 non-palpable breast lesions with surgical correlation in lesions with cancer or atypical hyperplasia. Radiology 193:91, 1994.
183. Jackman RJ, Nowels KW, Shepard MJ, et al. Histologic correlation of non-palpable breast lesions showing cancer or atypia by using stereotaxic large-core needle biopsy with subsequent excisional biopsy. Presented at 79th RSNA meeting. November 1993, Chicago. Radiology 189P: 221 (abstract), 1993.
184. Evans WP III. Stereotactic core breast biopsy. In: JR Harris, ME Lippman, M Morrow, S Hellman, eds. Diseases of the Breast. Philadelphia: Lippincott-Raven, 1996, pp 144–152.
185. Sickles EA, Parker SH. Appropriate role of core breast biopsy in the management of probably benign lesions. Radiology 188:315, 1993.
186. Schmidt R, Morrow M, Bibbo M, et al. Benefits of stereotactic aspiration cytology. Admin Radiol 9:35, 1990.
187. Lindfors KK, Rosenquist CJ. Needle core biopsy guided with mammography: a study of cost-effectiveness. Radiology 199:217, 1994.
188. Nguyen M, McCombs MM, Ghandehari S, et al. An update on core needle biopsy for radiologically detected breast lesions. Cancer 78:2340–2345, 1996.
189. Sullivan DC. Needle core biopsy of mammographic lesions. AJR 162:601–608, 1994.
190. Yim JH, Barton P, Weber B, et al. Mammographically detected breast cancer: benefits of stereotactic core versus wire localization biopsy. Ann Surg 233(6):688–700, 1996.
191. Mokbel K, Ahmed M, Nash A, Sacks N. Reexcision operations in non-palpable breast cancer. J Surg Oncol 58:225–228, 1995.

192. Lee CH, Carter D. Detecting residual tumor after excisional biopsy of impalpable breast carcinoma: efficacy of comparing preoperative mammograms with radiography of the biopsy specimen. AJR 164:81–86, 1995.

193. Solin LJ, Fowble B, Martz K, et al. Results of re-excisional biopsy of the primary tumor in preparation for definitive irradiation of patients with early stage breast cancer. Int J Radiat Oncol Biol Phys 12:721–725, 1986.

194. Tafra L, Guenther JM, Guiliano AE. Planned segmentectomy: a necessity for breast carcinoma. Arch Surg 128:1014, 1993.

195. Ngai JH, Zelles GW, Rumore GJ, et al. Breast biopsy techniques and adequacy of margins. Arch Surg 126:1343–1347, 1991.

4

Breast Imaging with Positron Emission Tomography

Hans Bender, Holger Palmedo, and Hans J. Biersack
University of Bonn, Bonn, Germany

Axel Schomburg
Roentgeninstitut, Dusseldorf, Germany

I. INTRODUCTION

A. Historical Background

Positron emission tomography (PET) is a cross-sectional, nuclear medicine imaging technique that provides functional images of the body (e.g., by visualization of metabolic processes, expression of transporters, receptors, etc.). PET combines a series of characteristics/abilities that could not be realized in standard nuclear medicine applications:

1. Quantitation: While gamma rays can not be focused like visible light, the collimator technology allows a sufficient but limited substitute. The major limitation is due to the fact that gamma rays can not be stopped but only attenuated. By this way, the assumed volume of an imaged lesion is related to the accumulated activity. Thus, the higher the accumulated activity within a defined volume, the larger it appears on the display unit.

2. Resolution: The above-mentioned physical limitation of single-gamma ray imaging does not only limit true/accurate volume estimates but also limits the resolution of the system. In addition, deeply located and small lesions are significantly masked by attenuation and scatter, while the detected size seems to increase with the distance of the object from the collimator.

3. Production of biologically identical tracers: Certain positron emitters (^{11}C, ^{15}O, ^{13}N) are the building blocks of organic compounds as they are used in

living organisms. Substitution of the stable isotope by its radioactive form allows the production of biologically identical substances, which are substrate and tracer of a pertaining and highly specific metabolic pathway at the same time. If substances are employed that enter a main metabolization pathway but are side-channeled at a later metabolization step, active accumulation can be achieved with high target-to-background ratios.

The basis of PET is a coincidence measurement of two γ-rays which are simultaneously detected in opposite detector pairs. As a result of radioactive decay of certain radionuclides, a positron (positively charged electron) is emitted and annihilates with an electron, producing a pair of 511-keV γ-rays. The pair of γ-rays fly off in almost opposite direction, penetrate the surrounding matter (e.g., tissue), and can be recorded by scintillation detectors placed around (e.g., ring) the decay site. The event of the annihilation can be identified by the electronic circuit of the scanner, by recording only the arrival of γ-ray pairs activating opposite detector pairs within a defined time window. This type of measurement/recording is termed coincidence measurement and presents a kind of "electronic" collimation. The location of the annihilation can be estimated more easily and significantly more accurately than single gamma-ray detection. Nonetheless, the decay site is the more inaccurate the higher the energy of the emitted positron, due to the travel path of the positron from the emission to the annihilation site, thus having an impact on absolute quantitation.

Due to the above-mentioned characteristics, PET has been primarily employed to study and quantitate biochemical and physiological mechanisms of brain and heart and, only lately, for selected diseases in these organs [1] as well as for questions arising in oncology (see reviews after Reference list).

Like all nuclear medicine procedures, PET visualizes physiology in the context of known or expected anatomy and morphology. PET is able to do this more quantitatively and with a considerable higher contrast than other nuclear medicine tests [2]. Even though CT and MRI have superior resolution characteristics, visualization of physiology and providing in addition an exceptional set of anatomical landmarks is becoming a unique advantage of PET. This is especially true when PET is applied to cancer allowing to differentiate mass lesions as viable tumor vs. scar, identifying mildly or normal-size lymph nodes as tumor-infested vs. nonmalignant processes, detecting tumor lesions >1 cm, and predict whether cancer will respond or monitor the response to therapy. Nevertheless, best results can probably be expected only after simultaneous application of morphological (CT/MRI) and functional (PET) imaging modalities.

The basis of tumor imaging with PET, as well as any other nuclear medicine procedure, is radiopharmaceuticals exerting specific accumulation mechanisms. Potential radiopharmaceuticals can be chosen based on known differences in physiology, metabolisms, expression of membrane structures (antigens, receptors, transporter systems, etc.), gene expression, etc., between tumors and normal tissues.

The use of a cyclotron to produce short-lived positron-emitting radionu-

Table 1   Radionuclides and Examples of PET Substances Useful for In Vivo Imaging

Use	Radionuclide	$T_{1/2}$ (min)	Substance
Glucose utilization	F-18	109	Fluorodeoxyglucose
	C-11	20	Glucose
Perfusion	O-15	2	Water
	Rb-82	1.5	RbCl
	Rb-81	298	
Blood volume	O-15, C-11		Carbon dioxide
Oxygenation	O-15		Oxygen
Hypoxia	F-18		Fluoromisonidazole
Protein synthesis	C-11		Methionine, leucine
	N-13	10 min	Glutamate
DNA synthesis	C-11		Thymidine
	F-18		Fluorodeoxyadenosine
Drugs	F-18		5-Fluorouracil
	C-11, N-13		BCNU
	N-13		Cisplatin
Estrogen receptors	F-18		Fluoroestradiol
Progestin receptors	F-18		Fluoronorprogesterone
Somatostatin receptors	G-68	68	Octreotide
Tumor antigens	Y-86	14 h	Antibodies
	I-124	4 days	

clides, which are the elements of biochemical substances (Table 1), has allowed the synthesis of a wide array of labeled and biologically identical compounds, which is usually not the case with SPECT tracers. Noteworthy, due to the short half-life of most of the positron emitters, production and usage are mostly limited to cyclotron sites and thus limit the clinical application and importance.

Typically tumors show some common alterations in physiology which can be employed for PET imaging including alteration in perfusion [3–9], oxygen consumption [8,9], increased growth rate [10], associated with enhanced rate of DNA/RNA and protein synthesis [11,12], and, consequently, upregulated amino acid transport and energy, e.g., glucose consumption. Interestingly, the greatest practical application, which has boosted PET as a clinical tool for tumor imaging, is the observation that tumors have greater rates of anaerobic and aerobic glycolysis than most normal tissues [13], a phenomenon first noted by Warburg [14,15]. In addition, increased expression and higher affinity of glucose transporter molecules, e.g., Glut-1 [47] on the tumor cell surface [16], increased levels and activity of hexokinase [17], and reduced levels of glucose-6-phosphatase [18–20] has been reported in cancer cells than in normal tissues. Subsequently, initial studies suggest that FDG uptake is strongly related to the proliferative activity of tumor cells [21].

Other strategies for tumor imaging employ increased perfusion [5,6,8,9], oxygen extraction [8,9], or detection of hypoxia [8] as nonspecific changes, as well as receptor or antigen overexpression as more specific alterations [22,23].

B.   Rationale for Clinical Use

Breast cancer (BC) is considered the most frequent malignant tumor in women of the Western world with an increasing incidence. It is understood that BC is curable if diagnosed in its earliest form, but this tumor represents a diagnostic problem in several specific settings. Detection of primary cancers can be difficult in younger women with dense breasts, while mammograms which show dense glandular tissue can obscure the tumors. At the same time, the specificity of mammography is relatively low, with a larger fraction of mammographic abnormalities being found to represent nonmalignant processes rather than cancer, thus open biopsies are often needlessly performed [24]. The same is true for MRI [25] and conventional sonography [26].

In many cases, BC is a systemic disease at the time of primary diagnosis. Metastases appear early in the course of tumor progression [27,28]. The size of the primary tumor seems to be correlated with the number and size of axillary lymph node metastases. For example pT1 tumors have a 15% risk of axillary lymph node involvement, which present mainly as micrometastases [29]. While the presence and extent of metastases to the axilla represent the single most important prognostic factor for patients with breast cancer (27), axillary recurrence is associated with unacceptably high morbidity and mortality. Thus, accurate staging is a prerequisite of optimal cancer management. Currently, the only reliable method to determine the spread to regional lymph nodes is their surgical resection and histopathological examination [30]. On the other hand, identification of tumor involvement in some lesions, e.g., soft tissues, can be difficult with current methods.

It is unquestioned that early detection of tumor recurrence and presence of metastases have significant influence on therapy: local recurrence and restricted axillary lymph node involvement would be treated by surgical revision and often radiation and/or neoadjuvant therapy, while clavicular, mediastinal lymph nodes or distant metastases (lung, liver, bone) would require chemotherapy and/or local radiation therapy [27,28].

Currently, for tumor screening, palpation of the breast and local lymph node regions, mammography, sonography, and serum tumor markers are used. Pathological findings are substantiated by sonography, CT, MRI, MIBI scintigraphy, and/or biopsy. In case of cancer verification, primary tumor staging and follow-up examinations employ physical examination, axillary lymph node sonography, mammography, CT, MRI, bone scintigraphy, and/or serum tumor markers [2,3,27,28]. The same is true if a recurrence is suspected.

While FDG-PET is a new, promising imaging modality, it offers the potential to evaluate primary, regionally metastatic, and systemic metastases and recurrence of breast cancer. In addition, PET may allow monitoring of therapy response (scar versus viable tumor tissue), early prediction of therapy outcome, and therapy success.

II. CHARACTERISTICS OF THE RADIOPHARMACEUTICAL

A. Chemistry

Chemical name: 2-[^{18}F]fluoro-2-deoxy-D-glucose ([^{18}F]FDG)
Chemical formula: $C_6H_{11}O_5F$
Structural formula:

α - D - glucose   2 - deoxy - D - glucose   [^{18}F] 2 - fluoro -
                                                          2 - deoxy - D - glucose

B. Dosimetry

The usual application dose in adults varies from 5 to 20 mCi (185 to 740 MBq) with most centers using 5 to 10 mCi (185 to 370 MBq). In children, a dose reduction has been proposed, but no optimal dose has been suggested. The interval between two injections should be at least long enough to allow complete physical decay (roughly 10 half-lives) and/or biological elimination. If no-carrier added FDG is used, a dose of 10 mCi (370 MBq) consists of 0.2 to 2 μg (1 to 10 pM) FDG, depending on the decay period. While plasma glucose levels are in the range of 5.5 mM (100 mg%), no effects of FDG (DG) on glucose metabolism can be expected. In patients, infusion of deoxyglucose in doses of 50 mg/kg yielded side effects comparable to hypoglycemia [31]. This dose is in an amount roughly 50,000 times the amount of FDG that could be administered to a patient receiving ^{18}F-DG.

   Systemic application is performed by an intravenous bolus injection and can be described by a triexponential elimination curve. FDG distributes uniformly to the kidneys, heart, brain, lungs, and liver and clears rapidly from all tissues except the heart, where it remains constant for at least 2 hours, and to a lesser extent, in the brain, where it decreases slowly from 1 to 2 hours [32].

Myocardial uptake is variable and depends on the fasting state of the patient. Since the heart has a insulin-sensitive glucose transporter, the myocardial uptake is enhanced in the presence of insulin, e.g., after eating. The same is true for skeletal muscle. Therefore, overnight fasting is recommended by FDG-PET studies for cancer as this lowers insulin levels and also generally reduces blood sugar levels [33,34].

FDG is primarily excreted with the urine following glomerular filtration and incomplete tubular reabsorption [15,35,36]. Within 30 min, approximately 4% of the injected dose can be measured in the urine; after 2 hours, >20% are present in the urine.

The intracellular accumulation of FDG is mediated by tissue-specific transporter mechanisms, which are partially insulin-dependent (myocard, muscle, fat tissue) and thereafter is phosphorylated by hexokinase. This phosphorylation to 2-FDG-6-phosphate results in a polar intermediate which does not cross the cell membrane and is trapped in the cells. Dephosphorylation occurs relatively slowly, particularly in cancer cells, which usually lack glucose-6-phosphatase (18–20).

Its retention by the heart and brain results from the metabolic trapping mechanism and reflects glucose utilization. FDG behaves similarly to glucose in its transport from plasma to tissue and in its phosphorylation. The rate of phosphorylation, under a steady state for glucose, is equal to the utilization rate of exogenous glucose.

^{18}F decays by positron ($\beta+$) emission (97%) and electron capture (3%) with a half-life of 110 min to ^{18}O. The positron annihilates together with an electron to a pair of 511-keV gamma rays. Critical organs are bladder wall, heart, and brain with around 170, 65, and 26 μSv/MBq, respectively [37–39]. In all other organs, dose estimates are around or below 20 μSv/MBq, including ovaries and testicles.

Estimates of the effective equivalent dose range from 21 to 27 μSv/MBq, which adds up to a radiation exposure of 7.8 to 10 mSv following an injection of 10 mCi (370 MBq) FDG [39]. This is well in the range of the natural annual radiation exposure in middle Europe (2 to 6 mSv/year)

C. Radiolabeling

FDG is a structural analog of 2-deoxyglucose (2-DG). ^{18}F is attached to the 2-position of this molecule and thus behaves similar to 2-DG. ^{18}F is introduced by nucleophilic substitution of 1,3,4,6-tetra-O-acetyl-2-O-trifluoromethyl-sulfonyl-β-D-mannopyranose (mannose triflate) under stereospecific S_N2 reaction conditions. The acetyl groups are removed from the molecule by acidic hydrolization, and FDG can be purified by chromatographic methods with buffered saline solution. After filtration through a 0.22-μm filter, a sterile, isotonic, neutral 2-[^{18}F]-FDG solution is obtained, which is ready for intravenous injection, following quality control and dose calibration. The product is a no-carrier added solution with >95% of the radioactivity represented by 2-[^{18}F]-fluoro-2-deoxy-D-glucose [41]. The specific activity ranges from 27 to 2700 mCi/µmol (1 to 100 GBq/µmol). Noteworthy, ^{18}F-FDG is usually produced employing semi- or fully automated synthesis modules in a dedicated radiopharmacy.

D.   Quality Control

Quality control usually includes:

Total volume and radioactive concentration.

Radionuclide purity: gamma ray spectroscopy using a sodium iodide detector and a multichannel analyzer.

Radiochemical purity: high-pressure liquid chromatography (HPLC) against an FDG standard using refractive index and gamma ray detectors.

Chemical purity: thin-layer chromatography against a Kryptofix 222 standard.

Radionuclide identity: decay counting of the final product over a 10-min period in a dose calibrator to verify the radionuclide half-life.

pH: narrow range pH strip and compared to pH=6 and pH=7 buffers.

Sterility: incubation of final product in culture media; the medium is inspected for bacterial growth during a 14-day incubation at 30 to 35°C and 20 to 25°C. Due to the short half-life, sterility is obtained by sterile filtration (0.22-µm filter). Control samples can be stored at –20/70°C, which allows sterility testing in doubtful cases, any time later.

Bacterial endotoxins: limulus amebocyte lysate (LAL) against standard endotoxin.

E.   Experiences in Animal Model

Comparatively few studies have been performed using tumor-bearing animals. Early investigations were able to demonstrate high FDG uptake in human ovarian adenocarcinoma cells [41], colon cancer [41], choriocarcinoma [41], bladder cancer [41], renal cell carcinoma [41], neurablastoma [41], melanoma [41], small cell lung carcinoma [41], human head and neck carcinoma cell lines [42], and breast carcinoma [43]. FDG uptake shows a strong correlation with the number of viable tumor cells in vitro as demonstrated in human ovarian adenocarcinoma cells [44] and head and neck tumors [42]. Also in breast carcinoma, FDG uptake reflects mainly tracer uptake in proliferating cancer cells in vivo in xenotransplanted rats [43] as well as in patients [46].

One major issue is the effect of blood glucose levels on FDG uptake, which has been investigated by Wahl et al. [47] employing subcutaneously growing human mammary adenocarcinomas in rats. Their data demonstrated an inverse relationship of glucose level on FDG. Mainly, in tumor, brain, small bowel, and ovaries, tracer accumulation is significantly reduced (2.7- to 9.7-fold) comparing hyperglycemic versus normoglycemic animals. Thus, blood sugar levels should be monitored and a euglycemic status is preferred prior to FDG injection.

In order to improve detection of probable lymph node metastases, e.g., micrometastases, FDG had been injected subcutaneously (SC) versus intravenously (IV) in normal and tumor-bearing rats [48]. SC injection yielded a high lymph node accumulation and long tracer retention also in normal lymph nodes, which was not true after IV injection. Tumor-to-normal lymph node ratios were significantly higher after IV application than SC injection. Thus, SC injection is of no benefit to enhance tumor detection in lymph nodes.

III.   TECHNICAL ASPECTS

A.   Patient Preparation

Based on the above-mentioned animal data, patients should be fasted for at least 4 hours and probably best overnight, which is used by us routinely. Under these conditions, we have found that diabetic patients usually present with a blood sugar levels well below 180 mg%. Prior to FDG injection, blood sugar levels should be determined. Patients with levels >200 mg% are usually not enrolled in our facility. High blood sugar levels have been reported to decrease FDG uptake in proven tumors [33,34]. Furthermore, acute normalization of a high blood sugar by injection of insulin is not advisable due to uncontrolled uptake of FGD in normal tissue (muscle) and the risk of producing false-negative results [34,47].

B.   Injection Dose and Route of Injection

Intravenous injection of 5 to 10 mCi proved to be an efficient dose to obtain images with a high contrast. Most centers employ a bolus injection via an IV line (butterfly) to avoid paravasation. In addition, the arm opposite the suspected lesion should be preferred.

In our experience, degradation of image quality is mainly due to body weight. Patients with a body weight >80 kg show usually increasing scatter artifacts as a function of body weight. Injection of a higher FDG dose (e.g., 10 mCi/80 kg BW) did not improve image quality significantly. Thus we assume that body weight-dependent scatter correction algorithms are needed.

After injection, patients are kept in a resting position for at least 45 min (usually 45 to 60 min) employing a quiet and darkened room and are asked to drink 1 L of water. Prior to acquisition, patients are asked to void the bladder.

C. Imaging Acquisition

1. General Considerations

For assessment of primary breast tumors, patients are studied in the prone position with pending breasts and the arms over the head. At least two bed positions are studied covering the axillary region and the breasts.

For tumor staging, mainly in the assessment of recurrent disease, patients are studied in the supine position with the arms at their side. In order to reduce artifacts due to activity in the bladder, the move-out mode is selected with the pelvis being the first and the neck being the last bed position.

2. Transmission Scan

In order to allow quantitation, a transmission scan of the regions of interest is required. For most accurate results, the transmission should be performed prior to FDG injection, and the patient should not be moved during the following accumulation period and emission scan. Some institutions perform the transmission scan directly after the emission scan. Yet it is not clear to what extent artifacts are introduced.

For practical reasons, in our institution all patients receive a transmission scan of the body trunk (from neck to pelvis) for 10 min per bed position and a total of five or six beds. Patients are marked with three points at the start, middle, and endpoint, which allows sufficiently accurate repositioning. Qualitative assessment of patients, who have been moved after the transmission scan as compared to patients who had not been moved, did not reveal evident differences (unpublished data). Thus, patients are moved for FDG injection and the accumulation period. Overall, it is not yet clear whether a transmission scan is needed for routine clinical use, since the images are predominantly analyzed qualitatively. Yasuda et al. [49] studied 32 patients with 106 true-positive lesions. All of these lesions were identified on transmission-corrected images, whereas 104 were identified by emission scans (98%); one lesion in close contact with a large tumor mass and one deep lesion beside the spine were missed without transmission correction. In addition, semiquantitative (e.g., ratio considerations) or quantitative (e.g., SUV) approaches seem to improve the specificity and accuracy of PET [50–52] by a more objective differentiation of borderline cases.

3. Emission Scan

Emission scans are usually started 45 to 60 min after FDG injection and run for 10 min per bed position. Delayed scans (90 to 120 min) are possible and might reduce background activity, but no systemic studies have been performed substantiating the benefit of delayed scans.

4.   Data Acquisition

FDG-PET data should be acquired with a dedicated PET scanner in order to achieve high resolution, good counting statistics, and an acceptable investigation time. In our institution we employ an ECAT EXACT 927/47 (Siemens-CTI, Knoxville, TN) with a field-of-view of 16.2 cm producing 47 simultaneous transaxial slices at each longitudinal bed position with a slice thickness of 3.2 mm in the transaxial projection. Actual resolution lies in the range of 7 to 8 mm.

The use of super-high-energy collimators or coincidence detection in combination with standard gamma cameras seems to be a cheap option, but their application is still limited by actual resolution and sensitivity in the detection of small lesions, and thus cannot be recommended.

5.   Data Processing

Emission data are usually reconstructed by filtered back-projection with a Hanning filter, a cut-off frequency of 0.4 without scatter correction. Scans are corrected for attenuation based on the measured transmission data. Results are displayed on computer screen as three orthogonal images and allow interactive choice of slice localization by the investigator. Images can be documented in transaxial, coronal, sagittal view, and pathological findings as a "three orthogonal image view." Iterative reconstruction algorithms seem to be beneficial, but are not yet part of routine software packages.

6.   Data Analysis

All PET images are evaluated primarily by visual inspection on a high-resolution display monitor. FDG uptake is currently scored qualitatively as follows: uptake markedly higher than liver or mediastine: intense = malignancy—typical; uptake comparable to liver or mediastine: moderate = malignancy—suspect/inflammatory; uptake lower than liver or mediastine but higher than background: low = inflammatory/unspecific; none = no evidence of disease. Images are usually read by two experienced nuclear medicine physicians who are not blinded to available data. All PET studies are part of ongoing prospective studies, which are retrospectively analyzed and compared to standard imaging modalities (X-ray, CT/MRI, ultrasound, mammography, bone scintigraphy) and final institutional diagnosis (gold standard) based on histological and/or clinical outcome.

IV.   CLINICAL APPLICATION

A.   Personal Experience

Between 1995 and 1997 more then 2000 patient studies have been performed in our institution, with roughly 70% of the cases presenting with oncological questions. Around 150 patients suffering from breast carcinoma have thus been referred either to obtain more information in equivocal findings or for reasons of staging/restaging.

1. Primary Breast Cancer

Till now, we have studied only a small number of patients (n = 22) with primary breast cancer (unpublished data). All patients had a documented lesion (mammography, palpation) and were scheduled for surgery (Fig. 1). Of 17 proven positive lesions, only 12 were identified by PET with an overall sensitivity of 71%. All lesions <10 mm were missed. Three of five false-negative lesions showed only minimal/moderate uptake. The three false-positive cases were due to fibroadenoma (n = 1), inflammation (n = 1), and artifacts (n = 1). In three patients (18%), unsuspected axillary lymph node involvement was detected.

In a limited prospective study, Palmedo et al. [53] compared the efficacy of FDG-PET and MIBI in the detection of primary breast carcinoma in 20 patients. In 12 of 13 histologically positive lesions (12 palpable), PET and MIBI were positive. One lesion (<8 mm) was false-negative, and one lesion (fibroadenoma) false-positive, in both methods. No evident advantage of FDG-PET over MIBI was observed, at least in palpable breast lesions.

2. Local Recurrence

We have evaluated 75 patients with suspected recurrent breast carcinoma or restaging of recurrent carcinoma [54]. Table 2 summarizes all FDG-PET results and relevant diagnostic safety evaluation.

In 16 patients (21%) local recurrence was verified, but in four patients (5%)

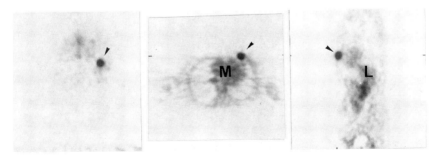

Figure 1   Case 1: A 37-year-old woman with a palpable mass in the left breast. Mammography and a MIBI study were indicative for a breast carcinoma. FDG-PET showed an intense tracer uptake (arrow), which was considerably higher than mediastine (M) and liver (L). Histology confirmed the presence of a 2.5-cm ductal carcinoma. No lymph node or distant metastases were found. Right: coronal; middle: transversal, and left: sagittal view.

TABLE 2   Assessment of FDG-Positive Lesions and the Diagnostic Safety in the Staging of Recurrent Breast Carcinoma (n = 75)

Tumor site	True-positive	False-positive	True-negative	False-negative	Sensitivity	Specificity	Accuracy
Local recurrence	16	2	53	4	80	96	92
Lymph nodes	28	4	42	1	97	91	93
Bone	15	1	59	0	100	98	99
Lung	5	2	67	1	83	97	96
Liver	2	2	71	0	100	97	97

Source: Data according to Bender et al. [54].

proven tumor was missed, probably due to small size (<8 to 10 mm) of the lesion, and two cases were false-positive. All true-positive lesions showed intense FDG uptake. Overall sensitivity and accuracy was 80% and 92%, respectively.

In contrast, CT/MRI (n = 63) showed a sensitivity and specificity of 93% and 97%, respectively. We have not yet fully assessed the reasons for this difference, but, so far, our data indicate that CT/MRI are more suited for the evaluation of local recurrence (Table 3).

TABLE 3   Comparison of Histologically or Clinically Proven Lesions as Detected by FDG-PET Versus CT/MRI (n = 63) in Recurrent Breast Carcinoma

Tumor site	True-positive	False-positive	True-negative	False-negative	PET+ CT/MRI+	PET+ CT/MRI−	PET− CT/MRI+	PET− CT/MRI−
Local recurrence	11/14[a]	2/1	46/47	4/1	7	4	2	2
Lymph nodes	21/17	3/2	38/40	1/6	17	5	0	0
Bone	13/6	2/1	48/49	0/7	6	7	1	0
Lung	5/5	2/2	55/55	1/1	5	0	0	0
Liver	2/1	1/1	72/20	0/1	1	0	0	0

Source: Data according to Bender et al. [54].
[a]Number of lesions detected by FDG-PET/CT-MRI.
PET+ = FDG-PET-positive lesions.
PET− = FDG-PET-negative lesions.
CT/MRI+ = CT/MRI-positive lesions.
CT/MRI− = CT/MRI-negative lesions.

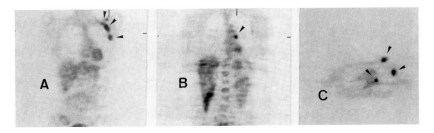

FIGURE 2   Case 2: A 41-year-old woman with dense breasts and a questionable mass in the left breast in combination with small axillary lymph nodes. Mammography and MRI were indicative for breast carcinoma. Multiple, pathologically enlarged axillary and one para-aortal lymph node were described by MRI. FDG-PET showed intense tracer uptake (arrows) in the breast lesion, axillary and para-aortal lymph nodes. Histology confirmed intraductal and scirrhos carcinoma. No distant metastases (lung, liver, bone) were found. (A) Coronal view of the axillary region; (B) coronal view of the para-aortic region; (C) transversal view.

3.   Lymph Node Involvement

In 15 of 75 patients (20%), no evidence of disease was found by PET, which was confirmed by negative histology and/or follow-up results over a period of at least 6 months (Table 2). In 28 patients (37%) solitary or multiple lymph node metastases were found (Figs. 2 and 3); in four patients (5%) false-positive lesions, and

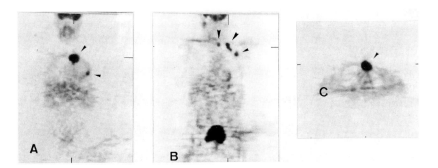

FIGURE 3   Case 3: 52-year-old woman with are intraductal carcinoma of the left breast 5 years ago (pT2NoMo). Due to rising tumor markers and pain in the sternoclavicular region, she was referred for an FDG-PET study. Bone scintigraphy showed a diffuse tracer uptake in this region but no metastases in typical pattern. FDG-PET revealed a massive tracer accumulation (arrows) parasternally and multiple clavicular and axillary lesions (lymph nodes) and a small lesion in the left breast (local recurrence), which was not palpable. (A) Coronal view of the parasternal and ventral region; (B) coronal view of the axillary region; and (C) transaxial view of the parastenal region.

in one case (1.3%) no uptake (false-negative). Sensitivity and accuracy in lymph node metastases proved to be 97% and 93%, respectively.

Direct comparison of FDG-PET vs. CT/MRI results (Table 3) in 63 patients suggested a disease-free status in nine (14%) patients. Overall, 17 out of a total 25 (68%) identified lesion sites were positive in FDG-PET and CT/MRI, with with no false-positive or false-negative finding. In addition, five (20%) true-positive lesion sites were only identified by FDG-PET, whereas none were identified by CT/MRI only. On the other hand, three lesions (12%) (FDG-positive/CT-MRI-negative) proved to be nonmalignant tissue. No lymph node manifestation was missed. Overall, our data indicate that FDG-PET is the most sensitive modality to detect lymph node metastases and, in conjunction with CT/MRI, provides an excellent tool for lymph node staging. It might be especially useful in the evaluation of parasternal/mediastinal lymph nodes if the primary tumor is localized in the mesial quadrants of the breast.

4.   Distant Metastases

One of the major advantages of FDG-PET is the ability to use this method for whole-body staging. In the above-mentioned patient cohort (n = 75), we were able to identify in 15 patients (20%) bone (Fig. 4), in five lung (7%), and in two, liver metastases (Fig. 5), with an overall sensitivity of 100%, 83%, and 100%, respectively and an accuracy of 97%, 87%, and 90%, respectively (Table 2).

When these results were compared with CT/MRI (Table 3), significantly more lesions were found in the bone (confirmed by conventional bone scintigraphy) by FDG-PET (comparing only fields-of-view), whereas in the lung, no difference was observed. While the number of these tumor sites is small, more data are needed to confirm this trend. Nevertheless, our data indicate that in breast carcinoma a complete tumor staging seems to be possible with one investigation, allowing revelation of a significant number of lesions, which would have been missed by conventional imaging modalities. This has therapeutic relevance in many cases in the face of new drugs and aggressive treatment schemes.

B.   Review of Medical Literature

1.   Primary Breast Carcinoma

More than 450 patients suffering from breast carcinoma have been evaluated [2,11,52–71]. Data are summarized in Table 4.

In the first feasibility studies [55,57] patients with advanced primary and metastatic disease were included, which were readily apparent by other techniques. Nevertheless, the data demonstrated high sensitivities (100%) and specificities (100%) in tumors >3 cm and thus proved the potential of the technique also in breast cancer patients. Later studies with larger patient numbers were able

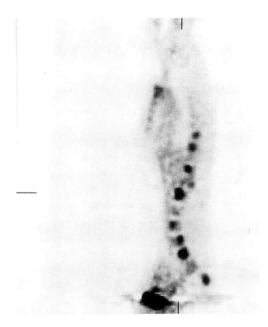

FIGURE 4   Case 4: Example of bone metastases in a 27-year-old woman with ductal breast carcinoma in the left breast, which had been removed 1 month prior to the PET study. Patient complained of pain in sternum and spine. Sagittal view through the spine with multiple lesions showing intense tracer uptake. Multifocal tracer uptake also in the sternum.

to confirm these first observations, with lower but still acceptable sensitivities (67% to 95%) and specificities (70% to 90%). Nevertheless, various investigators report a detection limit around 1 to 1.2 cm [51,59,61,71], with lesions <1 cm being often/always false-negative [51,62], noting a sharp decline of sensitivity as a function of tumor volume. Lesions <10–8 mm or in less aggressive tumors tend to have lower sensitivities [51,52,71]. To our understanding, it is not yet clear whether the detection of lesions <1 cm is due to physical detection limits or due to rather "normal" glucose utilization in small lesions. Glucose utilization might become more pathological only after further tumor progression; e.g., in larger tumor lesions more clones are being favored which are less oxygen-dependent and thus show higher anaerobic glycolysis.

Nevertheless, in a certain fraction of patients (10% to 40%), primary tumor sites could be identified which would have been missed with conventional imaging modalities [51,58,67,73], underscoring the potential of FDG-PET in the clinical setting and demanding an optimization of diagnostic algorithms.

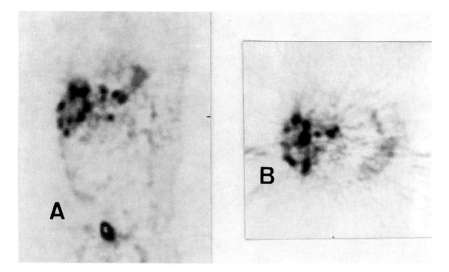

FIGURE 5   Case 5: Example of multiple liver metastases of an intraductal carcinoma. (A) Coronal and (B) transversal view through a representative liver area.

Introduction of semiquantitative methods (tumor-to-normal; tissue ratios, and/or SUV) seems to increase sensitivity and specificity [49,50,52].

2.   Benign Breast Lesions

One major diagnostic problem is the differentiation of benign lesions, especially in fibrocystic and radiodense breasts. While the primary focus of FDG-PET was the detection of malignant lesions, the experience in the differentiation of benign processes is comparatively small. Adler et al. [60] have described five benign cysts, which were visualized as rather photopenic areas. Fibroadenoma (n = 10) were usually true-negative [52,53,61,67]. Palmedo et al. [53] have observed one fibroadenoma which showed FDG and SESTAMIBI uptake. Fibrocystic changes (n = 11) did not show significant FDG uptake [52,53,67], with the exception of one case [52]. The same was true for inflammatory processes, with three of five being correctly identified [52,61,67].

Detection of breast cancer after augmentation mammoplasty is critical due to the radiodensity of a silicone implant, which can obscure tumor visualization. Wahl et al. [74] have reported two patient studies which accurately detected FDG uptake in suspicious lesions representing tumors <1.5 cm in the augmented breasts

TABLE 4   Clinical Studies on FDG-PET in the Assessment of Primary Breast Carcinoma

Source	Patient/ Lesion	Sensitivity (%)	Specificity (%)	Comment
Kubota et al. [55]	1/1	NA[a]	NA	
Wahl et al. [57]	1/3	NA	NA	
Wahl et al. [58]	10/12	100	100	all lesions > 3 cm
Tse et al. [59]	14/14	86	100	smallest lesion 7 × 10 mm
Wahl et al. [60]	11/NA	100		all lesions > 3 cm/therapy-monitoring
Adler et al. [61]	28/35	96	100	
Nieweg et al. [62]	11/11	91	NA	lesion < 1.2 cm missed
Hoh et al. [63]	15/17	88	NA	
Wahl et al. [74]	2/2	NA	NA	lesion detected (silicon implant)
Dehdashti et al. [67]	32/24	88	87/100	lesions 1–10 cm
Bruce et al. [66]	14/15	93	NA	
Holle et al. [52]	50/NA	67	82	(SPECT) all true-positive lesions > 2, 3 cm
Crowe et al. [65]	28/37	96	100	
Bassa et al. [70]	16/NA	75	100	therapy-monitoring
Scheidhauer et al. [68]	30/23	91	86	
Avril et al. [51]	71/95	74	98	false-negative lesions < 1 cm
Utech et al. [71]	124/NA	100	NA	all lesions > 1 cm
Chaiken et al. [64]	4/4	100	100	therapy-monitoring
Palmedo et al. [53]	9/9	89	83	all lesions palpable; no benefit to SESTAMIBI

[a]NA = Not available.

without displacement. This is in contrast to the need to perform adequate mammograms. We have studied three patients with augmented breasts by silicon implants and were able to confirm these results (unpublished data) (Fig. 6).

These preliminary data do not yet allow generalized conclusions. Further research is necessary to determine the ability to allow for distinction between carcinoma on one side and fibroadenoma, adenomas, or fibrocystic disease on the other side.

3.   Axillary Lymph Nodes

While detection of malignant breast lesions is very competitive due to multiple detection modalities, much emphasis has been put on detection of axillary lymph node involvement [29,52–54,57–59,61,62,65,68,71]. More than 300 patient stud-

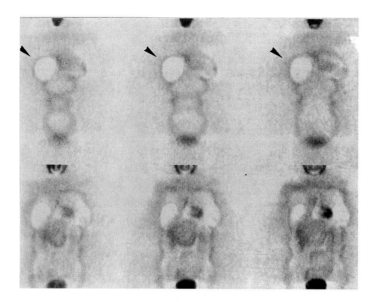

FIGURE 6   Case 6: Example of a follow-up study in a 50-year-old woman with a carcinoma in the right breast (1994) and silicon implant mammoplasty A series of coronal slices shows the lack of tracer uptake in the silicon implant (arrow) on the right side as compared to the normal left breast tissue, thus allowing a good differentiation in the case of tumor recurrence.

ies have been evaluated with sensitivities ranging from 73% to 100% and specificities from 93% to 100% (Table 5). Detection of small lesions has been assumed to be a major problem, but could so far not be substantiated by controlled studies. The overall experience, rather, indicates that far less than 5% of FGD-PET-negative studies are falsely negative. Due to the resolution of FDG-PET, the actual number of lesions is smaller as counted after surgery [29], which might limit its use concerning prognostic assessment. In addition, the rate of lymph node detection depends on the size of the primary tumor. Avril et al. [29] observed that in pT1 (<2 cm) breast carcinoma, axillary lymph node metastases consist usually of micrometastases, which are missed by PET (sensitivity 33%). In contrast, in primary tumors >2 cm, axillary lymph node involvement is detected with a sensitivity of 94%. This study was substantiated by Utech et al. [71], demonstrating a sensitivity of 100% in the detection of axillary lymph nodes, studying primary breast carcinoma >1 cm.

In this study, the primary drawback was a high rate of false-positive lymph

TABLE 5   Clinical Studies on FDG-PET in the Assessment of Axillary Lymph
Node Involvement

Source	Patient/ Lesion	Sensitivity (%)	Specificity (%)	Comment
Wahl et al. [57]	1/3	NA[a]	NA	
Wahl et al. [58]	4/NA	100	100	
Tse et al. [59]	14/7	57	100	
Adler et al. [61]	28/35	90	93	28 of 95 lymph nodes detected by PET
Nieweg et al. [62]	5/5	NA	NA	smallest lesion 8 mm
Crowe et al. [65]	20/10	90	100	
Holle et al. [52]	12/NA	75	NA	all false-negative lesions < 8 mm
Scheidhauer et al. [68]	18/18	100	89	
Avril et al. [29]	51/NA	73	33	false-negative lesions < 10 mm
Utech et al. [71]	124/64	100	69	20 of 64 lymph nodes false-positive
Palmedo et al. [53]	3/3	100	100	more lymph nodes detected by PET than MIBI
Bender et al. [54]	75/51	97	91	5 of 23 lymph nodes detected only by PET

[a]NA = Not available.

nodes (20 of 64; 31%) (Fig. 8). Overall, there was a high correlation between the number of individual abnormal nodes detected with FDG-PET and by axillary node dissection, underscoring the potential benefit of FDG-PET in selected patient groups. The data suggest that in this way a certain number of axillary lymph node dissections may be avoided.

4.   Distant Metastases

FDG-PET is increasingly used for whole-body or body truck scanning. Few studies have demonstrated the feasibility of the detection of lung, liver, lymph node, and bone metastases [54,56–58,67,68,75], underscoring the potential of FDG-PET for tumor staging (Table 6). Its clinical and therapeutic relevance has still to be established, but our data indicate that high-risk patients are often understaged by conventional staging.

5.   Monitoring of Therapy Response Versus Outcome Prediction

Current evaluation of therapy response relies on the qualitative or quantitative assessment of tumor size or volume. Since the majority of cells within a tumor mass are in a resting state, reduction of tumor volume requires time and might be

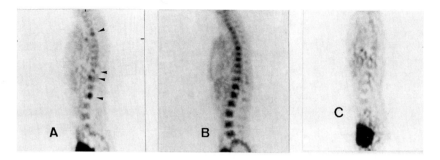

FIGURE 7   Case 7: Example of therapy monitoring in a 27-year-old woman with systemic spread of disease (lymph nodes, bone). Tumor vitality was assessed prior to (A), 7 days after (B), and 3 months after (C) high-dose chemotherapy. Prior to chemotherapy, tumors show intense uptake in multiple sites (A) of the spine (arrows). Seven days after the first treatment cycle, unspecific bone marrow activation masks the known tumor sites (B), but 3 months after completion of chemotherapy, no vital tumor lesions could be observed (C). Follow-up over 1 year suggests a complete remission of disease.

masked by unspecific effects—e.g., edema as a result of necrosis. In contrast, cellular FDG uptake is a function of cell vitality [43,45,76] and seems to be associated with the speed of cell turnover. Thus, it is conceivable that reduction of cell vitality as a result of therapeutic interventions (e.g., radiation, chemotherapy) could be monitored by FDG uptake. Few studies have substantiated this concept [60,64,66,70,75,78] assessing roughly 50 patients (Table 7). In general, signifi-

TABLE 6   Clinical Studies on FDG-PET in the Assessment of Distant Metastases in Breast Cancer

Source	Patient/lesion	Sensitivity (%)	Specificity (%)	Comment
Minn et al. [56]	17/NA[a]	88	NA	(planar imaging) lymph nodes, lung, liver, bone
Wahl et al. [57]	1/3	NA	NA	bone
Wahl et al. [58]	3/NA	100	100	bone, pleura
Dehdashti et al. [67]	19/45	89	100	metast. n=13; recurr. n=4
Jansson et al. [75]	16/NA	NA	NA	lymph nodes, liver, pleura
Bender et al. [54]	75/21	80	97	lymph nodes, bone, lung, liver
Scheidhauer et al. [68]	30/NA	NA	NA	lung, brain, bone, liver, soft tissue, adrenal gland

[a]NA = Not available.

TABLE 7   Clinical Studies on PET in the Assessment of Therapy Outcome in
Breast Carcinoma

Source	Patient/lesion	Sensitivity (%)	Specificity	Comment
Wahl et al. [60]	11/NA[a]	NA	NA	FDG uptake decreasing in responding lesions
Chaiken et al. [64]	4/4	NA	NA	FDG uptake only in recurrence
Huovinen et al. [78]	8/NA	NA	NA	^{11}C-methionine uptake decreasing in responding lesions
Bruce et al. [66]	14/15	93	NA	decrease in tumor-to-normal breast ratio
Jansson et al. [75]	16/NA	NA	NA	FDG uptake decreasing in responding lesions
Jansson et al. [75]	16/NA	NA	NA	^{11}C-methionine uptake decreasing in responding lesions
Bassa et al. [70]	16/NA	75	100	FDG uptake decreasing in responding lesions

[a]NA = Not available.

cant reduction of FDG uptake following therapeutic intervention as compared to
pretherapy values is most often associated with stable disease or tumor regression. Unchanged or enhanced FDG uptake indicates tumor progression. Wahl et
al. [60] observed continuously decreasing FDG accumulation as a function of
time (8 to 63 days after therapy) in responding tumors. Our own results in five
patients with systemic spread of breast carcinoma indicate that outcome prediction might be possible as early as 48 hours after the first chemotherapy application
(unpublished data). Decrease of FDG uptake by >35% (tumor-to-normal tissue

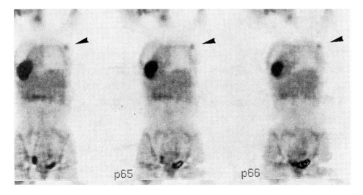

FIGURE 8   Case 8: Example of "unspecific" FDG uptake in the axillary region (arrow) due
to lymph node biopsy 7 days prior to the PET study. Histology confirmed no evidence of
cancer in the resected lymph nodes.

ratios) seems to be associated with tumor response, but final assessment is under way (Fig. 7).

Preliminary studies have also indicated that serial quantitative FDG imaging may permit assessment of tumor responsiveness during treatment [60,70], but more serial FDG studies are necessary to define the earliest time point that allows accurate outcome prediction and excludes regenerative processes (invasion of leukocytes), which could mask effective therapy response.

Noteworthy, ^{11}C-labeled methionine (physical half-life 20 min) has shown good uptake in primary breast cancer >3 cm [11,70,77] and soft-tissue metastases [78]. Uptake was correlated with number of cells in S phase (11). Sequential imaging prior to and posttherapy demonstrated decreasing accumulation in stable or regressing tumors, while enhanced uptake is associated with tumor progression [75,78].

6.   Assessment of Estrogen Receptors

Measurement of estrogen receptors (ER) status in vitro is a standard procedure allowing prediction of the response to hormonal therapy and the prognosis in patients. Imaging with ^{18}F-labeled progesterone yielded discouraging results with a sensitivity of 50% [50]. Later studies, employing ^{18}F-labeled estrogen analogs showed acceptable uptake in primary [2,67] and recurrent tumors [67] and in lymph node metastases [67,79] including approximately 50 patients. Specificity of estrogen uptake was proved by diminished accumulation under antiestrogen therapy [79].

Sensitivities of 93% have been reported (79), as well as good correlation of FES uptake and in vitro receptor status [2,67,79]. Interestingly, no correlation of ER uptake and FDG utilization has been observed [67]. Lately, several studies have focused on ^{18}F-labeled tamoxifen as tracer with promising results, at least in rats [80,81].

If further studies substantiate the potential of FES for determination of ER status in vivo, this technique could improve the assessment of the overall receptor status, thus allowing a kind of in vivo receptor staging. Currently receptor status is assumed to be the same in metastases and the primary tumor, while only the primary tumor is actually determined. This additional information may have a therapeutic impact solely by improved selection of patients who have a higher chance to profit from hormone therapy.

V. SUMMARY

Even though FDG-PET can be considered the most sensitive and accurate functional imaging modality currently available for detection of primary breast carcinoma, its unacceptably low sensitivity in lesions <1 cm limits its use for screening. Besides, due to high study costs (radionuclide and scanning units) as well as limited availability of PET scanners, and a relatively low patient through-put, it also lacks the "hardware" bases. Indications to perform FDG-PET in the case of primary tumors are (1) the need to provide additional (functional) information in lesions >1 cm complementary to conventional imaging modalities and as part of preoperative staging of high-risk patients; (2) in tumors >2 cm, the data indicate that FDG-PET is useful in providing functional information of the primary tumor in selected cases such as mammographic dense breasts, fibrocystic changes, and maybe in the staging of (axillary) lymph node involvement and exclusion of distant metastases. Identification of lymph node involvement might initiate neoadjuvant chemotherapy while negative results may avoid axillary lymph node dissection. The latter issue is still controversially discussed [82] and prospective, multicenter trials are needed to support this concept.

In recurrent disease, FDG-PET is mostly applicable in detection of lymph node involvement and verification/exclusion of distant metastases (bone, liver, brain, lung), but selection criteria of eligible patients, e.g., rising tumor markers, unexplained pain, have not been established.

The same is true for prediction of therapy outcome and monitoring of therapy success. While the concept has been established, demonstrating decreasing FDG accumulation in responding tumors in contrast to stable or increasing values in progressive lesions, more specific parameters—e.g., best time of scanning after therapy or most robust and easiest method of analyzing the lesions (SUV, tumor-to-normal tissue ratios)—have to be evaluated by prospective studies. This is even more pressing concerning new tracers such as ^{11}C-methionine and ^{18}F-estrogens, which have shown promising characteristics in preliminary studies.

On the other hand, FDG-SPECT using super-high-energy collimators or coincidence measurement seems to open up second-line screening and monitoring options. Nonetheless, while dedicated PET scanners lack sufficient spatial resolution, the group of eligible patients may be significantly smaller for this imaging modality. While FDG combines a series of preferable tracer characteristics, e.g., active accumulation and trapping mechanisms, the development of dedicated breast imaging cameras with higher spatial resolution is pressing and might solve some of the limitations encountered by using dedicated PET scanners. In addition, fusion of morphological and functional data is envisioned to boost sensitivity and specificity of the relevant imaging capabilities [83].

REFERENCES

1. Phelps ME, Mazziotta JC, Schelbert HR (eds.). Positron emission tomography and autoradiography. In: Principles and Applications for the Brain and Heart. New York: Raven, 1986.

2. Mintun MA, Welch MJ, Siegel BA; Mathias CJ, et al. Breast cancer: PET imaging of estrogen receptors. Radiology 169:45–48, 1988.

3. Kallinowski F, Schlenger KH, Runkel S, et al. Blood flow, metabolism, cellular microenvironment, and growth rate of human tumor xenografts. Cancer Res 49:3759–3764, 1989.

4. Kallinowski F, Schlenger KH, Kloes M, Stohrer M, Vaupel P. Tumor blood flow: the principle modulator of oxidative and glycolytic metabolism, and of the metabolic millieu of human tumor xenografts in vivo. Int J Cancer 44:266–272, 1989.

5. Cherry SR, Carnochan P, Babich JW, Serafini F, Rowell NP, Watson IA. Quantitative in vivo measurements of tumor perfusion using rubidium-81 and positron emission tomography. J Nucl Med 31:1307–1315, 1990.

6. Schelstraete K, Simons M, Deman J, et al. Uptake of ^{13}N-ammonia by human tumours as studied by positron emission tomography. Br J Radiol 55:797–804, 1982.

7. Wilson CB, Lammertsma AA, McKenzie CG, Sikora K, Jones T. Measurements of blood flow and exchanging water space in breast tumors using positron emission tomography: a rapid and noninvasive dynamic method. Cancer Res 52:1592–1597, 1992.

8. Beaney RP, Lammertsma AA, Jones T, McKenzie CG, Halnan KE. Positron emission tomography for in-vivo measurement of regional blood flow, oxygen utilisation, and blood volume in patients with breast carcinoma. Lancet 1:131–134, 1984.

9. Leenders KL. PET: blood flow and oxygen consumption in brain tumors. J Neurooncol 22:269–273, 1994.

10. Kim CG, Yang DJ, Kim EE, et al. Assessment of tumor cell proliferation using [^{18}F]fluorodeoxyadenosine and [^{18}F]fluoroethyluracil. J Pharm Sci 85:339–344, 1996.

11. Leskinen Kallio S, Nagren K, Lehikoinen P, Ruotsalainen U, Joensuu H. Uptake of ^{11}C-methionine in breast cancer studied by PET. An association with the size of S-phase fraction. Br J Cancer 64:1121–1124, 1991.

12. Leskinen Kallio S, Nagren K, Lehikoinen P, Ruotsalainen U, Teras M, Joensuu H. Carbon-11-methionine and PET is an effective method to image head and neck cancer. J Nucl Med 33:691–695, 1992.

13. D'Argy, Paul R, Frankenberg L. Comparative double tracer whole body autoradiography: uptake of ^{11}C, ^{18}F, and ^{3}H labeled compounds in rat tumors. Int J Rad Appl Ins B 15:577–585, 1988.

14. Warburg O. The Metabolism of Tumours. London: Constabel, 1930.

15. Warburg O. On the origin of cancer cells. Science 123:309–314, 1956.

16. Gallagher BM, JS Fowler, NI Gutterson. Metabolic trapping as a principle of radiopharmaceutical design: some factors responsible for the biodistribution of 2-deoxy-2-[^{18}F]fluoro-D-glucose. J Nucl Med 30:1154–1161, 1989.

17. Weber G. Enzymology of cancer cells. N Engl J Med 296:486–493, 1977.

18. Miyazaki M, Wahid S, Sato J. In vivo and in vitro test for growth potential of liver cells from rats during early stage of hepatocarcinogenesis by 3'-methyl-4-dimethylaminoazobenzene. J Cancer Res Clin Oncol 115:1–8, 1989.

19. Hacker HJ, Vollmer G, Chiquet Ehrismann R, Bannasch P, Liehr JG. Changes in the cellular phenotype and extracellular matrix during progression of estrogen-induced mesenchymal kidney tumors in Syrian hamsters. Virchows Arch B Cell Pathol Incl Mol Pathol 60:213–223, 1991.

20. Yang G, Dong Y, Du W, et al. Ultrastructural cytochemistry of human gastric cancer: electron microscopic observations of five organellae marker enzymes. Chin Med J Engl 108:859–863, 1995.

21. Haberkorn U, Strauss LG, Reisser CH. Glucose uptake, perfusion and cell proliferation in head and neck tumors: relation of positron emission tomography to flow cytometry. J Nucl Med 32:1548–1555, 1991.

22. Frost JJ. Receptor localization and quantification with PET. Radiology 169:273–24, 1988.

23. Smith Jones PM, Stolz B, Bruns C, et al. Gallium-67/gallium-68-[DFO]-octreotide— a potential radiopharmaceutical for PET imaging of somatostatin receptor-positive tumors: synthesis and radiolabeling in vitro and preliminary in vivo studies. J Nucl Med 35:317–325, 1994.

24. Hermann G, Janus CL, Schwarz IS, Kriviski S, Bier J, Rabinowitz G. Non-palpable breast lesions: accuracy of prebiopsy mammographic diagnosis. Radiology 65:323–326, 1987.

25. Gilles R, Guinebretiere JM, Lucidarme O, et al. Non-palpable breast tumors: Diagnosis with contrast-enhanced substraction dynamic MR imaging. Radiology 191:625–631, 1994.

26. Jackson VP. The role of ultrasound in breast imaging. Radiology 177:305–311, 1990.

27. Henderson IC, Harris JR, Kinne DW, Hellman S. Cancer of the breast. In: DeVita VT, Hellman S, Rosenberg SA, eds. Cancer. Principles and Practice of Oncology. Philadelphia: J. B. Lippincott, 1989.

28. Bastert G, Costa SD. Therapie des Mammakarzinoms. In: Zeller WJ, Zur Hausen H, eds. Onkologie. Grundlagen, Diagnostik, Therapie, Entwicklungen. Landsberg: Ecomed, 1995.

29. Avril N, Dose J, Janicke F, et al. Assessment of axillary lymph node involvement in breast cancer patients with positron emission tomography using radiolabeled 2-(fluorine-18)-fluoro-2-deoxy-D-glucose. J Natl Cancer Inst 88:1204–1209, 1996.

30. Moore MP, Kinne DW. Is axillary lymph node dissection necessary in the routine management of breast cancer? Yes. Important Adv Oncol 19:245–250, 1996.

31. Thomas DG, Duthie NL. Use of 2-deoxy-D-glucose to test for the completeness of surgical vagotomy. Gut 9:125–128, 1968.

32. Gallagher BM, Fowler JS, Gutterson NI, MacGregor RR, Wan CN, Wolf AP. Metabolic trapping as a principle of radiopharmaceutical design: some factors responsible for the biodistribution of 2-deoxy-2-[^{18}F]fluoro-D-glucose. J Nucl Med 19:1154–1161, 1978.

33. Minn H, Leskinen Kallio S, Lindholm P, et al. [^{18}F]fluorodeoxyglucose uptake in tumors: kinetic vs. steady-state methods with reference to plasma insulin. J Comput Assist Tomogr 17:115–123, 1993.

34. Lindholm P, Minn H, Leskinen Kallio S, Bergmann J, Ruotsalainen, Joensuu H. Influence of the blood glucose concentration on FDG uptake in cancer—a PET study. J Nucl Med 34:1–6, 1993.

35. Gallagher BM, Ansari A, Atkins H, et al. ^{18}F-labeled 2-deoxy-2-fluoro-D-glucose as a radiopharmaceutical for measuring regional myocardial glucose metabolism in vivo: tissue distribution and imaging studies in animals. J Nucl Med 18:990–996, 1977.

36. Woosley RL, Kim YS, Huang KC. Renal tubular transport of 2-deoxy-D-glucose in dogs and rats. Pharmocol Exp Ther 173:13–20, 1970.
37. Dowd MT, Chin Tu C, Wendel MJ, Faulhaber PJ, Cooper MD. Radiation dose to the bladder wall from 2-[18F]-fluoro-2-deoxy-D-glucose in adult humans. J Nucl Med 32:707–712, 1991.
38. Mejia AA, Nakamura T, Mastoshi I, Hatazawa J, Masaki M, Shoichi W. Estimation of absorbed doses in humans due to intravenous administration of fluorine-18F-fluorodeoxyglucose in PET studies. J Nucl Med 32:699–706, 1991.
39. Meyer GJ, Waters SL, Coenen HH, Luxen A, Maziere B, Langstrom B. PET radiopharmaceuticals in Europe: current use and data relevant for the formulation of summaries of product characteristics (SPCs). Eur J Nucl Med 22:1420–1432, 1995.
40. Hamacher K, Coenen HH, Stoecklin G. Efficient stereospecific synthesis of no-carrier-added 2-[18F]fluoro-D-glucose. J Nucl Med 27:235–238, 1986.
41. Wahl RL, Hutchins GD, Buchsbaum DJ, Liebert M, Grossmann HB, Fisher S. 18F-2-deoxy-2-fluoro-D-glucose uptake into human tumor xenografts. Cancer 67:1544–1550, 1991.
42. Minn H, Clavo AC, Wahl RL. In vitro comparison of cell proliferation kinetics and uptake of tritiated 2-fluoro-2-deoxy-D-glucose and L-methionine in squamous cell carcinoma of the head and neck. J Nucl Med 36:252–253, 1995.
43. Brown RS, Leung JY, Fisher SJ, Frey KA, Ethier SP, Wahl RL. Intratumoral distribution of tritiated fluoro-deoxyglucose in breast carcinoma. I. Are inflammatory cells important. J Nucl Med 36:1854–1861, 1995.
44. Higashi K, Clavo AC, Wahl RL. Does FDG uptake measure proliferative activity of human cancer cells? In vitro comparison with DNA flow cytometry and tritiated thymidine uptake. J Nucl Med 34:414–419, 1993.
45. Zincke M, Avril N, Dose J, et al. PET imaging of breast cancer: comparison between FDG uptake vs. histology and expression of the glucose transporter protein GLUT-1. J Nucl Med 38:250A, 1997.
46. Brown RS, Wahl RL. Overexpression of Glut-1 glucose transporter in human breast cancer. An immunohistochemical study. Cancer 72:2979–2985, 1993.
47. Wahl RL, Henry CA, Ethier SP. Serum glucose: effect on tumor and normal tissue accumulation of 2-[F-18]-fluoro-2-deoxy-D-glucose in rodents with mammary carcinoma. Radiology 183:643–647, 1992.
48. Wahl RL, Kaminski MS, Ethier SP, Hutchins GD. The potential of 2-deoxy-2-[18F]fluoro-D-glucose (FDG) for the detection of tumor involvement in lymph nodes. J Nucl Med 31:1831–1835, 1990.
49. Yasuda S, Ide M, Tagaki S, et al. Cancer detection with whole-body FDG-PET images without attenuation correction. Kaku Igaku 33:367–373, 1996.
50. Dehdashti F, McGuire AH, Van Brocklin HF, et al. Assessment of 21-[18F]fluoro-16 alpha-ethyl-19-norprogesterone as a positron-emitting radiopharmaceutical for the detection of progestin receptors in human breast carcinomas. J Nucl Med 32:1532–1537, 1991.
51. Avril N, Dose J, Janicke F, et al. Metabolic characterization of breast tumors with positron emission tomography using F-18 fluorodeoxyglucose. J Clin Oncol 14:1848–1857, 1996.

52. Holle LH, Trampert L, Lung Kurt S, et al. Investigations of breast tumors with fluorine-18-fluorodeoxyglucose and SPECT. J Nucl Med 37:615–622, 1996.
53. Palmedo H, Bender H, Grünwald F, et al. Comparison of fluorine-18 fluorodeoxyglucose positron emission tomography and technetium-99m methoxyisobutylisonitrile scintimammography in the detection of breast tumors. Eur J Nucl Med 24:1138–1145, 1997.
54. Bender H, Kirst J, Palmedo H, et al. Value of ^{18}F-fluoro-deoxyglucose positron emission tomography in the staging of recurrent breast carcinoma. Anticancer Res 17:1687–1692, 1997.
55. Kubota K, Matsuzawa T, Amemiya A, et al. Imaging of breast cancer with [^{18}F]fluorodeoxyglucose and positron emission tomography. J Comput Assist Tomogr 13:1097–1098, 1989.
56. Minn H, Soini I. [^{18}F]fluorodeoxyglucose scintigraphy in diagnosis and follow up of treatment in advanced breast cancer. Eur J Nucl Med 15:61–66, 1989.
57. Wahl RL, Cody R, Hutchins G, Mudgett E. Positron-emission tomographic scanning of primary and metastatic breast carcinoma with the radiolabeled glucose analogue 2-deoxy-2-[^{18}F]fluoro-D-glucose [letter]. N Engl J Med 324:200, 1991.
58. Wahl RL, Cody RL, Hutchins GD, Mudgett EE. Primary and metastatic breast carcinoma: initial clinical evaluation with PET with the radiolabeled glucose analogue 2-[F-18]-fluoro-2-deoxy-D-glucose. Radiology 179:765–770, 1991.
59. Tse NY, Hoh CK, Hawkins RA, et al. The application of positron emission tomographic imaging with fluorodeoxyglucose to the evaluation of breast disease. Ann Surg 216:27–34, 1992.
60. Wahl RL, Zasadny K, Helvie M, Hutchins GD, Weber B, Cody R. Metabolic monitoring of breast cancer chemohormonotherapy using positron emission tomography: initial evaluation. J Clin Oncol 11:2101–2111, 1993.
61. Adler LP, Crowe JP, al Kaisi NK, Sunshine JL. Evaluation of breast masses and axillary lymph nodes with [F-18] 2-deoxy-2-fluoro-D-glucose PET. Radiology 187:743–750, 1993.
62. Nieweg OE, Kim EE, Wong WH, et al. Positron emission tomography with fluorine-18-deoxyglucose in the detection and staging of breast cancer. Cancer 71:3920–3925, 1993.
63. Hoh CK, Hawkins RA, Glaspy JA, et al. Cancer detection with whole-body PET using 2-[^{18}F]fluoro-2-deoxy-D-glucose. J Comput Assist Tomogr 17:582–589, 1993.
64. Chaiken L, Rege S, Hoh C, et al. Positron emission tomography with fluorodeoxyglucose to evaluate tumor response and control after radiation therapy. Int J Radiat Oncol Biol Phys 27:455–464, 1993.
65. Crowe JP Jr, Adler LP, Shenk RR, Sunshine J. Positron emission tomography and breast masses: comparison with clinical, mammographic, and pathological findings. Ann Surg Oncol 1:132–140, 1994.
66. Bruce DM, Evans NT, Heys SD, et al. Positron emission tomography: 2-deoxy-2-[^{18}F]-fluoro-D-glucose uptake in locally advanced breast cancers. Eur J Surg Oncol 21:280–283, 1995.
67. Dehdashti F, Mortimer JE, Siegel BA, et al. Positron tomographic assessment of estrogen receptors in breast cancer: comparison with FDG-PET and in vitro receptor assays. J Nucl Med 36:1766–1774, 1995.

68. Scheidhauer K, Scharl A, Pietrzyk U, et al. Qualitative [^{18}F] FDG positron emission tomography in primary breast cancer: clinical relevance and practicability. Eur J Nucl Med 23:618–623, 1996.

69. Yasuda S, Ide M, Takagi S, et al. [Cancer detection with whole-body FDG PET images without attenuation correction.] Kaku Igaku 33:367–373, 1996.

70. Bassa P, Kim EE, Inoue T, et al. Evaluation of preoperative chemotherapy using PET with fluorine-18-fluorodeoxyglucose in breast cancer. J Nucl Med 37:931–938, 1996.

71. Utech CI, Young CS, Winter PF. Prospective evaluation of fluorine-18 fluorodeoxyclucose positron emission tomography in breast cancer for staging of the axilla related to surgery and immunocytochemistry. Eur J Nucl Med 23:1588–1593, 1996.

72. Jacobs M, Mantil J, Peterson C, et al. FDG-PET in breast cancer. J Nucl Med 35:142P, 1995.

73. Inoue T, Kim EE, Wong FC, et al. Comparison of fluorine-18-fluorodeoxyglucose and carbon-11-methionine PET in detection of malignant tumors. J Nucl Med 37:1472–1476, 1996.

74. Wahl RL, Helvie MA, Chang AE, Andersson I. Detection of breast cancer in women after augmentation mammoplasty using fluorine-18-fluorodeoxyglucose-PET. J Nucl Med 35:872–875, 1994.

75. Jansson T, Westlin JE, Ahlstrom H, Lilja A, Langstrom B, Bergh J. Positron emission tomography studies in patients with locally advanced and/or metastatic breast cancer: a method for early therapy evaluation? J Clin Oncol 13:1470–1477, 1995.

76. Brown RS, Leung JY, Fisher SJ, Frey KA, Ethier SP, Wahl RL. Intratumoral distribution of tritiated-FDG in breast carcinoma: correlation between Glut-1 expression and FDG uptake. J Nucl Med 37:1042–1047, 1996.

77. Leskinen Kallio S, Huovinen R, Nagren K, et al. [^{11}C]methionine quantitation in cancer PET studies. J Comput Assist Tomogr 16:468–474, 1992.

78. Huovinen R, Leskinen Kallio S, Nagren K, Lehikoinen P, Ruotsalainen U, Teras M. Carbon-11-methionine and PET in evaluation of treatment response of breast cancer. Br J Cancer 67:787–791, 1993.

79. McGuire AH, Dehdashti F, Siegel BA, et al. Positron tomographic assessment of 16 alpha-[^{18}F]fluoro-17 beta-estradiol uptake in metastatic breast carcinoma. J Nucl Med 32:1526–1531, 1991.

80. Yang D, Kuang LR, Cherif A, et al. Synthesis of [^{18}F]fluoroalanine and [^{18}F]fluorotamoxifen for imaging breast tumors. J Drug Target 1:259–267, 1993.

81. Yang DJ, Li C, Kuang LR, et al. Imaging, biodistribution and therapy potential of halogenated tamoxifen analogues. Life Sci 55:53–67, 1994.

82. Avril N. Nuklearmedizinische Diagnostik des Mammakarzinoms. Nuklearmediziner 19:251–258, 1996.

83. Weinberg I, Majewski S, Weisenberger A, et al. Preliminary results for positron emission mammography: real-time functional breast imaging in a conventional mammography gantry. Eur J Nucl Med 23:804–806, 1996.

REVIEWS

1. Bakir MA, Eccles S, Babich JW, et al. c-erbB2 protein overexpression in breast cancer as a target for PET using iodine-124-labeled monoclonal antibodies. J Nucl Med 33:2154–2160, 1992.

2. Hawkins RA, Hoh C, Glaspy J, Rege S, Choi Y, Phelps ME. Positron emission tomography scanning in cancer. Cancer Invest 12:74–87, 1994.
3. Adler DD, Wahl RL. New methods for imaging the breast: techniques, findings, and potential. AJR 164:19–30, 1995.
4. Beaney RP. Positron emission tomography in the study of human tumors. Semin Nucl Med 14:324–341, 1984.
5. Budinger TF, Brennan KM, Moses WW, Derenzo SE. Advances in positron tomography for oncology. Nucl Med Biol 23:659–667, 1996.
6. Cook GJ, Maisey MN. The current status of clinical PET imaging. Clin Radiol 51:603–613, 1996.
7. De Landsheere C, Lamotte D. [Methods and clinical applications of positron emission tomography in endocrinology.] Ann Endocrinol Paris 51:148–154, 1990.
8. Glaspy JA, Hawkins R, Hoh CK, Phelps ME. Use of positron emission tomography in oncology. Oncology Huntingt 7:41–46, 1993.
9. Khalkhali I, Mena I, Diggles L. View of imaging techniques for the diagnosis of breast cancer: a new role of prone scintimammography using technetium-99m sestamibi [see comments]. Eur J Nucl Med 21:357–362, 1994.
10. Kubota K. [Diagnosis of early cancer with positron emission tomography.] Nippon Rinsho 54:1263–1267, 1996.
11. Kubota K. [Cancer diagnosis with positron emission tomography (PET).] Kaku Igaku 33:207–212, 1996.
12. Lagrange JL, Maublant J, Darcourt J. [Positron-emission tomography: role of ^{18}F-fluorodeoxyglucose (^{18}FDG) imaging in oncology.] Bull Cancer Paris 82:611–622, 1995.
13. Strauss LG, Conti PS. The applications of PET in clinical oncology. J Nucl Med 32:623–648, 1991.
14. von Gumppenberg RM, Strauss LG. [Clinical indications for PET in oncology.] Schweiz Rundsch Med Prax 82:919–923, 1993.
15. Wahl RL. Nuclear medicine techniques in breast imaging. Semin Ultrasound CT MR 17:494–505, 1996.
16. Dose J, Avril N, Graeff H, Jänicke F. Positron emission tomography for diagnosis of breast tumors. Onkolgie 20:190–195, 1997.

5

Breast Imaging with Radiolabeled Antibodies

Lamk M. Lamki
*University of Texas Medical School and Hermann Hospital at Houston,
Houston, Texas*

Bruce J. Barron
University of Texas Medical School, Houston, Texas

I. INTRODUCTION

To date, there is not a radiolabeled antibody that is FDA approved and commercially available in the U.S. for specific imaging of breast cancer. There are, however, a few radiolabeled monoclonal antibodies which are commercially available in the U.S. as they are FDA approved for imaging of other cancers and are, incidentally, also useful in breast cancer imaging. They are therefore clinically used by many nuclear physicians diagnostically. Research into breast cancer imaging with monoclonal antibodies has been going on for several years and, in some respect, earlier than radioimmunoscintigraphy of other organs. For various reasons, breast imaging with monoclonal antibodies has not found its niche in clinical practice. Some very useful monoclonal antibodies to breast cancer have been discovered and tested clinically—both murine antibodies and bioengineered antibodies, though none has been fully accepted with a definite clinical role in patient management. Some do have a focused clinical part to play, and that will be discussed in this chapter. These antibodies are directed against various antigens found in breast cancer, specific and nonspecific. There are also some polyclonal antibodies which react with breast cancer and have been used for imaging purposes [1–3] but are rarely used today.

A. Historical Background

The use of labeled antitumor antibodies for the detection of human cancer began with the attempts of David Pressman in 1949 [4,5]. The first antitumor antibodies he used were able to localize a mouse osteogenic sarcoma [5].

There were several other workers involved in polyclonal imaging of tumors between then and the mid-1970s when monoclonal antibody imaging came to being. The history of monoclonal antibody imaging goes back to the discovery of monoclonal antibodies by Kohler and Milstein [6]. These workers describe production of monoclonal antibodies (Mab) from hybrid cells made of mouse spleen cells and myeloma cells. The hybrid cells can be cultured in vitro in test tubes or they can be grown in peritoneal cavities of mice as hybridomas. Highly specific monoclonal antibodies can now be produced from various types of hybridomas on commercial basis. In the late 1970s and early 1980s, nuclear medicine and oncology researchers started radiolabeling the newly discovered monoclonal antibodies for the purposes of imaging various cancers, including breast cancer. Thus, radioimmunoscintigraphy came of age, and the initial results were exciting [7–20] because they were better than earlier results with polyclonal antibodies. While there may still be a specific role for polyclonal antibodies, this is very limited and the future lies with the monoclonal antibodies, both for diagnosis and for therapy. Early Mab studies in oncology concentrated on colon cancer [21–27], melanoma [28–33,29], ovaries [14,34,35], prostate, but less so on the breast. It was not until the late 1980s and early 1990s that work on breast cancer got on the way [36–42]. This started with efforts on breast-specific antibodies, but this changed as it became clear that anti-CEA Mabs react with breast cancer. The improvement in labeling techniques and the success in Tc-99m labeling, in particular, opened new doors for breast cancer immunoscintigraphy.

B. Rationale for Clinical Use

To develop monoclonal antibodies to breast cancer, workers had to find antigens that are more common in breast cancer than in normal breast tissue. In addition, those antigens have to be of low density in benign breast tumors and inflammatory tissues. So far, the winning antigen has been CEA [43]. Most breast cancers produce CEA (even though the serum levels of CEA may not reflect this). Another winner is the ubiquitous TAG-72, in addition to some other antigens, which include mucin and epithelial antigens, milk fat globule membranes, cell surface receptors, oncogene products, cytokeratin, or epidermal growth factors [35,44–62]. The development of Mabs to these antigen has allowed workers to identify multiple target epitopes of certain tumor-associated antigens such as CEA. Thus, several different Mabs can be identified with the same antigen but directed to different epitopes, and they display different characteristics [63,64]. A list of antibodies used for breast cancer detection is presented in Table 1.

II. RADIOPHARMACEUTICALS

A. Radionuclides and Radiolabeling

1. Radioiodine: I-131 and I-123

One of the earliest radionuclides used for labeling monoclonal antibodies is radioiodine (I-131). Prior to the advent of monoclonal antibodies, I-131 was used

TABLE I   Antibodies and Antigens Used for Breast Immunoscintigraph

Antibody	Antigen	Isotope	Comments
Bw431/26	CEA	Tc-99m	Intact Fab (Lind Kareimo)
CYT-380	CEA	Tc-9m	Fragment (Nabi HA, Rosner D)
BC2C114	CEA	Tc-99m	Intact IgG (Duran JC)
Arcitumomab	CEA	Tc-99m	Fragment (Goldenberg; Barron, Abstracts, Nabi, Tumor Targeting)
ZCE-25	CEA	In-111	Intact igG (Patt; Haseman)
ZCE-25	CEA	In-111	Fragment (Lamki)
MN-14	CEA	I-131	IgG Intact fragment (treatment)
IORCEA1	CEA	Tc-99m	IgG Intact (Duran)
NP-2	CEA	In-131	Polyclonal Goat (Deland)
B72.3	TAG 72	In-111	Intact IgG (Lamki, Thor)
155HF	TAG	In-111	Longenecker, Springer, MacLean, McEwan
170H.82	Thomsen	In-111, Tc-99m	Intact IgG (Longenecker, Springer, MacLean, McEwan
	Friedenreich Ag (TAG)		(aka Thomsen Friedenreich Ag)
B6.2	TAG-72	I-125	Intact IgG (Stephens, Thor, Nieroda)
12H12	Mucin glycoprotein TAG-12	Tc-99m, I-125, I-131	Intact IgG (Brummerdorf)
BM-2	Mucin glycoprotein TAG-12	Tc-9m	Fragment (Brumgrardorf 1994)
Anti-HMFG1	Mucin/epithelial	I-123	Intact IgG to human milk fat globule (breast epithelial) (Taylor-Papadimitriou, Burchell, Major, Arklie, Rosner)
Anti-HMFG1	Mucin/epithelial	In-111	Fragment (Kalofonos)
Anti-HMFG2	Mucin/epithelial	I-123	Fragment (Espenetos))
MA5	Mucin/epithelial	In-111	Intact IgG (Major)
SM3	Ca-15-3	Tc-99m	Fragment (Granowski)
BM-7	Mucin	Tc-99m	Intact IgG (Brummendorf)
BrE-3 (HMFG1)	Mucin, BEM	In-111	Breast epithelial mucin (Kramer) intact IgG
3C6F9	37-kD surface Ag	I-123	IgG2a ILS (Mandeville)
RCC-1	Membrane/cytoplasm	I-131	Intact IgG (Tjandra)
Anti-c-erb B-2	p-185	Tc	Ag is a gene product of proto-oncogene P-185 (Allan, Mangili)
3E1.2	Membrane/cytoplasm	I-131	IgM (Tsandra 1988)
34BE12	Keratins 1.5.10 and 14		(Josh, Lee) No Imaging
4D5	P185		(De Santes) HER-2/nu oncogene No imaging
7c2	P185 HER-2/neu oncogene		Fragment (Kennedy) No imaging

TABLE I   (Continued)

Antibody	Antigen	Isotope	Comments
16.88 (Human)	CTA 16.88 Keratin	In-111 Tc-99m	Intact IgM (lymphoscintigraphy) (Pecking) Some antibodies 88 BV 59
EBA-1	Nonspecific	In-111	Fragment-AG not specified F(ab')$_2$
BW250/183	Granulocyte/myelo-cyte	Tc-99m	For bone marrow, fragment (Korpii)

to label polyclonal antibodies for imaging cancer [1]. With the introduction of monoclonal antibodies, researchers continued using I-131 for diagnostic purposes. Soon, however, the use of radioiodine-131 was found to have several disadvantages, including the lack of ideal physical characteristics for imaging with modern gamma cameras. The high energy of the gamma emission at 364 keV is beyond the useful range of modern gamma cameras and results in degradation of image quality. Also, the presence of beta emissions and the long physical half-life (8.05 days) of I-131 tend to result in high radiation exposure to the patient, unless we limit the administered diagnostic dose, for example, to <5 mCi. In addition, it is difficult to block radioiodine uptake by the thyroid gland and the stomach completely, despite the concurrent use of Lugol's iodine solution or potassium perchlorate. The poor-quality images, high background activity, and high radiation exposure to the patient are compounded by yet another problem of endogenous dehalogenation, which results in the removal of the radioiodine label from the monoclonal antibodies. This further raises the high background activity and lowers target uptake [14,21]. Radioiodine-131, however, does have an advantage of relatively low liver uptake, resulting in less liver background interference when imaging the breast. Another advantage is the technical ease of radiolabeling proteins with iodine as there are several choices of iodination available, e.g., chloramine T, iodogen, and lactoperoxidase. The iodogen method, particularly, is easy to perform and results in very high specific activity and labeling yield of typically <90%. I-131 is still used to label Mab for purposes of therapy [7,65,66].

Another radiolabel that was historically used to overcome the problems associated with I-131 was iodine-123 (I-123), which is in many ways better than the 131 isotope, but they share many of the disadvantages, such as dehalogenation. The physical half-life of I-123 is shorter at 13.3 hours versus 8.05 days of I-131, and thus results in lower radiation exposure to the patient. Also, I-123 emits negligible amount of β-emission, thus resulting in patient radiation dosimetry lower than that of I-131. We can therefore use a larger dose and get better images. The high cost of I-123, limited availability to many nuclear medicine laboratories, and the above-mentioned disadvantages common to all iodine isotopes has forced those involved in radiolabeling Mabs to look into alternative radioisotopes.

2. Indium-111

The next radionuclide that was used to label monoclonal antibody is indium-111 (In-111) which was used extensively to label intact monoclonal antibodies in the 1980s with good results [8–10,12,21,23,25,26,36]. However, In-111 has a high liver uptake which often interferes with the imaging of metastatic liver disease and possibly the primary tumor, too. To some extent, this limits its use [67,68]. There is also a distinct possibility that In-111 may get detached from the antibody and interfere with the metastatic disease localization because of the resultant high background activity. Besides the unwanted localization in normal organs like liver, spleen, bowel, and bone marrow, there is a problem of nonspecific localization in other diseases and other nontarget areas [21]. In-111 in some ways behaves like gallium-67 and may localize nonspecifically in tumors. This reduces the specificity of the monoclonal antibody imaging. We have previously found that In-111-labeled antibodies localize in sites of infections, such as pneumonia, also in arthritic degenerative disease of lumbar spine [21], as well as in old bone fractures or other nonspecific localization as observed when we studied breast cancer using In-111-labeled antibodies [8,23,36]. Variation in radiolabeling techniques did change the biodistribution, but to a limited extent only. Bifunctional DTPA was the most popular technique for labeling Mabs with In-111 [11]; then came the GYK-DTPA modification [36]. In vivo labeling, as well as modification of the In-111 antibody complex by use of biotin and avidin and double antibodies methods, never became successful enough to be accepted by the nuclear oncologists.

3. Technetium-99m

The most successful radiolabel for diagnostic radioimmunoscintigraphy so far has been technetium-99m. It can overcome several of the problems related to radioimmunoimaging with In-111 and I-131/I-123 [21,69–74]. European workers have used Tc-99m earlier than their American counterparts. One of the early problems with the use of Tc-99m for immunoscintigraphy has been related to the technique of radiolabeling. This is now fairly well mastered by several workers in both the U.S. and Europe [43–75]. Besides the problem of radiolabeling, Tc-99m also has a potential disadvantage of free Tc-99m activity detached from the antibody-Tc-99m complex or Tc-99m bound to subfragments from the metabolism of the Fab or Fab' fragments. These are relatively minor disadvantages compared to the several advantages associated with the use of Tc-99m. Tc-99m has almost ideal gamma emission energy at 140 keV, which is well suited for modern gamma camera imaging both planar and SPECT imaging. Also, the physical half-life ($T_{1/2}$ of 6 hours) is nearly ideal for imaging radiolabeled fragments of monoclonal antibodies, since the physical $T_{1/2}$ of Tc-99m matches the biological $T_{1/2}$ of Mab fragments. The short half-life lack of beta and other particulate emissions results in very low radiation exposure to the patient. This permits us to administer a generous diagnostic dosage (20 to 30 mCi) with the accompanying advantages in image quality. This favorable radiation dosimetry together with the excellent physical properties has led to the popularity of Tc-99m label, despite the initial hurdles in radiolabeling experienced by workers on both sides of the Atlantic. Tc-99m-labeled monoclonal antibodies are now available in kit form that can be readily radiolabeled with Tc-99m for instant use. Besides the advantages of Tc-99m related to its near ideal physical properties, it is also readily available in every nuclear medicine department from a molybdenum-Tc-99m generator at a low cost, making it particularly attractive.

The radiolabeling technique for Tc-99m has a long history dating back to the chelate method and the N_2S_2 methods in the 1980s, followed by direct conjugation methods in the early 1990s [69,76]. The advantage of the direct conjugation method is that it is rapid, is stable, and requires no postlabeling purification [11,74]. Variations of the direct conjugation method are the current standard of practice.

B. Antibodies and Antigens

1. Monoclonal Versus Polyclonal

Polyclonal antibodies have been used much earlier than monoclonal, but unfortunately, they have a problem of diminished specificity and higher incidence of hypersensitivity reaction to the antibody injections. When radiolabeled polyconal antibodies are used in imaging, they may go to sites of inflammation or infection, as well as a variety of nontargeted tumors and normal tissue. The advent of hybridoma technology enabled the production of the more specific monoclonal antibodies. However, monoclonal antibodies may also crossreact with antigens shared by other tumors, though less commonly than polyclonal. Compared to polyclonal, Mabs have a lower incidence of hypersensitivity reactions and HAMA production. Further advances in immunology have enabled the production of human or humanized Mab fragments and subfragments, which have practically eliminated these reactions.

2. Intact IgG Versus Fragments and Subfragments

Initial work with immunoscintigraphy was based on intact antibodies (usually IgG and rarely IgM), which were labeled with indium-111 or iodine-131. However, with the development of Tc-99m labeling techniques, it became more attractive to explore the use of fragments of the IgG Mab. The biological half-life of the whole IgG matched that of the I-131 and In-111 radiolabels, but, with the shorter $T_{1/2}$ of technetium-99m, we were able to better match the shorter biological half-life of the fragments of IgG (Fig. 1). The whole IgG antibody can be enzymatically digested in vitro to produce Fab, Fab', or F(ab')₂ fragments. The use of fragments as opposed to the intact antibody is now universally accepted as a better choice at least for diagnostic purposes [75,77–79]. Among other disadvantages of the intact antibodies are that they are more immunogenic with a resultant high incidence of human antimouse antibodies (HAMA) [80]. The Fc fragment can be removed from the IgG (either by pepsin or papain action) (Fig. 1) to result in Fab,

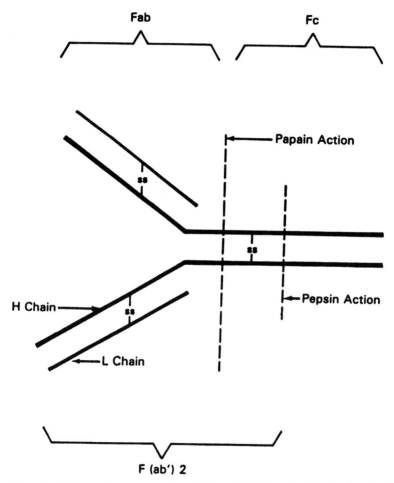

FIGURE 1   Diagnostic representation of the intact IgG molecule showing that it can be digested enzymatically by papain to result in three parts of about 50,000 daltons each (two Fab and one Fc fragment); or by pepsin to produce F(ab')₂ and Fc fragments. From Ref. 21.

Fab', or (Fab')$_2$ fragments, or the fragments can be genetically engineered. In either case, the absence of the Fc portion in these fragments reduces significantly the immunogenicity of the Mab used. This is a major step in immunoscintigraphy from the clinical point of view. The incidence of HAMA is significantly lower with the use of fragments than intact IgG. There are several other advantages to fragments, including shorter imaging periods, lower background activity, and therefore easier-to-identify lesions. Body distribution of fragments is also different from the intact IgG.

Because intact antibody is a protein, it is more likely to be localized and metabolized in the liver, thus resulting in interference of imaging. This makes fragments and subfragments more desirable, especially when one is looking for liver metastases. Also the long half-life of the whole IgG antibody makes it a poor match for Tc-99m and better suited for labeling with less ideal isotope, e.g., In-111 or I-131. On the other hand, the fragments are cleared from the bloodstream more rapidly, resulting in low background imaging. They also have greater penetrating capacity than the intact IgG [81]. Thus there are several advantages of using fragments or subfragments over the whole IgG antibody. There are differences between the fragments themselves; Fab or Fab' are monovalent, while (Fab')$_2$ is divalent, having double the capacity to bind antigen. However, the sensitivity of (Fab')$_2$ is not significantly better than Fab or Fab'.

The next consideration in the choice of an antibody is the avidity and the affinity of the antibody. The attraction and the strength between the antibody and the antigen and the bond with the radiolabel may determine the success of immunoscintigraphy. The significance of avidity and affinity in imaging results has not been fully realized clinically. However, in theory and in in vitro experiments, these two factors do matter in the outcome of immunoscintigraphy. Another important consideration is the labeling efficiency and bonding between the isotope and the antibody both in vitro after labeling procedure and in vivo after intravenous injection. The impact of dehalogenation of iodinated antibodies after injection has already been discussed. This occurs in vivo independent of labeling efficiency, and contributes to high background activity and poor images. Detailed discussion of these and other factors related to labeling and antibody properties that can affect biodistribution are beyond the scope of this chapter. Likewise, strep-avidin and biotin have been used by several workers to improve labeling and targeting, but discussion of that has to be deferred to specialized texts.

Bioengineering can produce a variety of murine Mabs, chimeric or humanized antibodies which are part human and part mouse. Likewise, bioengineering can produce hyperhumanized antibody by making it predominantly human with only minimal mouse component in the antigen-binding end of the Fab fragment. The future of immunoscintigraphy lies in genetic engineering of these antibodies and biosynthesis of the fragments, subfragments, single chains, and peptides for imaging [82]. Peptides are discussed elsewhere in this book. At this stage there has not been a major clinical trial of the humanized fragments or single chains for

breast imaging to be certain on the precise role of that technique in patient management, present or future.

C. Dosimetry and Quality Control

With the increasing use of fragments versus intact IgG the use of iodine-131 and
indium-111 has significantly fallen, while that of Tc-99m has risen, making radiation exposure less of a major consideration in immunoscintigraphy. The dose estimate results (effective dose equivalent and organ dosimetry data) of Tc-99m anti-
CEA fragment (Arcitumomab) and of In-111 anti-TAG intact IgG (Satumomab) as
example of the two extremes are summarized in Table 2. Absorbed doses are given
in rads/20 mCi (mGy/740 MBq) for the Tc-99m-labeled fragment example and
rads/5 mCi (mGy/185MBq) for the In-111-labeled intact IgG example. The kidneys are the critical organ with Tc-99m labeled Fab and Fab' fragments, since these
fragments are primarily excreted in the kidneys. In contrast, the intact IgG is han-
dled mainly by the liver. The combination of intact IgG and In-111, a radioisotope
that physiologically concentrates in the liver, together can result in a high radiation
exposure to the liver. On the other hand, $F(ab')_2$ goes to both the liver and kidney,
and the dosimetry partly depends on the radioisotope used—radiation exposure
being lower for Tc-99m than In-111 [22]. In general, all organ doses are within
acceptable limits in immunoscintigraphy, even when In-111 is used [79]. Generally, the dosimetry will fall between the two examples shown in Table 2.

D. Biodistribution

Biodistribution depends on the antibody used; e.g., anti-CEA antibody shows a
distribution half-life is about 1 hour, and the elimination half-life is about 13
hours, with 27% of the radiolabeled substance excreted via the urine in the first 24
hours postinjection. This is typical for a Fab' fragment, but much larger for $(Fab')_2$
and intact IgG. In the case of In-111-labeled B72.3 (IgG), we found the plasma
half-life to be between 33.3 and 41.2 hours, depending on the dosage of antibody
used. Biodistribution of all Mabs depends on whether IgG or fragments are used
and also what radiolabel is used, as already discussed. Typically Fab' fragments go
more to kidneys, because of their small size, while IgG goes more to the liver,
where it is metabolized with orthoproteins. The relative distribution of the Mab is
also influenced by the isotope used, e.g., when Tc-99 was used to label antimelanoma Fab' fragment, there was a significant myocardial uptake not seen with
other isotopes labeling of the same Fab' fragment [11,28].

Another factor that affects biodistribution is the development of HAMA.
HAMA to the anti-CEA IMMU-4 antibody (Arcitumomab) is very rare. We were
not able to document any cases in our experience with the Immu-4 fragment. In
contrast, the anti-TAG-72 (intact IgG) antibody has been shown to induce HAMA
response after a single injection in up to 40% of patients [36,83]. These two anti-

TABLE 2   Human Adult Organ Dosimetry Estimates for Tc-99m Anti-CEA and In-111-B72.3

Organ/tissue	Tc-99m arcitumomab		In-111 satumomab	
	Rad/20 mCi	mGy/740 MBq	Rad/5 mCi	mGy/185 MBq
Total body	0.340	3.404	2.7	27
Red marrow	0.736	7.360	2	120
Lung	0.572	5.720	4.9	49
Liver	0.770	7.700	15	150
Spleen	1.176	11.760	16	160
Kidney	7.424	74.240	9.7	97
Urinary bladder	1.232	12.320	2.8	28
Ovaries	0.568	5.680	2.9	29
Testes	0.330	3.300	1.4	14
Breast	0.112	1.120	—	—
Bone surfaces	0.588	5.880	3.3	33
Thyroid	0.208	2.080	1.5	15
Small intestine	0.416	4.160	3.0	30
Upper lg. intest.	0.408	4.080	3.1	31
Lower lg. intest.	0.346	3.460	2.5	25
Uterus	—	—	2.7	27
Pancreas	—	—	3.7	37
Other tissues	—	—	2.3	23

bodies illustrate the role that molecular size plays in the development of HAMA. HAMA incidence is far more common with the use of intact IgG compared to fragments. A rare patient can show the presence of human immunoglobin or immunoglobin-like substance that binds to injected murine monoclonal antibody even when there is no history of exposure to mouse antibody. HAMA levels, if significant, can interfere with biodistribution, because of immune-complex formation, and therefore diminish tumor:background ratios and give high splenic uptake.

III.   TECHNICAL ASPECTS

A.   Image Acquisition

Several techniques have evolved with respect to image acquisition in breast immunoscintigraphy. This partly depends on whether technetium-99m, indium-111, or iodine-labeled antibodies are used, and whether fragments or intact antibodies are used. Nevertheless, typical immunoscintigraphy involves acquisition of total body images to look for metastatic disease, if the antibody used has been shown to be useful for that purpose. Spot views for areas of interest are taken between 4 and 6 hours for technetium-labeled fragments and between 72 and 120 hours for indium-labeled intact IgG monoclonal antibodies. Earlier imaging, especially of the liver, may result in "cold" lesions, which eventually fill in. For the technetium-labeled anti-carcino embryonic antigen (anti-CEA) that we had used for the detection of breast cancer [84], we used between 1 and 2 mg of the antibody-labeled with 15 to 25 mCi of Tc-99m using the kit from the direct method (Immunomedics) for Tc-99m labeling. Anterior and posterior total body images are supplemented by static anterior planar spot views obtained for 7 to 10 min each, of the breast as well as cross-lateral view of the breast. In this special lateral view, the camera is on the lateral aspect of each breast, and the patient lies prone on a special table (Fig. 2), which has holes cut out for the breasts to be dependent one at a time for a good lateral image.

The limitation of this method is that we were unable to obtain a good image of the medial aspect of the breast. The special lateral view is repeated for each breast using the alternate cut-off areas of the table. Each spot view is acquired for 10 min at a matrix of 128* 128. This technique is generally referred to as scintimammography. This is then followed by SPECT imaging of the chest. We found SPECT to contribute significantly in most cases with antibody imaging. A typical SPECT is acquired using a dual-headed camera and a protocol of 60 stops at 30 sec/stop on 128×128 matrix at the 4 to 6 hours imaging time and 40 sec/stop at the 16 to 24 hours imaging session. Reconstruction is performed using a Hamming filter with a 0.9 cycle/cm high-frequency cut-off and Nyquist of 1:136. The high cut-off may need to be lowered to as low as 0.7 cycle/cm to achieve satisfactory smoothing of the back projected images taken at 24 hours, because of the low count.

B. Data Analysis

The data collected from the total body and from spot views are then analyzed qualitatively by visual inspection using the computer monitor so the windows contrast can be continuously varied to pick up small lesions rather than hard copies on film. Hard copies alone are often insufficient in most cases; at our institution, we never rely on them. The images are also semiquantitatively analyzed using regions of interest (ROI) and ratios of average count. The lesion average counts were compared to the surrounding normal breast tissue background and also to the contralateral breast. Spot views were repeated at 16 to 20 hours the next morning using the same planar technique, but longer exposure times. Analysis of the images includes the target:background ratio of the lesion as described and in addition the ratios of target-to-background ratios are compared, 4 hours versus the 16

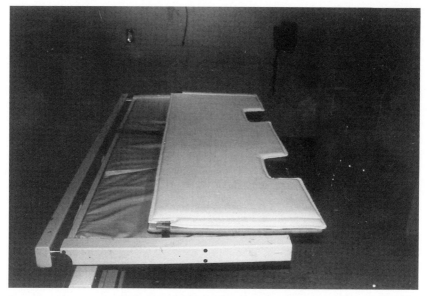

FIGURE 2   Photograph of the special overlay pad used for performing scintimammography. Note the two cut-out areas for the breasts—one at a time. Alternate lateral images of the alternate breasts dependent are obtained with a standard gamma camera in the lateral position. The overlay pad is secured on a regular nuclear table with straps. We used this table for both scans using Tc-99m anti-CEA and with Tc-99m sestamibi.

to 20 hours. As a reference point, we compared nipples and areola average counts versus background counts also at 4 hours as well as at 16 hours. The breast lesion-to-background ratio was up to 2.6:1.0 and axillary lesions up to 3.3:1.0 by planar imaging. SPECT ratios were higher for breast lesions and lower for the axillary lymph notes [36,84].

The above refers mainly to Tc-99m-labeled fragments. When we used In-111-labeled intact IgG B-72.3 monoclonal antibody in the detection and staging of breast cancer, a different imaging technique was used. Because of the nature of the isotope and because we used the intact IgG, early images taken at 4 hours were abandoned, as they did not contribute to the diagnosis. Best images were obtained when the background blood pool activity cleared at 72 hours. We found the plasma $t_{1/2}$ of In-111 B72.3 to be 41 hours for the small dose and 33 hours when high dose of Mab was used (2 to 10 mg). Again, total body images were taken, as well as spot images for the breast, including lateral and oblique views. ROIs were also used for this antibody, and we obtained higher target-to-background ratio (5.1:1.0 for breast lesions, but this dropped to lower ratios of 2.9:1.0 with higher Mab dosage. At that time, we did not have the specially designed table with the cut-out areas for the special lateral view of scintimammography as we did for the Tc-anti-CEA study, and for the other, more recent studies, such as sestamibi scintimammography. Only 0.0011% to 0.0025% of injected dose (ID) was taken up by a 1-g lesion.

IV. CLINICAL TRIALS OF MABS IN BREAST CANCER

A.   Anti-CEA Antibodies

1. Historical Aspect

A useful antibody for breast cancer is the anti-CEA antibody, initially as a polyclonal product and now as monoclonal. CEA is a tumor-associated antigen first discovered by Gold and Freedman [85]. Since then, at least two CEA antigens have been described, the classical one being the 200,000-dalton molecule described by Krupey [86]. The other form has a molecular weight of 180,000 daltons and has been called various names, including meconium antigen, normal cross-reactive antigen II, normal fecal antigen, and CEA low. Thus the CEA molecule is a glycoprotein having molecular mass of between 180,000 and 200,000 daltons [87,88]. It was initially considered to be a fetal antigen because it was found at high tissue levels in the fetal gastrointestinal tract, but more sensitive assays have, since then, found CEA in the adult normal colon. The CEA content in normal colon is approximately 1 μg/g. In colon cancer, it is typically in the range of 5 to 10 μg/g tumor. When CEA is secreted by cancer cells into the extracellular fluid, it gains access to the blood; and serum CEA levels are normally in the 0 to 2.5 ng/ml range, but this can be elevated with cigarette smoking and other lung injury, acute nonmalignant chronic inflammatory conditions of the gastrointestinal tract [89], breast cancer, and lung cancer. CEA levels may climb to over 15 ng/ml in patients with metastatic disease. In 1980, an NIH consensus panel concluded that serum CEA levels may be of value in the management of patients with lung, breast, and colon cancer [90].

Imaging of tumors with anti-CEA antibodies has been investigated since 1977 by scientists worldwide. The first antibody used was affinity-purified goat anti-CEA IgG antibody. In 1978, Goldenberg et al. administered affinity-purified I-131-labeled anti-CEA goat IgG to patients with advanced cancer [1]. These workers were highly impressed by the specificity of the antibody. Due to significant blood pool activities seen with these antibodies, a nonspecific blood pool marker such as Tc-99m albumin was used for computer subtraction of background to further improve the specificity. Early work with I-131-labeled antibodies demonstrated a resolution of 2 cm for CEA-producing neoplasms [90], and occult neo-plasms were also detected. In the 1980s there were development and characteriza-tion of a series of CEA murine monoclonal antibodies including the NP series of antibodies [63,91,92]. Patients were initially evaluated using an I-131-labeled NP-2 antibody. For detection of colorectal cancers there was a sensitivity of 90%, specificity of 88%, and an overall accuracy of 89%. Twenty percent of patients had at least one occult lesion uncovered by this antibody, but not previously sus-pected. It took up to 13 months for these occult lesions to be confirmed by other diagnostic imaging studies or by surgery. This gave great credibility to antibody imaging, even though CEA was used much earlier and resulted in a search of other tumor-associated antigens.

While most of the early investigations concerned the evaluation for colorec-tal carcinoma, the same antibodies have potential for imaging breast neoplasms, both occult and primary. When anti-CEA antibody is used to detect colon or breast cancer, it may pick up occult lesions up to 2 years before they become clinically obvious or detected by other imaging technique [93].

2. Current Anti-CEA Antibodies and Fragments Clinical Trials

Another anti-CEA antibody, designated as NP-4, demonstrated even greater speci-ficity for CEA, and it is now FDA approved and currently commercially available as CEA-Scan (Arcitumomab) for colon cancer. During the early clinical trials, it was also referred to as Immu-4. However, it is not yet FDA approved for the diag-nostic detection of breast cancer, only for the detection of colon cancer. Numer-ous clinical studies have been performed evaluating this agent for breast cancer detection [60,73,84,94–98]. This antibody, arcitumomab, previously called IMMU-4, is an anti-CEA antibody of the IgG_1 class, specific for the 200,000-dal-ton CEA molecule. Initially, the whole antibody was labeled with I-131 and images were not obtained for 24 hours or longer after injection. Wahl et al. found that ear-lier imaging could be obtained if the antibody fragments were used instead of the whole antibody [78]. This NP-4 antibody has excellent specificity and is nonreac-tive with blood and vascular elements and does not crossreact with "normal cross-reactive antigens," but is specific for the 200,000-dalton form of CEA. It does not complex significantly with circulating CEA. The Fab' fragment is produced from the intact IgG by pepsin cleavage which produces $F(ab')_2$, and further action of papain at the hinge region results in Fab' (Fig. 1). Currently, the commercially available anti-CEA antibody (arcitumomab) is a Fab' fragment.

Early Phase II studies evaluating this antibody were promising, with a 71.4% sensitivity for known lesions. A recently concluded Phase III study was also under-taken to determine whether these antibody imaging results can alter the patient's management and whether metastatic occult lesions or axillary lymph nodes can be found. Overall, at our center, there was a sensitivity of 93% to 100% for the primary lesions and 83% overall sensitivity (Figs. 3–9). There were also unknown (occult) lesions detected. Two out of four unknown lymph nodes were confirmed, and one took 2 years to become clinically evident. Three out of five occult breast lesions were also confirmed. This antibody was also helpful when detecting previously undetected liver metastases and lung metastases in two of the patients. In this study, 7/15 patients were either downstaged or upstaged based on imaging data. No primary tumor was missed. In fact, a 4-mm lesion was found in the contralateral breast of one patient. Our results were similar to a study performed by Nabi et al., in which 5/5 palpable lesions were detected and only 2/8 nonpalpable cancers, giving a positive predictive value of 78%. Seven of the eight nonpalpable masses were <1 cm. The negative predictive value was 100% with patients determined to have benign disease, such as fibrocystic changes, ductal hyperplasia, and fibroadenoma, for example.

The difference between our study and Nabi's initial study is that we performed SPECT on all our patients, and he did not. In our study, all primary tumors were detected by SPECT (100% sensitivity) (Figs. 5–8), while only 14/15 were positive by planar images (93% sensitivity). In addition, 7/7 known positive lymph nodes were detected by SPECT, while only 5/7 were seen on planar images. SPECT has clearly improved the sensitivity in our study. These two studies together gave great hope that Tc-arcitumomab has a potential for the detection of nodal disease, as well as the primary disease [84,92].

3. European and American Anti-CEA Studies

A variety of anti-CEA Mabs were studied by other workers on both sides of the Atlantic. Lind et al., in 1991 [56], utilized the preoperative intravenous administration of the Tc-99m-labeled IgG anti-CEA in 45 women with breast cancer. A sensitivity of 82% was obtained with the smallest detectable lesion by SPECT imaging being 7 mm. Only 17% of patients with breast cancer had elevated CEA levels detectable in serum. This further supports the notion that tumor markers such as CEA, although expressed in the tumor, do not necessarily translate into detectable serum levels.

Haseman et al. [87] used indium-111-labeled intact murine IgG anti-CEA monoclonal antibody ZCE-025 to detect occult lesions in 140 patients who had a negative or equivocal CT scan. This antibody is an intact murine IgG_1 antibody with a high affinity for CEA. A number of patients had a history of prior murine antibody injections and had an adverse reaction rate of 18%, vs. 1% of patients with no prior exposure. Nineteen out of 19 patients with liver metastases were diagnosed with SPECT. Seventeen of these were "hot" lesions; however, the number of breast cancer patients in this series was extremely small. In this study, 75/95 patients with occult cancer (disease not detected by CT) were correctly identified. This further supports the utility of anti-CEA monoclonal antibody imaging of cancer patients, looking for occult disease.

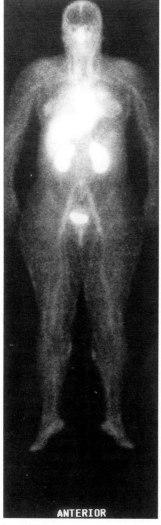

ANTERIOR   A

FIGURE 3   (A) Anterior whole-body image at 4 hours postinjection of Tc-99m anti-CEA antibody demonstrating physiologic uptake in the blood pool, liver, kidneys, and both breasts diffusely. Focal abnormal increase in activity is seen in the primary tumor in the left upper and inner quadrant. (B,C) 4.5-Hour anterior and lateral planar images demonstrating focal uptake in the left breast tumor and diffuse uptake in both breasts. No lymph node uptake was noted, and all resected nodes were negative for tumor. (D,E) Marker images showing "hot" nipple marker and marker around areolas. (F) Scintimammogram showing focal uptake in the left breast. The right breast (not shown) was normal. (G,H) Left mammogram showing the primary tumor; right mammogram showing a dense breast without focal abnormality.

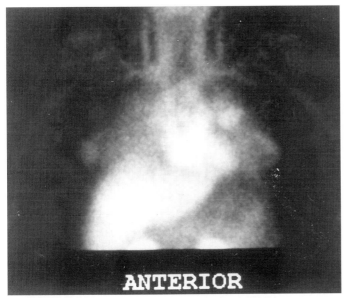

B

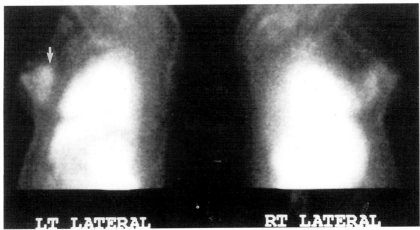

C

FIGURE 3   Continued

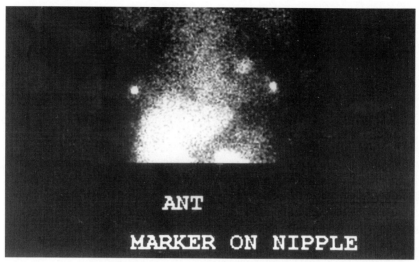

D

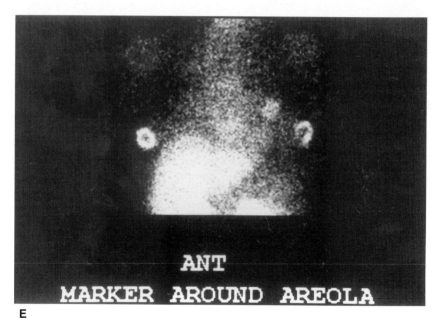

E

FIGURE 3   Continued

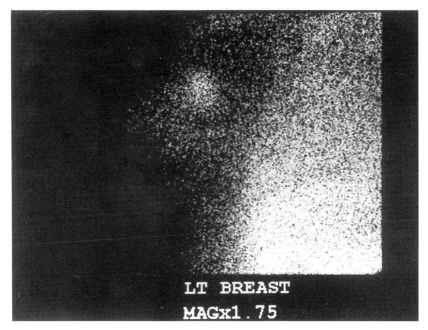

LT BREAST
MAGx1.75

F

FIGURE 3   Continued

Nabi et al. also studied patients using yet another Tc-99m-labeled anti-CEA fragment, CYT-380, to evaluate its utility in detection of lymph node involvement and residual disease after excisional biopsy. Radioimmunoscintigraphy demonstrated positive localization in 4/4 primary carcinomas, with the smallest lesion seen being 1 cm in size. In two patients with prior definitive surgery, no abnormal uptake was noted. Two small axillary lymph nodes were not detected in one patient. CYT-380 was useful in ruling out the presence of involved lymph nodes and residual disease after excisional biopsy. However, smaller nodes have been detected with Tc-arcitumomab and SPECT imaging. At this point, however, given the small number of patients imaged with CYT-380, an accurate comparison is not possible [60]. Riva used yet another monoclonal anti-CEA antibody FO23C5 injected intraperitoneally. Sensitivity and specificity for identifying hepatic metastases was improved after intraperitoneal injection [99]. De Castiglia et al. [71] and Duran et al. [72] separately reported using B2C114, an anti-CEA antibody in the detection of murine mammary carcinoma. Results revealed good detection of these tumors, although not any better than the labeled fragments [71,72].

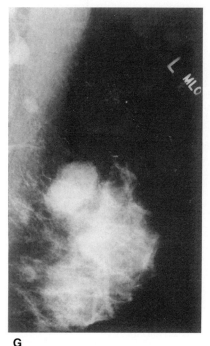

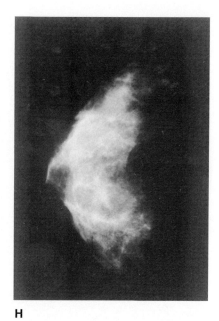

H

G

FIGURE 3   Continued

The above brief review of the literature reflects the interest in anti-CEA antibodies. This is because patients with recurrent disease often present with elevated serum CEA levels, negative or equivocal CT scans, and a prior history of a CEA-producing tumor. This poses a difficult challenge for the oncologist and the radiologist. MoAb scanning with anti-CEA antibodies can contribute significantly to the accurate diagnosis of these difficult patients. Earlier detection of metastases or recurrence permits early therapeutic intervention—surgical or conservative, whichever is more relevant. In patients with breast cancer, identification of nodal involvement or of satellite breast lesions may preclude or modify surgical intervention and also help in timing of chemotherapy and radiation therapy.

B.   B72.3 Antibodies (Anti-TAG 72)

I.   Historical Aspect

Besides antibodies to CEA, radiolabeling of other breast cancer antigens, such as tumor-associated glycoprotein and breast epithelial antigen (mucin), have also

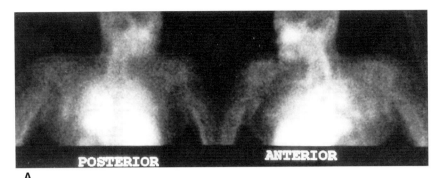

A

FIGURE 4   (A) Planar images of the chest at 7 hours postinjection demonstrating uptake in the left breast primary and in axillary nodes. The lesion can be seen even from the posterior views. Breast lesions and axillary nodes can be confused from a posterior view. (B) Planar scintimammography (special table listed view) of another patient taken at 24 hours after injection of Tc-99m arcitumomab demonstrating extensive area of abnormal tracer accumulation. (C) Bilateral mammograms showing a left spiculated mass with nipple retraction, consistent with carcinoma.

proven successful. Monoclonal antibody B-72.3 is an IgG subclass which reacts with a 200,000- to 400,000-molecular-weight tumor-associated glycoprotein (TAG-72) antigen [37]. Using immunohistologic methods, up to 80% of human breast cancers were found to be reactive with the antibody B72.3 [100].

We ran the early clinical trials of this antibody for breast cancer and obtained very good results for the primary lesion (Figs. 10–12). Two milligrams of this antibody was labeled with 5 mCi of In-111 using the site-directed GYK-DTPA method (at carbohydrate moiety). This antibody is now FDA approved and commercially available in the U.S. (under the trade name Oncoscint and the generic name satumomab), but approved only for colon cancer and ovarian cancer investigation, not for breast cancer.

Using this antibody, we imaged the patients up to 96 hours after injection of the In-111-labeled intact IgG Mab. We acquired both special axillary views from anterior and oblique views and with arms up and down for best view of axillary lymph nodes (Fig. 13), and anterior, lateral, and oblique views of the breast and also total body. The planar spot views were acquired using 125 × 125 matrix or 256 × 256 matrix for 7 to 10 min each. SPECT is acquired for 360° using dual-head gamma cameras. Typically for SPECT, we use 30 sec per stop for 64 stops using stop-and-shoot technique. Blood samples are taken before injection of antibody to screen for HAMA levels, and for pharmacokinetics, in the research setting, HAMA test was also repeated at 1 week and at 1 month or as called upon by individual protocols. There are now, however, new studies involving fragments of

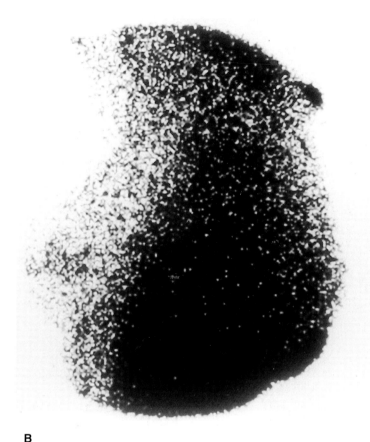

B

FIGURE 4   Continued

this antibody about to be started in Great Britain [101]. This should result in lower HAMA incidence than we had with the intact IgG. Hopefully, the fragments may also have better sensitivity for the axillary nodes detection.

2.   Anti-TAG-72 Clinical Trials Results

We have [3] used In-111-labeled B72.3 monoclonal antibody in 16 patients to detect and stage breast cancer; 0.2, 2, or 20 mg of the antibody was In-111 GYK-DTPA labeled with 5 mCi of indium. The 2-mg dose was optimal. The pan carcinoma antibody is a murine Mab of the IgG class, directed against the TAG-72 antigen. It had been shown to react with 80% of needle biopsy aspirates of breast cancer but not with normal tissue [91,102]. Other cancers also express TAG-72 antigen, including 96% of small cell cancers of the lung, 100% of epithelial ovar-

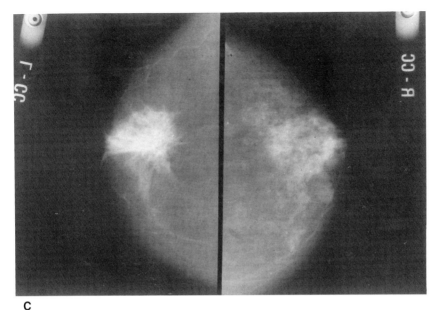

C

FIGURE 4   Continued

ian cancers, and 80% of colon cancers, among others. Fourteen of 16 patients in our study were found to have primary breast cancer at the time of surgery. All 14 primary breast lesions were detected by the antibody using In-111-B72.3 (100% sensitivity). Normal nipple was visualized in about half of the patients and may have been related to the timing relative to the menstrual cycle. Seven patients had proven axillary lymph node metastases but were not detected by the radioimmunoscintigraphy. This is in contrast to higher percentage of lymph node metastases detected by the Immu-4 anti-CEA antibody fragment labeled with Tc-99m. While the sensitivity of B72.3 Mab in our laboratory was 100% for detection of the primary tumor (14/14), the negative findings in axillary nodes were a major setback in that study. We did not detect the four patients' proven axillary lymph nodes metastases. There were two benign breast lesions which were not detected by the radioimmunoimaging, in keeping with good specificity. The size of the primary lesions ranged from 1.2 to 2.5 cm, while the size of the lymph nodes resected was 0.3 to 1.5 cm. Three occult lesions were discovered and all were confirmed. There were three distant metastatic lesions; one each to the skin, bone, and lymph node (Fig. 14) were detected and were previously not known. All of these were found to be true positives on subsequent follow-up of these patients. Two of the 12 patients tested for HAMA had a positive response. HAMA incidence is actually higher in other studies.

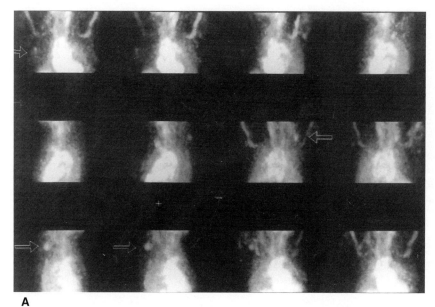

A

FIGURE 5   (A) Three-dimensional (3-D) reprojection of the transverse SPECT slices can dramatically demonstrate abnormal uptake in both the breasts and axillary or other lymph nodes. In this patient there is abnormal uptake in a right supraclavicular node and in the primary lesion in the right breast (arrows). The 3-D images are sequentially rotated. (B,C) A close-up display of the 3-D images showing the supraclavicular lesion (B) from anterior and lateral projections and the breast lesion (C). The right supraclavicular node did not become clinically evident for 6 months. (D) Mammogram of the right breast demonstrating diffuse reticular markings, consistent with diffuse inflammatory carcinoma.

3.   Other Anti-TAG-72 Antibodies

Other antibodies have been produced against a variety of tumor-associated glycoproteins (TAGs). B6.2 is one of these antibodies used by several investigators [103,104]. These consist of cell surface glycoproteins and glycolipids altered during malignant transformation [96]. However, the results using these antibodies are not an improvement over the original B72.3 (Oncoscint) that we had tested. There is, however, a potential for fragments of this antibody, which will be tested in the near future.

C.   Other Breast Monoclonal Antibodies

1.   Anti-HMFG and Antimucin Antibodies

Human milk fat globulin antigens (HMFGs) are found in a number of epithelial tumors. Antibodies to HMFG have been used in several clinical trials for a variety

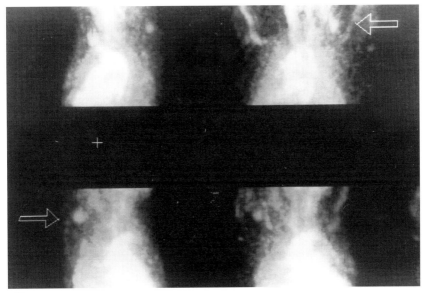

B

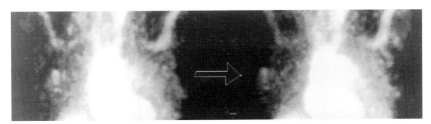

C

FIGURE 5   Continued

of tumors [40,61,62,105–108]. Early clinical imaging using these antibodies was by Epenetos [20] and then Gykalofonos [106]. Rosner et al. [40] were able to demonstrate successful imaging in 5/5 patients with Tc-99m anti-CEA antibody and 5/7 using HMFG labeled with I-123. They concluded that antihuman milk fat globulin may be useful as a diagnostic agent for the evaluation of primary or recurrent breast cancer. Several other workers have studied the anti-HMFG and antimucin antibodies for breast imaging. Brummendorf et al. [109] found good tumor to background in mice using Tc-99m-radiolabeled antimucin antibodies and [46] to imagine human mammary cancer xenografts. Athanassiou used an antibody targeting HMFG1 or HMFG2. Injecting this labeled antibody subcutaneously for immunolymphoscintigraphy or intravenously did not result in good

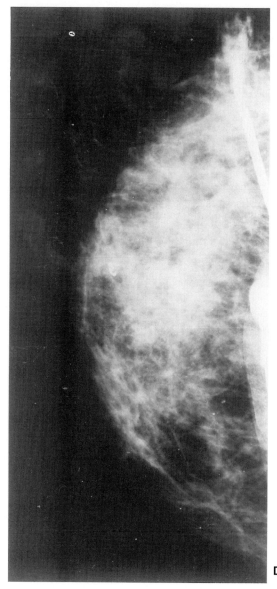

D

FIGURE 5   Continued

tumor localization [59]. Conversely, Nabi et al., studying 13 patients with I-123 HMFG1, identified recurrences in 3/3 patients—bone metastases in one patient, and primary operable cancer in 2/3. A lesion measuring 0.8 cm was not detected by the scan [60].

Major et al. investigated other labeled antibodies directed against the epithelial membrane antigen MA5. Variable degree of uptake was noted in those primary lesions or metastases >3 cm, while smaller lesions were not detected. Limited amount of antigen expressed at the tumor surface may explain the lack of significant [105] uptake. Kramer et al. [41] investigated In-111-(MX-DTPA)-BrE-3, an antibody detected against another breast epithelial mucin found in the human milk fat globulin in 15 patients. The expression of the epitope recognized by this antibody was first checked using immunohistochemical staining of previously obtained tumor specimens. Seventy-two separate sites of disease were identified by conventional diagnostic modalities. These included 43 skeletal, seven chest wall, eight lymph nodes, six liver, and eight other lesions. Overall, 62 (86%) of the lesions, including 2/6 liver metastases, 3/4 lung metastases, and 7/8 lymph node metastases, were detected by In-111 BrE-3. In addition, 39/43 skeletal lesions were detected (91% sensitivity). Radiation dosimetry performed for this agent showed that the liver and spleen received the highest doses, as expected for an In-111-labeled whole antibody. The doses were 1.30 ± 0.46 rads/mCi and 1.48 ± 0.85 rads/mCi, respectively. The average whole-body dose was 0.45 ± 0.11 rads/mCi. The ability of this antibody to detect skeletal and lymph node metastases is encouraging and may have a future application in therapy. The antibody was also ester-labeled with Yttrium-90 for therapeutic trials.

2. Miscellaneous Antibodies

Besides the anti-CEA (arcitumomab, CEA scan) and B72.3 (satumomab, Oncoscint), other antibodies have been used successfully for breast cancer imaging. The antimucin and anti-HMFG are already discussed above but are not in the market yet. These are directed against a variety of antigens (Table 1). The antibody 170H.82 appears to have a good detection rate and lower false-negative rate for soft-tissue lesions. In McEwan's study, 6/7 breast lesions and 17/19 lymph node metastases were correctly detected [70,110]. There was also a good detection of bone metastases detected, a finding not supported by most other investigators. For this antibody a 9% HAMA response has been reported.

Two antibodies against Thomson-Friedenreich antigen, a tumor-associated glycoconjugate, have been tried. This antigen is expressed on cell surface early in malignant transformation of cells or even preneoplastic phase; 155HF and 170H.82 were labeled with In-111, while 170H.82 has also been labeled with Tc-99m and used in 15 patients with an overall sensitivity of 90% to 96%. McEwan used this antibody in patients with primary or metastatic breast cancer and 25/32

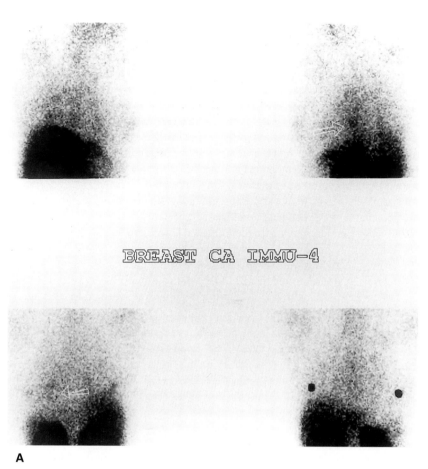

BREAST CA IMMU-4

A

FIGURE 6   (A) Planar images of Tc-99m anti-CEA antibody images taken at 24 hours show the abnormal chest wall uptake (arrow). Note the nipple markers. (B,C) Coronal SPECT slices in alternate inverted color presentations show the focal lung metastases, most pronounced posteriorly. This is better seen in the black-on-white than in the white-on-black presentation in this case, but not in all patients. (D) Transverse SPECT slides further delineating the posterior chest metastasis. (E) Lateral skull images showing subtle abnormal uptake in the right side of the head, consistent with brain metastases.

soft-tissue metastatic sites were detected but only 1/5 bone mets [111]. Further evaluation by McEwan showed that 18/20 breast lesions, 36/40 lymph nodes, and 23/28 bone metastases were detected. A sensitivity of 90% for localization of soft-tissue disease and a specificity of 93% were reported [111]. A recent trial involving Tc-99m-labeled anti CA-15-3 antibody SM3 demonstrated that while

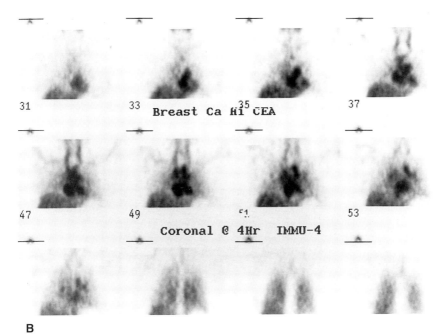

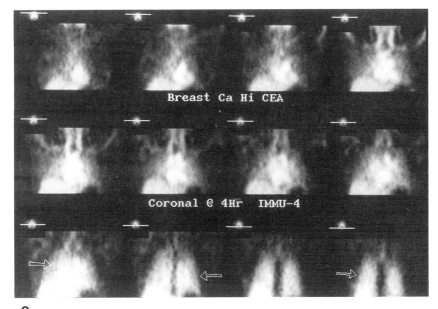

FIGURE 6   Continued

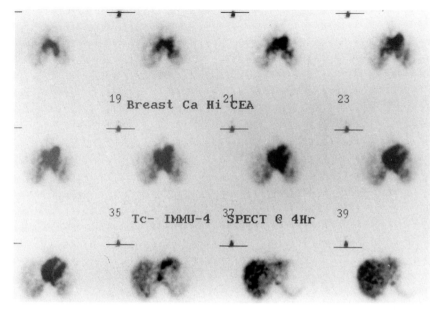

19 Breast Ca Hi CEA 21   23

35 Tc- IMMU-4 37 SPECT @ 4Hr 39

D

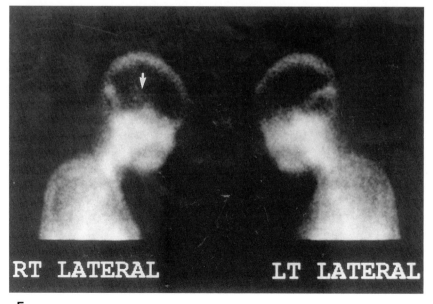

RT LATERAL   LT LATERAL

E

FIGURE 6   Continued

planar imaging was unsuccessful, axillary node involvement was correctly determined in 11/13 patients; 6/7 true negatives and 5/6 true positives. This antibody also has potential for early detection of breast cancer and for presurgical staging [38]. Few reports have been published on antibodies which target proto-oncogenous products such as ICR. Allan et al. [58] used the gene product of C-erb B2 [112] as the target antigen. Epenetos used 1-123-labeled tumor-associated monoclonal antibodies to ovarian, breast, and gastrointestinal tumors [20]. Rosner et al. [94] proposed using this antibody to screen for potential lesions and indeterminate mammograms prior to biopsy, similar to the current clinical usage of Tc-99m sestamibi. This has potential for reducing the number of unnecessary biopsies being performed in 75% of women who have abnormal pathology on conventional mammography—but not cancerous.

D. Primary Versus Metastatic Imaging

Mabs are not only for detection of the primary breast tumor or axillary nodes but can be used to detect distant metastasis as well, e.g., liver, lung, bone marrow, brain, and soft tissue. As a rule, most workers have been more successful in imaging the primary tumor versus metastases, as already discussed. Korpi et al. [113] investigated bone marrow involvement by breast cancer metastases using the two most popular monoclonal antibodies. Several other workers have detected distant metastasis using a variety of Mabs [114–121], but there is no convincing large series which shows that antibody staging of breast cancer has come of age.

Mangili et al. [118] used immunohistochemical staining to determine whether multiple different antibodies could lead to improved imaging detection. The authors evaluated CEA, c-erb B-2 protein, and TAG-72 expression in 100 cases of breast cancer using FO23C5 anti-CEA, B72.3 anti-TAG-72, and anti-c-erb-B-2 protein monoclonal antibodies. The results showed immunoreactivity for c-erb in 39/99 cases, B72.3 in 41/100 cases, and CEA in 15/100 cases. Multifocal lesions demonstrated positivity for c-erb in 6/16, B72.3 in 11/16, and anti-CEA in 1/16 cases. For lymph node metastases the immunoreactivity was positive for c-erb in 12/33, for B72.3 in 21/33, and for CEA in 8/33. When all three antibodies were considered together, the sensitivity improved to 60% for primary tumors, 78% in lymph nodes, and 81.2% in multifocal lesions.

E. Radioimmuno-Guided Surgery

Radioimmuno-guided surgery (RIGS) utilizes a gamma probe intraoperatively to more precisely localize metastatic lesions prior to surgical removal. It has been shown to be useful in patients with colon cancer. Several hours after IV injection of Tc-99m-IMMU-4, patients are taken to surgery, and the probe is used to identify involved lymph nodes and margin of disease. The combination of preop imaging plus intraoperative probe seems to have a very promising role in surgical

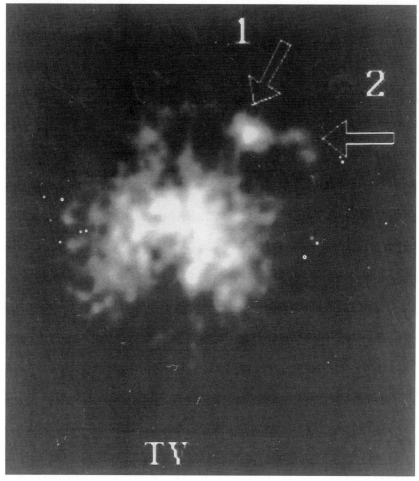

A

FIGURE 7   SPECT imaging of Tc-99m labeling antibody can demonstrate lesions, which are not clearly seen on planar. These are images of four different patients illustrating four examples of the utility of SPECT. (A) Transverse SPECT slice showing a second, smaller lesion not seen in planar imaging. (B) Coronal SPECT slices show deep mediastinal nodal involvement not seen in planar images. (C) These 3-D reprojection images from the SPECT transverse slices show a large left breast lesion and a second, smaller axillary node which was only suspected in planar images. There is also a lesion in the right breast, as well—a finding in support of the utility of antibody imaging for multicentric disease. (D) This is a frame from the 3-D reprojection of Tc-99m anti-CEA SPECT slices. These images, when put in a cine mode, were able to decipher the neoplasm (larger focus) in the left breast, a smaller lesion (4 mm) in the right breast, as well as the two nipples (arrows). Sometimes the motion of the cine mode contributes significantly to SPECT examination.

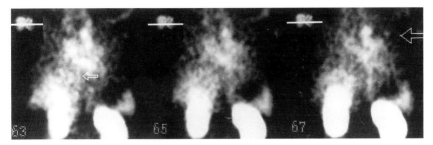

B

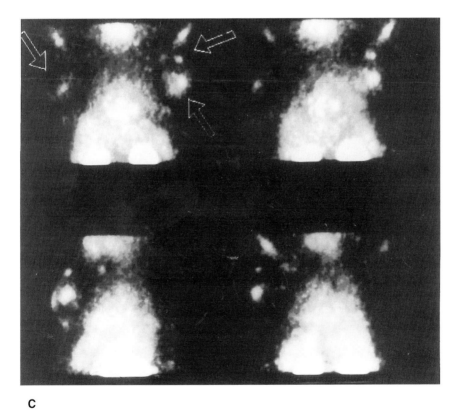

C

FIGURE 7   Continued

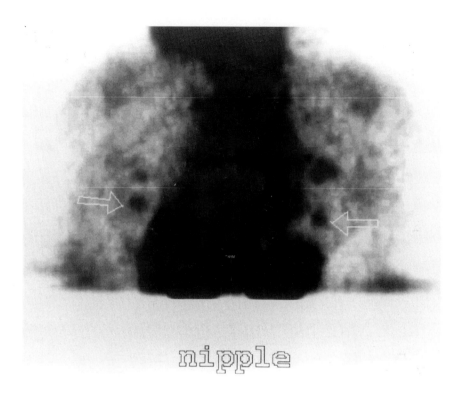

D

FIGURE 7   Continued

oncology. This system has potential for the detection of ipsilateral and contralateral lymph nodes and may be helpful in preventing a second surgical exploration. The probe system consists of the carrier substance, such as the Tc-IMMU-4, a radionuclide detector, data processor, and an audible and numerical output. There are probes designed for In-111 Tc-99m and iodine, often simply by changing the collimator head.

Nieroda described nonspecific localization in tumor-negative nodes by using I-125-labeled B72.3 and a hand-held intraoperative gamma detector. High counts were detected in tumor-free axillary nodes in 3/14 patients. This may have been a result of the presence of antigen shed in the tumor-negative nodes, a pitfall of which we have to be acutely aware.

Stephens et al. [116] conducted similar studies on patients with colon cancer and also reported false-positive uptake. The authors proposed that false-positive nodes may be due to immunologically mediated complexing of the cancer with the B72.3 monoclonal antibody. A well-collimated probe reduces the incidence of false positives from bladder activity and other physiological accumulations that can interfere.

F. Liposomes and Antibodies

Nonspecific oncotropic indicators such as gallium-67 citrate have shown an affinity for neoplastic tissues. This affinity is based in part on increased vascularity, tissue permeability, and cellular proliferation. Because they are taken up by numerous tumors, they are not specific enough to be used for tumor detection or staging of most tumors. Immunoscintigraphy using anti-CEA, anti-CA 19-9 or 15-3, and anti-TAG72 labeled with Tc-99m, I-131, or In-111-DTPA are more specific but also have limitations. One of the limitations of this method is that the antibody's molecules bind only some of the radiotracer, allowing for a high radioactive background. The use of liposomes for immunoscintigraphy is a novel way of enhancing the amount of entrapped radiotracer molecules. Rombi et al. have used several Mab-labeled liposomes as artificial carriers for radioisotopes and drugs [122]. In one study, six patients (four with liver localization, one with brain, and one with lung localization) were included and immunoscintigraphy was carried out using unilayer I-131-charged liposomes or Tc-99m for brain localization, and labeled with specific monoclonal antibodies (anti-CA 15-3 and anti-TAG 72). Planar scintigrams were obtained at 12, 24, 48, and 96 hours after infusion of the tracer. Subtraction images of the various organs were performed. Images showed early diffuse uptake, becoming more localized by 48 to 96 hours. The study concluded that selective localization of metastases could be performed with less of radiotracer dose than required by standard immunoscintigraphy. Perhaps this method can be incorporated into delivery methods for both immunoscintigraphy and radioimmunotherapy.

G. Immunolymphoscintigraphy

Most women diagnosed with breast cancer do not have clinical evidence of lymph node metastases. However, approximately 30% with clinical stage I do have occult lymph node metastases. Diagnosing these is a major challenge for the imaging community. There have been fewer antibody imaging studies performed for the of detection of breast cancer to lymph nodes than there have been for other cancers such as colon or prostate. Most of the older studies involved either intravenous or subcutaneous injection of the radiolabeled MoAb, and variable results have been reported. The subcutaneous route of administration and even direct injection into the lymphatics have been used for lymphoscintigraphy. Several methods of lymphoscintigraphic detection of breast cancer nodal metastases have been described using various colloids such as Tc-99m-rhenium colloid or antimony colloid, or human serum albumin [123]. The advent of labeled antibodies had stirred some interest in utilizing these for lymphoscintigraphy. One of the earliest studies was

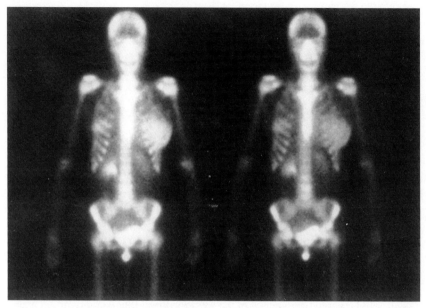

A

FIGURE 8   (A) Whole-body Tc-99m MDP bone scan demonstrating abnormal, diffuse left breast uptake. (B) 21-hour anti-CEA antibody scan showing similar, intense uptake in the left breast. In addition, focal abnormal uptake in a *right* supraclavicular node is noted. The node became clinically identifiable only after 2 years postscan as metastatic disease. (C) 3-D images reprojected from SPECT transverse slices showing an additional focal uptake in a lymph node above the left breast, which was not seen on planar imaging. (D) Bilateral mammograms showing malignant lesion involving the entire left breast with associated left axillary adenopathy. The right breast is unremarkable.

performed by Deland's group, who studied nine patients using an I-131 anti-CEA goat antibody. Interdigital injection of the antibody resulted in axillary accumulation in all eight patients with surgically confirmed disease. The ninth patient had no uptake and no axillary disease. This provided the impetus for future work in this area. Studies involving radiolabeled antibodies 3E1.2 [121] and 3C6F9 [124] reported similar results. Kairemo et al. studied breast cancer patients using a Tc-99m-labeled CEA MoAb BW431/26and had a sensitivity of 90% with a specificity of 88% for lymphoscintigraphic detection of axillary metastases [75].

Tjandra et al. [125] also evaluated I-131-radiolabeled antibodies injected interdigitally to evaluate involved axillary lymph nodes. The antibodies used, 3E1.2 (IgM) and RCC-1 (IgG), react strongly with the membrane and cytoplasm breast carcinomas in approximately 90%, with very little cross reactivity with

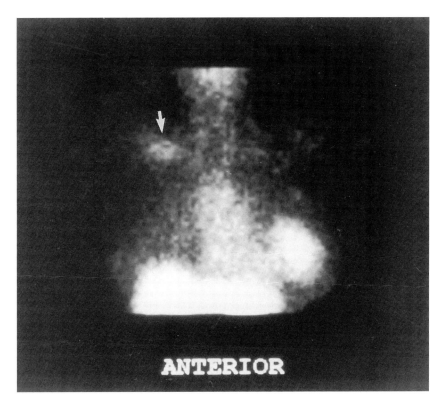

B

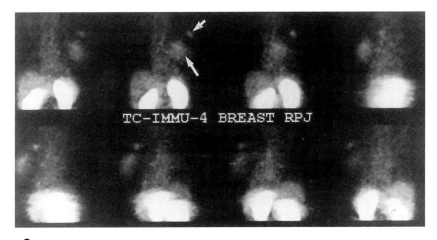

C

FIGURE 8   Continued

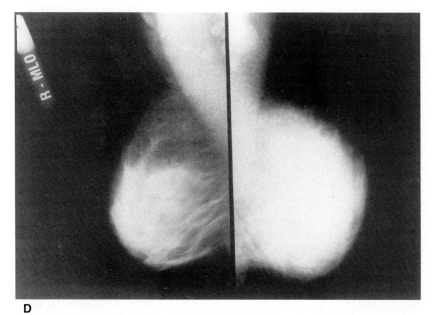

D

Figure 8   Continued

normal breast tissue. Forty patients with clinically suspected breast cancer were studied prospectively (36/40 eventually proved to have breast cancer). At 16 to 24 hours postinjection anterior scintigrams were taken of the chest and axillae. Lymph nodes that were resected were processed and 6-μm sections were stained. One patient who received 3E1.2 and one receiving RCC-1 developed HAMA antibodies.Correct prediction of the axillary node status was obtained in only 41% (9/22) of patients in the preoperative scan and 59% of patients (13/22) by preoperative clinical assessment. These results were not promising, as better prediction can be obtained after intravenous injection of antibodies, such as Tc-99m-IMMU-4: lymphoscintigraphy performed with I-131-RCC-1 resulted in a sensitivity of 86% and a specificity of 92% [84,93,15,125].

There are other antibodies that can nonspecifically localize in normal lymph nodes. Pecking et al. used an In-111-labeled human antibody directed against cytoplasmic antigen CTA 16.88, injected directly into the mammary glands. Simultaneous subcutaneous injections of ln-111-16.88 were also made in juxta-areolar sites. While the CTA-16.88 was detected in all of the primary tumors and involved lymph nodes tested, it was also positive in 89% of nodes with follicular hyperplasia. Overall, radioimmunolymphoscintigraphy had a sensitivity of 72.7%, specificity of 80.4%, and accuracy of 77.7% [117].

The detection rates of involved lymph nodes with radioimmunolymphoscintigraphy appear to be very good. However,this technique is not yet accepted universally, especially by the surgical oncology clinicians, and neither is immunoscintigraphy. Perhaps including lymphoscintigraphy as part of the workup of the patient may add credence to the findings of immunoscintigraphic imaging.

V. BREAST CANCER IMMUNOSCINTIGRAPHY: PRESENT AND FUTURE

A. Present Clinical Role

Because of the potential risk of HAMA formation or adverse reaction to the protein component and a debatable clinical role, immunoscintigraphy is not yet recommended as a primary method for screening or diagnosing primary breast cancer.However, its use in evaluating occult recurrences has great potential, and possibly also for distant metastasis in staging or restaging.

Radiolabeled monoclonal antibodies against tumor-associated antigens can indeed detect primary and metastatic tumors but may miss critical areas. TAG-72 is a good example for excellent detection of primary tumors, though it falls short in detecting involved lymph nodes [36]. The agent that so far seems to be the best compromise for detecting primary and metastatic lesions, including lymph nodes, is Tc-99m CEA scan (arcitumomab). This antibody is now commercially available for colon cancer, but can be used for breast cancer at the discretion of the physician.The big question is what can the role of this and the anti-TAG Oncoscint (satumomab) antibodies really be? Though radioimmunodetection of breast cancer has a definite potential for a contributory role in management of this disease, that is still not clarified and there is no consensus. Thus far, there has been no approved antibody agent that can accurately stage lymph nodes. Surgical sampling of nodes is still needed, as radiotherapy of nodes still has a 3% recurrence rate [114].

In patients with suspicious mammographic abnormalities or inconclusive mammographic findings, e.g., dense or fatty breasts, Mab could be used for scintimammography similar to Tc-99m sestamibi to separate benign from malignant lesions. However, many clinicians feel that patients should not be subjected to this testing with the possibility of developing HAMA or allergic reactions, albeit a very small possibility. So far, this has not been the case and it is doubtful whether these issues should be limiting factors. There are no studies demonstrating the role of this agent in screening scintimammography. Based on our experience, the sensitivity for detection of primary tumors is very good. In fact, several lesions that were detected by this scan did not become clinically evident for 2 months to 2 years afterward. This fact was also noted by Kramer et al., using the BrE-3 anti-

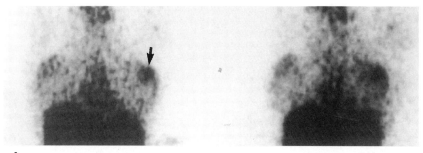

A

FIGURE 9 (A) Anterior anti-CEA planar images demonstrating normal physiologic uptake of antibody by breast tissue bilaterally. In addition, focal, intense uptake is seen in the left breast, consistent with a malignant lesion. The upper-outer quadrant lesions are the most common and easier to detect. (B) Anterior arcitumomab image demonstrating focal increase in the inferior and medial aspect of the breast, consistent with the tumor seen on the mammogram. Lesions in the medial region are harder to detect on planar and scintimammographic images. (C) Right mammogram of a 56-year-old with fibrocystic disease showing a focal mass with a "comet tail" suggesting malignancy. (Figures 9B and 9C with permission from Dr. David Goldenberg, Immunomedics, Inc.)

body [41]. The potential problem comes in the area of specificity, since this is not fully established in a multicenter trial, like sestamibi. A trial similar to the sestamibi breast trial would be helpful in further defining the role of this or other labeled antibodies, prior to performing a biopsy.)

Another issue is related to the utility in accurately staging the patient before radical or sparing surgery. Again, in our experience, radiolabeled antibodies have detected unsuspected multifocality of disease in several patients, thus postponing surgery to allow initiation of adjuvant chemotherapy, because of this upstaging. Immunoscintigraphy might play an important role in defining the multicentricity of disease systemically or in clarifying mammographic findings locally. It may also help identify the extent of disease, such as carcinoma in situ, and thus possibly prevent the need of surgery or modify the surgical approach. Radioimmunoscintigraphy has also been helpful to the surgeon in knowing what to expect regarding axillary involvement.

A third consideration in discussing is the utility of radiolabeled antibodies to determine the adequacy of chemotherapy and its response before doing surgery, especially regarding lymph nodes. If there is a good response to surgery, based on a reduction of tracer localization on a follow-up scan, the surgeon would be more likely to agree to perform a curative operation. On the other hand, if the scan did not show any improvement, further chemotherapy or a switch of therapeutic agents may be desired. This role is well established for sestamibi scanning of the breast. The last unexplored areas involve using radiolabeled antibodies to look for occult

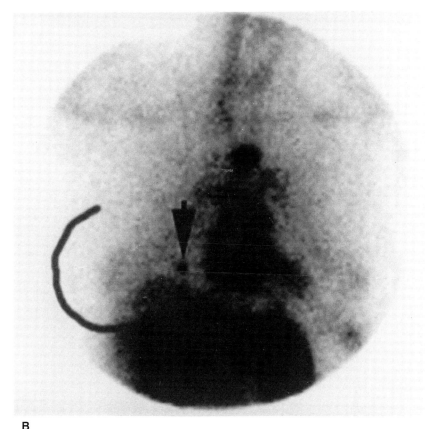

B

FIGURE 9   Continued

metastases in someone with a rising CEA level or for routine follow-up imaging. Radiolabeled anti-CEA has been fairly successful in finding occult tumors in patients with a history of colon cancer [22,23,74]. Its utility in detecting occult breast metastases has not been adequately studied. Nor has the potential of these agents to find the primary lesion in patients with adenocarcinoma of unknown origin. All these potential roles need to be explored, as does the role of Mab in detecting a second primary in the other breast.

B.   Complementary Roles of Mammography and Malignancy

The anti-CEA antibody (arcitumomab), which has been approved by the FDA for clinical use in the detection of occult colorectal cancer recurrence, can be very useful in detecting occult breast cancer. There is preliminary evidence that Tc-

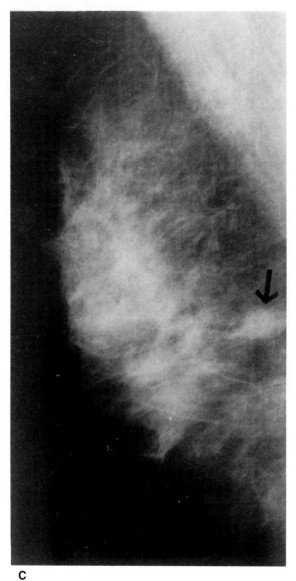

C

Figure 9   Continued

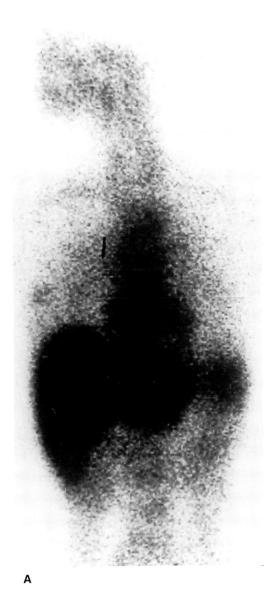

A

FIGURE 10   Indium-111 B72.3 (A) Total-body image 48 hours postintravenous injection of In-111-labeled B72.3 Mab. Note the abnormal focus of increased uptake in the right breast malignant tumor. (B) Anterior chest image of the same patient taken at 72 hours. Note the higher concentration of the labeled Mab in the right breast lesions. Also note the high blood pool which is still present even at 72 hours—quite common with In-111-labeled intact IgG Mab.

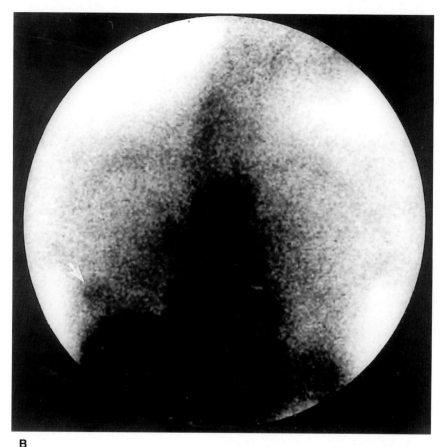

B

FIGURE 10   Continued

99m-arcitumomab (CEA-Scan) can disclose tumors missed by mammography [73,84].

Mammography has a high rate of detection of nonpalpable breast carcinoma, but cannot always reliably differentiate benign from malignant lesions. A substantial number of breast biopsies for benign conditions result. The utility of Tc-sestamibi in differentiating malignant from benign breast disease is discussed elsewhere in this book. However, a similar use of Tc-99m CEA scan may prove more specific. Rosner et al. evaluated the utility of Tc-arcitumomab in 72 patients with nonpalpable, indeterminate, or suspicious mammographic lesions. In 13 patients with early, nonpalpable primary breast cancer, six were detected by

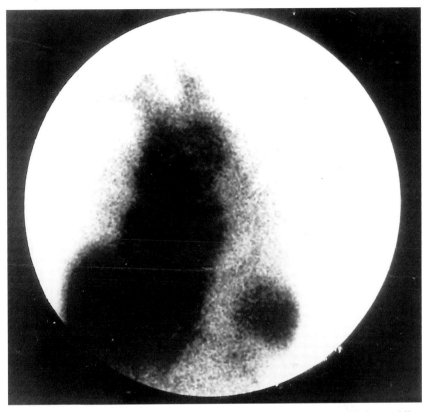

FIGURE 11   Another patient with a large inflammatory breast cancer. This is an oblique view taken 72 hours after intravenous In-111 B72.3 (satumomab). Note the intense uptake of In-111 B72.3 (now also referred to as oncoscint) by the breast cancer.

scintigraphy, while seven were falsely negative. Of these 7/13, five were not thought to be low-probability or indeterminate, while five were thought to be suspicious by immunoscintigraphy. Of the 59 patients with benign disease, 57 scans were negative, while two were falsely positive. This resulted in a specificity of 97%, better than the 75% reported for mammography. The false-negative rate in patients with low-probability, indeterminate mammograms was 4.1%, vs. 10.2% for mammography [95]. It can also help differentiate between benign, abnormal hyperplasia with atypia, and carcinoma, thus having higher specificity than mammography [74]. Unfortunately, this potential cannot be widely utilized, since the antibody is not FDA approved for that use in the U.S.

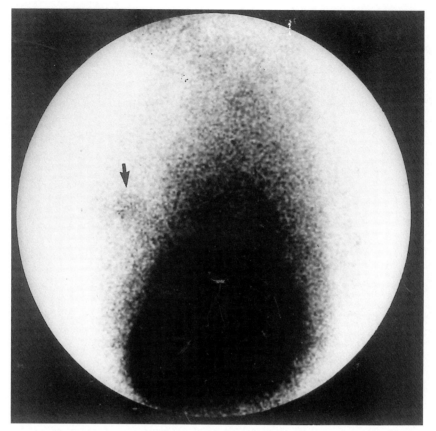

FIGURE 12 A lateral view in this patient shows the heterogeneity of the uptake of In-111 B72.3 in the breast lesion. This image was acquired at 72 hours after 5-mCi injection—a 10-min planar image.

C. Future Prospects

Clinical considerations that will determine the usage of these agents are discussed above. However, there are several other factors, such as acceptance by third-party payers, insurers, and managed care, as well as FDA approval of the agents with an indication for breast cancer detection. FDA approval is essential before managed care organizations can incorporate radiolabeled antibody imaging into their diagnostic protocol algorithms.

Based on our experience and that of others over several years, we believe radioimmunodetection with anti-CEA antibody can save money for the health care system. However, more work needs to be done. Upstaging patients by diag-

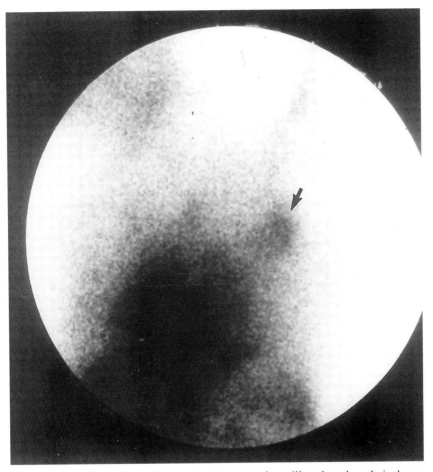

FIGURE 13   A rare example of metastatic disease to the axillary lymph node is demonstrated in this axillary view (anterior oblique with arrows up). It shows the axillary lymph nodes uptake—often missed by this antibody.

nosing widespread disease may lead to postponement or cancelation of surgery, thus saving the patient unnecessary surgery.In addition, by detecting lymph node involvement, surgery may be switched from a limited procedure to a more radical one. One can use the immunoscintigraphy to follow the progress of chemotherapy, as already discussed. All of these potential uses await the approval of the Mabs for breast cancer. Lastly, the radiolabeled antibodies may have the capability of early detection of breast cancer, especially in patients with high risk factors, but this has not been established.

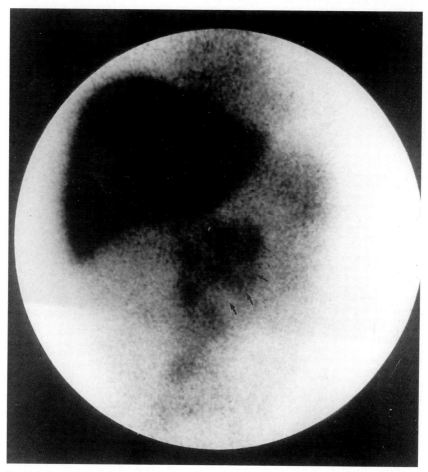

FIGURE 14   This anterior abdominal image at 72 hours postinjection shows significant metastatic lesions in the abdominal lymph nodes. Note the high liver uptake of the ln-111 B72.3 (oncoscint) antibody, which is a common finding with ln-111-labeled intact IgG antibodies.

Other potential uses of the radiolabeled antibodies in breast cancer management include radioimmuno-guided surgery with a gamma probe. While there have been some studies demonstrating the utility of RIGS in colorectal surgery, the utility of intraoperative detection of involved lymph nodes, in patients with breast cancer, has yet to be evaluated. Intraoperative probe for detection of concentration of radiolabeled antibody in lymph nodes is now available and already being used by many breast surgeons. This can make the surgery more complete, with removal of all diseased nodes.

One area that will contribute significantly to the potential future clinical role of Mabs in breast cancer management is the developments in the technical aspect of bioengineering of Mabs. Better fragments of old antibodies, such as B72.3, are already in the making. Antibodies to more specific antigens and epitopes for breast cancer for diagnosis and therapy will be developed [55,111,105,120,126–128]. Human or humanized antibody fragments are in clinical trials. Improvement in radiolabeling techniques for both diagnosis and therapy are being explored.

When the ideal radioimmunoconjugate that localizes in high concentration in a large percentage of tumors is identified, the potential for radioimmunotherapy will become compelling. Radioimmunoimaging will play a crucial role in determining eligibility for radioimmunotherapy and for determining dosimetry. Therapeutic trials with the murine antibody BrE-3 and with the humanized anti-CEA antibody are already under way.

REFERENCES

1. Goldenberg DM, DeLand FH. Use of radiolabeled antibodies to carcinoembryonic antigen for the detection and localization of diverse cancers by external photoscanning. NEJM 298:1384–1388, 1978.
2. Goldenberg DM, Larson SM. Radioimmunodetection in cancer identification. J Nucl Med 33:803–814, 1992.
3. Goldenberg DM, Kim EE, DeLand FM, Bennett S, Primus FJ. Radioimmunodetection of cancer with radioactive antibodies to carcinoembryonic antigen. Cancer Res 40:2984–2992, 1980.
4. Pressman D. The zone of activity of antibodies as determined by theuse of radioactive tracers. Ann NY Acad Sci 11:203–206, 1949.
5. Pressman D, Korngold L. The in vivo localization of anti-Wagner osteogenic sarcoma antibodies. Cancer 6:619–623, 1953.
6. Kohler G, Milstein C. Continuous cultures of fused cells secreting antibody of predefined specificities. Nature 256:495–504, 1975.
7. Lamki L, Kim EE, Haynie TP. Tumor Immunoscintigraphy Using Monoclonal Antibodies. In: Roth J, ed. Monoclonal antibodies in cancer: advances in diagnosis and treatment. Mount Kisco, New York: Futura Publishing Co.: 259–288, 1986.
8. Murray JL, Rosenblum MG, Sobol RE, Bartholomew RM, Plager CE, Haynie TP, Jahns MG, Glenn HJ, Lamki L, Benjamin RS, Papadopoulos N, Boddie AW, Fincke JM, David GS, Carlo DJ, Herch EM. Radioimmunoimaging in malignant melanoma with In-111 labeled monoclonal antibody 96.5. Cancer Res 45:2376–2381, 1985.
9. Murray JL, Rosenblum MG, Lamki L, Glenn HJ, Krizan Z, Hersh EM, Plager CE, Bartholomew RM, Unger MW, Carlo DJ. Clinical parameters related to optimal tumor localization of indium-111 labeled mouse antimelanoma monoclonal antibody ZME-018. J Nucl Med 28:25–33, 1987.

10. Babaian FJ, Murray JL, Lamki L, Haynie TP, Hersh EM, Rosenblum MG, Glenn HJ, Unger MW, Carlo DJ, Von Eschenbach AC. Radioimmunological imaging of metastatic prostatic cancer with 111Indium-labeled monoclonal antibody PAY 276. J Urol 137:439–443, 1987.

11. Hansen HJ, Jones AL, Grebenau R, Kunz A, Goldenberg DM. Labeling of anti-tumor antibodies and antibody fragments with Tc-99m. (Review Article). Cancer Treatment 7 Research. 51:233–244, 1990.

12. Murray JL, Lamki L, Shanken LJ, Blake ME, Plager CE, Benjamin RS, Schweighardt, S, Unger MW, Rosenblum MG, Murray JL, Lamki L, Shanken LJ, Blake ME, Plater CE, Benjamin RS, Schweighardt S, Unger MW, Rosenblum MG. Immunospecific saturable clearance mechanisms for Indium-111 labeled anti-melanoma monoclonal antibody 96.5 in humans. Cancer Res 48:4417–4422, 1988.

13. Murray JL, Rosenblum MG, Lamki L, Haynie TP, Glenn HJ, Plager CE, Unger MW, Carlo DJ, Hersh EM. Radioimmunoimaging in malignant melanoma patients with the use of Indium-111 labeled antimelanoma monoclonal antibody (ZME-018) to high molecular weight antigen. NCI Monograph (3):3–9, 1987.

14. Lamki LM, Kasi LP, Kim EE, Podoloff DA, Haynie TP. Radioimmunoscintigraphy of cancer. Cancer Bull 40:143–1150, 1988.

15. Carrasquillo JA, Sugarbaker P, Colcher D. Radioimmunoscintigraphy of colon cancer with iodine-131 labeled B72.3 monoclonal antibody. J Nucl Med 29:1022–1030, 1988.

16. Thor A, Ohuchi N, Szpak CA, Johnson WW. Distribution of oncofetal antigen tumor associated glycoprotein TAG-72 defined by monoclonal antibody B72.3. Cancer Res 46:3118–3124, 1986.

17. Smedley HM, Finan P, Lennox ES, Ritson A, Takei F, Wraight P, Sikora K. Localisation of metastatic carcinoma by a radiolabelled monoclonal antibody. Br J Canc 47(2):253–259, 1983.

18. Tjandra JJ, McKenzie IF. Murine monodlonal antibodies in breast cancer, an overview. Br J Surg 75(11):106–177, 1988.

19. Thor A, Weeks MO, Schlom J. Monoclonal antibodies and breast cancer. Sem Oncol 13(4):393–401, 1986.

20. Epenetos A, Britton KE, Mather S, Granowska M, et al. Targeting of I-123 labeled tumor associated monoclonal antibodies to ovarian, breast and gastrointestinal tumors. Lancet 2(8306):999–1005, 1982.

21. Lamki L. Radioimmunoscintigraphy of cancer: problems, pitfalls andprospects. In: "Nuclear Medicine Annual, 1990." Freeman L, ed. New York: Raven Press, 113–150, 1990.

22. Lamki LM, Patt YZ, Rosenbllum MG, Shanken LJ, Thompson L, Sweighward S, Frinckl JM, Murray JL. Metastatic colorectal cancer: radioimmunoscintigraphy with a stabilized In-111-labeled F(ab')2 fragment of an anti-CEA monoclonal antibody. Radiology 174:147–151, 1990.

23. Patt YZ, Lamki LM, Shanken J, Jessup JM, Charsangavej C, Ajanu JJ, Levin B, Merchant B, Halverson C, Murray JL. Imaging with Indium-111-labeled anticarcinomembryonic antigen monoclonal antibody ACE-025 of recurrent colorectal or CEA-producing cancer in patients with rising serum carcinoembryonic antigen and occult metastases. J Clin Oncol 8(7):1246–1254, 1990.

24. Doerr RJ, Abdel-Nabi H, Merchant B. indium-111 ZCE 025 immunoscintigraphy in occult recurrent colorectal cancer with elevated carcinoembryonic antigen level. Arch Surg 125:226–229, 1990.

25. Abdel-Nabi H, Doerr RJ, Chan HW. Safety and role of repeated administration of In-111 labeled anticarconoembryonic antigen monoclonal antibody ACE 025 in the postoperative follow-up of colorectal carcinoma patients. J Nucl Med 33:14–22, 1992.

26. Divgi CR, McDermott K, Johnson DK. Detection of hepatic metastases from colorectal carcinoma using Indium-111 (111In) labeled monoclonal antibody (mAb): MSKCC experience with mAb 111In-C110. Nucl Med Biol 18:705–710, 1991.

27. Doerr RJ, Abdel-Nabi H, Baker JM, Steinberg S. Detection of primary mcolorectal cancer with indium-111 monoclonal antibody B72.3. Arch Surg 125:1601–1605, 1990.

28. Lamki LM, Zukiwski AA, Shanken LJ, Legha SS, Benjamin RS, Plager CE, Salk DF, Schroff RW, Murray JL. Radioimaging of melanoma using 99m-Tc-labeled Fab fragment reactive with a high molecular weight melanoma antigen. Cancer Res 50(Suppl): 904s–908s, 1990.

29. Murray JL, Lamki LM, Rosenblum MG. Radioimmunoimaging of malignant melanoma with monoclonal antibodies. In: Cancer treatment and research, malignant melanoma: biology, diagnosis, and therapy. Nathanson L, ed. Dordrecht, Netherlands/Boston: Kluwer Academic Publishers, 123–153, 1988.

30. Murray JI, Lamki LM, Rosenblum MG, Haynie TP, Glenn HJ, Hersh EM. Clinical use of monoclonal antibodies in cancer therapy and imaging: current status, controversies, and future direction. Martinis Nijhofs, Publishing Co., Boston, Mass.

31. Lamki L, Murray JL, Rosenblum M, Patt YZ, Babaian R, Unger M. Effect of unlabelled monoclonal antibody (MoAb) on biodistribution of 111-Indium labelled MoAb. Nucl Med Commun 9:553–564, 1988.

32. Mardirossian G; Wu C; Rusckowski M; Hnatowich DJ. The stability of 99Tc-m directly labelled to an Fab' antibody via stannous ion and mercaptoethanol reduction. Nucl Med Com 13(7):503–512, 1992.

33. Wahl RL, Swanson NA, Johnson JW, Natale RB, Petry NA, Mallette S, Kasina S, Reno J, Sullivan K, Abrams P. Clinical experience with Tc-99m labeled (N2S2) anti-melanoma antibody fragments and single photon emission computed tomography. Am J Physiol Imag 7(2):48–58, 1992.

34. Crippa F, Buraggi GL, Di Re E, Gasparini M, Seregeni E. Radioimmunoscintigraphy of ovarian cancer with the Mov18 monoclonal antibody. Eur J Cancer 27(6):724–729, 1991.

35. Kim EE, Podoloff DA, Moulopoulos I et al. Magnetic resonance Imaging, positron emission tomography and radioimmunoscintigraphy of Breast cancer. Cancer Bull 45:500–505, 1993.

36. Lamki L, Buzdar AU, Singletary SE, Rosenblum MG, Bhadkamkar V, Esparza L, Podoloff DA, Zukiwski A, Hortobagyi GN, Murray JL. Indium-111 labeled B72.3 monoclonal antibody in the detection and staging of breast cancer: a phase I study. J Nucl Med 32(7):1326–1332, 1991.

37. Colcher D, Horan-Hand P, Nuti J, Schlom M. A spectrum of monoclonal antibodies reactive with human mammary tumors. Proc Natl Acad Sci USA 78:3199–3203, 1981.

38. Granowska M, Biassoni L, Carroll MJ, Howell R, Mather SH, Ellison D, Granowski

A, Briwwon KE. Breast cancer 99mTc SM3 radioimmunoscintigraphy. Acta Oncol 35(3):319–321, 1996.

39. Murray JL, Macey DJ, Grant EJ, Rosenblum MG, Kasi LP, Zhang HZ, Katz RI, Riger PT, LeBherz D, Bhadkamkar V. Enhanced TAG-72 expression and tumor uptake of radiolabeled monoclonal antibody CC49 in metastatic breast cancer patients following alpha-interferon treatment. Cancer Res 55(23 Suppl):5925s–5928s, 1995.

40. Rosner D, Nabi H, Wild L, Nabi-Ortman J, Hreschyshyn MM. Diagnosis of breast carcinoma with radiolabeled monoclonal antibodies (MoAbs) to carcinoembryonic antigen (CEA) and human milk fat globulin (HMFG). Cancer Investigation 13(6):573–582, 1995.

41. Kramer EL, DeNardo SJ, Liebes L, Noz ME, Kroger L, Glenn SD, Furmanski P, Ceriani R. Radioimmunolocalization of breast cancer using BrE-3 monoclonal antibody. Adv Exper Med Biol 353:181–192, 1994.

42. Peterson JA, Ceriani RL. Breast mucin and associated antigens in diagnosis and therapy. Adv Exper Med Biol 353:1–8, 1994.

43. Steinstrasser A, Oberhausen E. Anti-CEA labeling kit BW 431/26: results of the European multicenter trial. Nuklearmedizin 34(6):232–242, 1995.

44. Christian RB, Couto JR, Peterson JA, Ceriani RL. Cloning and expression of cDNAs encoding the variable domains of the antibreast carcinoma antibody Mc5. Hybridoma 15(2):155–158, 1996.

45. Allan SM, Dean CJ, Eccles S, Sacks NP. Clinical radioimmunolocalization with a rat monoclonal antibody directed against c-erbB-2. Cell Biophysics 24–25:93–98, 1994.

46. Brummendorf TH, Kaul S, Schuhmancher J, Baum RP, Matys R, Klivenyi G, Adams S, Bastert G. Immunoscintigraphy of human mammary Carcinoma xenografts using monoclonal antibodies 12H12 Bs BM-2 labeled with 99mTc and radioiodine. Cancer Res 54(15):4162–4168, 1994.

47. Yemul S, Leon JA, Pozniakoff T, Esser PD, Estabrook A. Radioimmunoimaging of human breast carcinoma xenografts in nude mouse model with 11In-labeled new monoclonal antibody EBA-1 and F(ab′)2 fragments. Nucl Med Biol 20(3):325–335, 1993.

48. Lind P, Hans-Jurgen G, Mikosch P, Kresnik E, Gomez I, Omann J, Dinges H-P, Boniface G. Radioimmunoscintigraphy with Tc-99m labeled monoclonal antibody 170H.82 in suspected primary, recurrent, or metastatic breast cancer. Clin Nucl Med 22:30–34, 1997.

49. Witters LM, Kumar R, Chinchilli VM, Lipton A. Enhanced anti-proliferate activity of the combination of tamoxifen plus HER-2. New Anti Br Canc Res Treat 42(1):1–5, 1997.

50. DiGiovanna MP, Carter D, Flynn SD, Stern DF. Functional assay for Her-2/neu demonstrates active signalling in a minority of Her-2/neu overexpressing invasive human breast tumours. Br J Canc 74(5):802–806, 1996.

51. Tosi E, Valota O, Canevari S, Adobati E, Casalini P, Perez P, Colnaghi MI. Anti-idogypic response to antigrowth factor receptor monoclonal antibodies. Eur J Canc 32A(3):498–505, 1996.

52. Charpin C, Bonnier P, Devictor B, Andrac L, Lavaut MN, Allasia C, Piana L. Immunodetection of Her-2/neu protein in frozen sections evaluated by image analysis: cor-

relation with overall and disease-free survival in breast carcinomas. Anticancer Res 13(3):603–612, 1993.

53. DeSantes K, Slamon D, Anderson SK, Shepard M, Fendly B, Maneval D, Press O. Radiolabeled antibody targeting of the Her 2/neu oncoprotein. Cancer Res 52(7):19916–1923, 1996.

54. Merino MJ, Monteagugo C, Neumann RD. Monoclonai antibodies for radioim-munoscintigraphy of breast cancer. Int J Rad App Instr—Part B, Nuc Med Bio 18(4):437–443, 1991.

55. DeNardo SJ, O'Grady LF, Macey DJ, Kroger LA, DeNardo GL, Lamborn KR, Levy NB, Mills SL, Hellstrom I, Hellstrom KE. Quantitative imaging of mouse L-6 mono-clonal antibody in breast cancer patients to develop a therapeutic strategy. Int J Rad Appl Instr—Part B, Nuc Med Bio 18(6):621–631, 1991.

56. Lind P, Smola MG, Lechner P, Ratschek M, Klima G, Koltringer P, Steindorfer P, Eber O. The immunoscintigraphy use of Tc-99m-labelled monoclonal anti-CEA antibodies (BW 431-26) in patients with suspected primary, recurrent and metastatic breast can-cer. Int J Cancer 47(6):865–869, 1991.

57. Thor A, Edgerton SM. Monoclonal antibodies reactive with human breast or ovarian carcinoma: in vivo applications. Sem Nucl Med 4:295–308, 1989.

58. Allan, SM, Dean C, Fernando I, Eccles S, Styles J, McCready VR, Baum M, Sacks N. Radioimmunolocalisation in breast cancer using the gene product of c-erbB2 as the target antigen. Brit J Canc 67(4):706–712, 1993.

59. Athanassiou A, Pectasides B, Pateniotis K, Tzimis L, Natsis P, Lafi A, Arapantoni P, Koutsiouba P, Taylor-Papadimitriou J, Epenetos A. Immunoscintigraphy with 131I-labelled HMFG2 and HMFG1 F(ab')2 in the pre-operative detection of clinical and subclinical lymph node metastases in breast cancer patients. Int J Canc 3(Suppl):89–95, 1988.

60. Nabi HA, Rosner D, Ortman-Nabi J, et al. Immunoscintigraphy of breast cancers with I-123 HMFG1 and 99m-Tc anti-CEA (CYT-380) monoclonal antibodies: initial clin-ical results and literature review. Tumor Targeting 1:223–231, 1995.

61. Taylor-Papadimitriou J, Peterson JA, Arklie J, Burchell J, Ceriani RL, Bodmer WF. Monoclonal antibodies to epithelium specific components of the human milk fat glob-ule membrane: production and reaction with cells in culture. Int J Canc 28(1):17–21, 1981.

62. Burchell J, Durbin H, Taylor-Papadimitriou J. Complexity of expression of antigenic determinants, recognized by monoclonal antibodies HMFG1 And HMFG2 in normal and malignant human mammary epithelial cells. J Immunol 131:508–513, 1983.

63. Primus FJ, Newell KD, Blue A, Goldenberg DM. Immunological heterogeneity of carcinoembryonic antigen: antigenic determinants on carcinoembryonic antigen dis-tinguished by monoclonal antibodies. Cancer Res 43(2):686–692, 1983.

64. Reynoso G, Chu TM, Haloyoke D, Cohen E, Nemoto T, Wang JJ, Chuang J, Guinan P, Murphy GP. Carcinoembryonic antigen in patients with different cancers. JAMA 220(3):361–365, 1972.

65. GL DeNardo, SJ DeNardo, LF O'Grady, NB Levy, GP Adams, SL Mills. Fractionated radioimmunotherapy of B-cell malignancies with 1311 lym-1. Cancer Res 50(3 Suppl):1014s–1016s, 1990.

66. Goldenberg DM, Horowitz JA, Sharky RM, Hall TC, Murthy S, Goldenbert H, Lee

RE, Stein R, Siegel JA, Izon DO. Targeting dosimetry and radioimmunotherapy of b-cell lymphomas with iodine-131 labeled LL2 monoclonal antibody. J Clin Oncol 9(4):548–564, 1991.

67. Goldenberg DM, Larson SM. Radioimmunodetection in cancer identification. J Nucl Med 33:803–814, 1992.

68. Nabi HA, Erb DA, Cronin VR. Superiority of SPECT to planar imaging in the detection of colorectal carcinomas with 111In monoclonal antibodies. Nucl Med Commun 16(8):631–639, 1995.

69. Griffiths GL, Goldenberg DM, Jones AL, Hansen HJ. Radiolabeling of monoclonal antibodies and fragments with technetium and rhenium. Bioconj Chem 3(2):91–99, 1992.

70. McEwan AJB, McLean GD, Hooper HR, Sykes T, McQuarrie SA, Golberg L, Bodnar DM, Lloyd SL, Noujaim AA. MoAb 170H.82: an evaluation of a novel panadenocarcinoma monoclonal antibody labelled with Tc-99m and In-111. Nucl Med Commun 13(1):11–19, 1992.

71. De Castiglia SG, Duran A, Fiszman G, Horenstein AL. 99mTc direct labeling of anti-CEA monoclonal antibodies: quality control and preclinical studies. Nucl Med Biol 22(3):367–372, 1995.

72. Duran AP, Asurmendi S, D'Orio E, Horenstein AL, DeCastiglia SG. Direct labeling of monoclonal antibodies with 99mTc and radioimmunodetection of a murine mammary carcinoma with 99mTc-B2C114. J Nucl Biol Med 38(4 Suppl 1):33–37, 1994.

73. Gulec SA, Serafini AN, Sfakianakis GN, Chirinos RE, Franceschi D, Moffat FL, Franceschi D, Crichton VZ, Subramanian R, Klein JL, DeJager RL. CEA-scan in diagnosis and staging of breast cancer. J Nucl Med 37(Suppl 5):238P(Abstr), 1996.

74. Goldenberg DM, Juweid M, Dunn RM, Sharkey RM. Cancer imaging with radiolabeled antibodies: new advances with technetium-99m-labeled monoclonal antibody Fab' fragments, especially CEA-scan and prospects for therapy. J Nucl Med Technol 1997; 25:18–23, 1997.

75. Kairemo KJ. Immunolymphoscintigraphy with Tc-99m-labelled monoclonal antibody (BW 431/26) reacting with carcinoembryonic antigen in breast cancer. Cancer Res 50(3 Suppl):949s–954s, 1990.

76. Hansen HJ, Jones AL, Sharkey RM, Grebenau R, Blazejewski N, Kuna A, Buckley MJ, Newman ES, Ostella F, Goldenberg DM. Pre-clinical evaluation of an instant Tc-99m labeling kit for antibody imaging. Cancer Res 50(3 Suppl):794s–798s, 1990.

77. Schultes BC, Reinsberg J, Wagner U, Schlesbusch H, Ritchter J, Krebs D, Biersack HJ. Idiotypic cascades after injection of the monoclonal antibody OC125: a study in the mouse model. Cell Biophysics 24–25:259–266, 1994.

78. Wahl RL, Parker CW, Philpott GW. Improved radioimaging and tumor localization with monoclonal F(ab')2. J Nucl Med 24:316–325, 1983.

79. Pinsky CM, Sasso NL, Mojsiak JZ, Hansen HJ, et al. Results of a multicenter Phase III clinical trial of ImmuRaid ®-CEA-Tc-99m imaging of patients with colorectal cancer. Proc Amer Soc Clin Oncol 10:136 (Abstr), 1991.

80. Torres G, Berna L, Estorch M, Juarez C, Martinez-Duncker D, Carrio. I. Preexisting human anti-murine antibodies and the effect of immune complexes on the outcome of immunoscsintigraphy. Clin Nucl Med 18(6):477–481, 1993.

81. Larson SM, Carrasquillo JA, Krohn KA, Brown JP, McGuffin RW, Fernens JM, Gra-

ham MM, Hill LD, Beaumier PL, Hellstrom KE, Hellstrom I. Localization of 131-I-labeled p97-specific Fab fragments in human melanoma as a basis for radiotherapy. J Clin Invest 72:2102–2114, 1983.

82. de Kruif J, Van der Vuurst AR, de Vries AR, Cilenti L, Boel E, van Ewijk W, Logtenberg T. New perspectives on recombinant human antibodies. Immunol Today 17(10):453–455, 1996.

83. Package Insert Oncoscint (Satumomab, In-111 B72.3).

84. Barron B, Lamki L, Pinero S, and Bull J. Clinical utility of Tc-99m-anti-CEA antibody (IMMU-4) in the evaluation of breast cancer. Clin Nucl Med 19:267(Abst), 1994.

85. Gold P, Freedman SO. Demonstration of tumor-specific antigens in human colon carcinomata by immunological tolerance and adsorption techniques. J Exp Med 21:439–462, 1965.

86. Krupey J, Wilson T, Freedman SO, Gold P. The preparation of purified carcinoembryonic antigen of the human digestive system from large quantities of tumor tissue. Immunochem 9:617–622, 1972.

87. Haseman MK, Brown DW, Keeling CA, Reed NL. Radioimmunodetection of occult carcinoembryonic antigen-producing cancer. J Nucl Med 33(10):1750–1756, 1992.

88. Chung JK, Jang JJ, Lee DS, Lee MC, Koh CS. Tumor concentration and distribution of carcinoembryonic antigen measured by in vitro quantitative autoradiography. J Nucl Med 35(9):1499–1505, 1994.

89. Hansen HJ, Snyder JJ, Miller E, Vandevoorde JP, Miller ON, Hines LR, Burns JJ. Carcinoembryonic antigen (CEA) assay. A laboratory adjunct in the diagnosis and management of cancer. Human Pathol 5(2):139–147, 1974.

90. Goldenberg DM, Neville AM, Carter AC, Go VLW, Holyoke ED, Isselbacher KJ, Schein PS, Schwartz M. CEA (carcinoembryonic antigen): its role as a marker in the management of cancer. J Canc Res Clin Oncol 101(3):239–242, 1981.

91. Stramignoni D, Bowen R, Atkinson Bm Schlom J. Differential reactivity of monoclonal antibodies with human colon adenocarcinomas and adenomas. Int J Canc 31:543–0552, 1981.

92. Nabi HA, Rosner D, Erb D, Panaro V, Doerr R. Evaluation of suspicious mammographic findings with CEA-Scans and correlation with histophatological results. J Nucl Med 37(Suppl):238p(Abstr), 1996.

93. Barron B, Lamki LM, Pinero S, Shepard P, Bull JM, Holoye P, Ephron VJ, MacFadyen B, Ingram L, Oggero K, Duke J. Clinical use of Tc-99m anti-carcinoembryonic antigen antibody in the evaluation of the breast. Radiology 193(P):424, 1994.

94. Rosner D, Abdel-Nabi H, Panaro V, Erb D, et al. Immunoscintigraphy (IS) may reduce the number of surgical biopsies in women with benign breast disease (BBD) and indeterminate mammograms: a novel approach. Anu Meet Am Soc Clin Oncol 15:A75, 1996.

95. Rosner D, Abdel-Nabi H, Panaro V, Goldenberg D. Personal communication.

96. Nabi HA. Antibody imaging in breast cancer. Sem Nucl Med 27(1):30–39, 1997.

97. Harwood SJ, Abdel-Nabi H. The use of monoclonal antibodies for radioscintigraphic detection of cancer. J Pharm Proc 7:93–116, 1994.

98. Nabi HA, Seldin D, Barron B, et al. CEA-SCAN radioimmunodetection of primary breast lesions: results of phase II multi center trial. Eur J Nucl Med 22(P):878 (abstr), 1995.

99. Riva P, Marangolo M, Tison V, Armaroli L, Moscatelli G, Franceschi G, Spineli A, Vecchietti G, Morigi P, Tassini R. Treatment of metastatic colorectal cancer by means of specific monoclonal antibodies conjugated with iodine-131: a phase II study. Int J Rad Appl Instr—Part B, Nucl Med Bio 18(1):109–119, 1991.

100. Nuti M, Teramato YA, Marian-Constantini R, Hand PH, Colcher D, Schlom J. A monoclonal antibody (B72.3) defines patterns of distribution of a novel tumor-associated antigen in human mammary carcinoma cell populations. Int J Canc 29(5):539–545, 1982.

101. Keith Britton. Personal communication,

102. Hayes BF, Zalutsky MR, Kaplan W, Noska M, Thor A, Colcher D, Kufe DW. Pharmacokinetics of radiolabeled monoclonal antibody B6.2 in patients with metastatic breast cancer. Cancer Res 46(6):3957–3163, 1986.

103. Thor A, Ohuchi N, Szpak CA, Johnston WW, Schlom J. Distribution of oncofetal antigen tumor-associated glycoprotein-72 defined by monoclonal antibody B72.3. Cancer Res 46(6):3118–3124, 1986.

104. Nieroda CA, Mojzisik C, Sardi A, Farrar WB, Hinkle G, Siddiqi MA, Ferrara PJ, James A, Schlom J, Thurston MO. Staging of carcinoma of the breast using a hand-held gamma detecting probe and monoclonal antibody B72.3. Surg Gyn Obs 169(1):35–40, 1989.

105. Major P, Wang TQ, Ishida M, Unger M, Rosenthall L. Breast cancer imaging with mouse monoclonal antibodies. Eur J Nucl Med 15(10):655–660, 1989.

106. Kalofonos HP, Sakier JM, Hatzistylianou M, Pervez S, Taylor-Papadimitriou J, Waxman JH, Lavender JP, Wood C, Epenetos AA. Kinetics, quantitative analysis and radioimmunolocalization using Indium-111-HMFG1 monoclonal antibody in patients with breast cancer. Br J Canc 59(6):939–942, 1989.

107. McKenzie IF, Xing PX. Mucins in breast cancer: recent immunological advances. Cancer Cells 2:75–78, 1990.

108. Arklie J, Taylor Papadimitrious J, Bodner W, Egan M, Millis R. Differentiation antigens expressed by epithelial cells in the lactating breast are also detectable in breast cancer. Int J Canc 28(1):23–29, 1981.

109. Brummendorf TH, Kaul S, Schulmacher J, Baum FP, Kliveny G, Matys R, Eichler A, Guckel B, Beldermann F, Bastert G. Immunoscintigraphy of breast cancer xenografts. 99m-Tc-labeled anti-mucin monoclonal antibodies BM-7 and 12H12. Nukearmedizin 34(5):197–202, 1995.

110. McEwan AJB, McLean GD, Goldberg L, Boniface G, Sykes T, McQuarrie S, Amyotte G, Noujaim A. Tc-99m-170H.82 (TRUSCINT®), A new monoclonal antibody for imaging breast cancer: a preliminary analysis. J Nucl Med 34(5):213p (Abstr), 1993.

111. McEwan A, MacLean GD, Golberg L, et al. Evaluating radioimmunoscintigraphy in patients with breast cancer. Eur J Nucl Med 21:748P (Abstr), 1994.

112. De Santes K, Slamon D, Anderson SK, Shepard M, Fendly B, Maneval D, Press O. Radiolabeled antibody targeting of the HER-2/neu oncoprotein. Cancer Res 52(7):1916–1923, 1992.

113. Korpi-Tommola ET, Kairemo KJ, Jekunen AP, Niskanen EO, Savolainen SE. Double-tracer dosimetry of organs in assessment of bone marrow involvement by two monoclonal antibodies. Acta Oncologia 35(3):357–365, 1996.

114. Fisher B, Redmond C, Fisher ER, Bauer M, Wolmark N, Wickerham DL, Deutsch M, Montague E, Margolese R, Foster. Ten-year results of a randomized clinical trial comparing radical mastectomy and total mastectomy with or without radiation. N Engl J Med 312(11):674–681, 1985.

115. Tijandra JJ Sacks NP, Thompson CH, Leyden MJ, Stacker SA, Liechtenstein M, Russell IS, Collins JP, Andrews JT, Pietersz GA, McKenzie IFC. The detection of axillary lymph node metastases from breast cancer by radiolabelled monoclonal antibodies: a prospective study. Br J Cancer 59(2):296–302, 1989.

116. Stephens AD, Punja U, Sugarbaker PH. False-positive lymph nodes by radioimmunoguided surgery: report of a patient and analysis of the problem. J Nucl Med 34(5):804–808, 1993.

117. Pecking AP, Bertrand FJ, Lokiec FM, et al. Pre-operative immunolymphoscintigraphy with human monoclonal antibody (16.88 lilo) to assess the nodal involvement in breast cancer. In: Cluzan RV Peckign AP, Loklec FM, eds. Progress in Lymphology XIII, Excerpta Medica 307–311, 1922.

118. Mangili F, Sassi I, DiRocco M, Leone BE, Garancini P, Santambrogio G. Breast carcinoma detection with a combination of radiolabeled monoclonal antibodies: promising results from immunohistochemical studies. Cancer 78(11):2334–2339, 1996.

119. Kairemeo KJ, Kiuru AJ, Heikkonen JJ. Image subtraction analysis with technetium-99m labeled monoclonal antibody and colloid for evaluation of liver lesions: phantom measurements and patient studies. Acta Oncologica 32(7–8):763–769, 1993.

120. Lind P, Lechner P, Kuttnig M, Klimpfinger M, Koltringer W, Cesnik H, Eber O. Differentiation in a patient with follicular thyroid and breast cancer. Nuklearmedizin 29(6):278–281, 1990.

121. Thompson CH, Lichtenstein M, Stacker SA, Leyden MJ, Salehi N, Andrews JT, McKenzie IF. Immunoscintigraphy for detection of lymph node metastases from breast cancer. Lancet 2(8414):1245–1247, 1984.

122. Rombi G, Cossu F, Melis G. MoAb-labeled liposomes in breast cancer cell targeting: therapeutics and diagnostic use of polyspecific artificial carriers. Ann N Y Acad Sci 698:429–435, 1993.

123. Terui S, Yamamoto H. New simplified lymphoscintigraphic technique in patients with breast cancer. J Nucl Med 1989; 30:1198–1204, 1989.

124. Mandeville R, Patiesky N, Philipp K, Kubista E, Dumas F, Grouix B. Immunolymphoscintigraphy of axillary lymph node metastases in breast cancer patients using monoclonal antibodies: first clinical findings. Anticancer Res 6(6):1257–1263, 1986.

125. Tjandra JJ, Russell IS, Collins JP, Andrews JT, Lichtenstein M, Binns D, McKenzie IF. Immunolymphoscintigraphy for the detection of lymph node metastases from breast cancer. Cancer Res 49(6):1600–1608, 1989.

126. Mackworth-Young CG. The Michael Mason Prize Essay: antiphospholipid antibodies and disease. Br J Rheum 34(11):1009–1030, 1995.

127. Diel IJ, Kaufmann M, Costa SD, Bastert G. Monoclonal antibodies to detect breast cancer cells in bone marrow. Important Adv Oncol 143–164, 1994.

128. DeLand F, Kim E, Corgan R, et al. Axillary lymphoscintigraphy in radioimmunodetection of carcinoembryonic antigen in breast cancer. J Nucl Med 20:1243–1250, 1979.

129. Longnecker BM, Willans DJ, MacLean GD, et al. Monoclonal antibodies and syn-

thetic tumor-associated glycoconjugates in the study of Thomson-Friedenreich-Like and Tn-Like antigens on human cancers. JNCI 78:489–496, 1987.

130. MacLean GD, McEwan AJ, Noujaim AA, et al. Two novel monoclonal antibodies have potential for gynecologic cancer imaging antibody. Immunoconj Radiopharm 4:297–308, 1991.

131. McEwan A, MacLean GD, Golberg L, et al. 99m-Tc 170H.82. A monoclonal antibody for the evaluation of patients with breast cancer. Eur J Nucl Med 19:8 (abstr), 1992.

132. Joshi MG, Lee AD, Pedersen CA, Schnitt S, Camus MG, Hughes KS. The role of immunocytochemical markers in the differential diagnosis of proliferative and neoplastic lesions of the breast. Mod Pathol 9(1):57–67, 1996.

133. Kennedy MJ. Metastatic breast cancer. Current opinion in oncology 8(6):485–490, 1996.

6

Breast Imaging with Radiolabeled Peptides

Eric P. Krenning, Marion de Jong, Roelf Valkema, and Casper H. J. van Eijck
University Hospital Rotterdam, Rotterdam, The Netherlands

I. INTRODUCTION

Since somatostatin and its analogs (and their receptors) are the most frequently discussed and used of all peptides in relation to breast cancer scintigraphy, their application is the main focus of this chapter.

After Schönbrunn and Tashjian first measured somatostatin receptors in 1978 using the clonal pituitary cell line GH4C [1], somatostatin receptors have been demonstrated on a variety of human tumors, using various iodinated somatostatin analogs in homogenate ligand binding assays or autoradiography on tissue sections [2,3]. Large numbers of binding sites with high affinity for somatostatin were found on most tumors with amine precursor uptake and decarboxylation (APUD) characteristics, as well as on meningiomas, well-differentiated brain tumors (astrocytomas), neuroblastomas, and human breast tumors [4–20]. Pharmacological studies have shown that the distribution of somatostatin receptors is often heterogeneous and that there are selective subtypes for both somatostatin (SS-14) and the precursor form prosomatostatin (SS-28). The biological activity of the two peptides generally correlates with their potency for receptor binding in most systems, suggesting that their selective actions result mainly from differential interaction with receptors [21–26].

Reubi et al. have identified pharmacologically different somatostatin receptor subtypes in rat and human brain by means of their differential affinity for certain somatostatin analogs [27–29]. At least five different human somatostatin receptor types have been cloned. All subtypes bind SS-14 and SS-28 with high affinity, while their affinity for the long-acting analog octreotide differs considerably (see below) [30–33]. The cloning of five human somatostatin receptor subtypes may provide the molecular basis for how somatostatin regulates differential functions, and this may lead to the development of selective analogs for a variety of clinical applications. Most somatostatin receptor-positive human tumors express the somatostatin receptor subtype 2 (sst$_2$); only a few have exclusively other somatostatin receptor subtypes.

A. Neuroendocrine Differentiation of Breast Cancer

Since expression of somatostatin receptors was a known feature of tumors of the nervous system, neuroendocrine tissues, and endocrine gastrointestinal tumors, Papotti et al. correlated the expression of neuroendocrine markers in human breast cancer with the presence of somatostatin receptors [18]. The presence of neuroendocrine cells in normal as well as in human breast cancer has been a matter of controversy for a long time. As early as 1947, Vogler demonstrated argyrophilic cells in normal breast tissue [34]. Later on, Freyter and Hartmann suggested, on the basis of silver impregnation, the endocrine nature of mucoid carcinomas ("carcinoids") of the human breast [35]. However, they were describing myoepithelial cells, which were not endocrine, as shown by several histochemical and electron-microscopic studies [36,37].

Between 1977 and 1982 several reports demonstrated a variety of argyrophilic breast tumors containing dense-core secretory granules and showing the typical features of carcinoids. Bussolati et al. also found argyrophilic chromogranin-positive cells immunocytochemically in part of human breast cancers with the mouse monoclonal antibody LK2H10 directed against human chromogranin [38]. Immunoreactivity for neuron-specific enolase, which is present in neurons, neuroendocrine cells, and tumors with neuroendocrine differentiation, was found in more than 30% of breast carcinomas. However, expression of this marker in mammary gland tissues does not appear to be always related to endocrine differentiation, as defined by ultrastructural demonstration of secretory granules. Other markers such as chromogranin A (CgA) and B and synaptophysin were later found to be more specific for neuroendocrine differentiation. In 391 patients with various tumors who underwent somatostatin receptor scintigraphy, we were recently able to make a comparison between serum values of CgA, neuron-specific enolase (NSE) and α-subunits of glycoprotein hormones (α-SU). Of 62 patients with breast cancer, elevated serum levels of CgA, NSE, and α-SU were found in 8%, 37%, and 10%, respectively; in 208 patients with various classical neuroendocrine tumors the mean figures were 50%, 43%, and 24%, respectively [39].

To correlate the existence of neuroendocrine differentiation with the presence of somatostatin receptors in breast carcinomas, Pappoti et al. stained a series of 100 cases with the Grimelius silver staining procedure, carried out immunocytochemistry with specific neuroendocrine markers, and compared the results with that of autoradiography for somatostatin receptors [18]. A highly significant correlation was established between the expression of neuroendocrine markers and high somatostatin receptor density. This occurred, however, in only seven of these 100 cases.

B.   Somatostatin Receptor Expression in Breast Cancer

In a large series Reubi et al. [16] evaluated the incidence of somatostatin receptors in a representative number of primary breast tumors. In a group of "small" tumor samples with a mean section surface of 14 mm^2, 21% of the tumors were somatostatin receptor-positive. However, in a group of "large" tumor samples with a mean section surface of 180 mm^2, 46% were somatostatin receptor-positive, and, especially in this group, often a nonhomogeneous distribution was seen, which means that tumor regions within somatostatin receptor-positive tumors were somatostatin receptor-negative. In their study they also showed that metastases of somatostatin receptor-positive primary tumors may often be somatostatin receptor-positive [16].

Binding capacities and apparent dissociation constants for somatostatin receptor were determined by Fekete et al. in 500 breast biopsy samples using multipoint membrane receptor assays [17]. In 36% of the tumor samples somatostatin receptors were present, and no correlation was found between somatostatin receptor binding sites and binding capacities of other receptors like estrogen, progesterone, and epidermal growth factor (EGF). A negative relationship between the expression of somatostatin receptor and EGF receptors in breast cancer samples was suggested by Reubi et al. [16].

C.   Genetic Characteristics and Somatostatin Receptor Expression in Breast Cancer

The study of breast cancer carcinogenesis is complicated by the heterogeneity of the disease. A way to reduce this problem is to delineate these tumors into clinically relevant subgroups. There are indications that breast carcinomas that express the somatostatin receptor are such a distinct subset. Clinical data assign better prognosis to patients with a somatostatin receptor-positive tumor [40].

Recently, we investigated whether somatostatin receptor-expressing breast tumors are also a distinct subgroup at the genetic level [41]. To this end a series of primary breast tumors were collected and tested for somatostatin receptor expression and for genetic alterations. For this survey we chose genetic markers that are frequently altered in both breast carcinomas and in neural or endocrine tumors such as neuroblastoma and small cell lung carcinoma. These are alterations of the retinoblastoma gene (RB1) and/or amplification of members of the *myc* family of oncogenes [42–47]. Amplification of the *neu* and *int*-2 oncogenes were also studied since these frequently occur in breast cancer.

In the course of the study it appeared that 58/87 (67%) of consecutively collected samples expressed the somatostatin receptor. This is higher than the 20% to 4% reported in the literature [13,16–18,40]. In an attempt to explain this observation, clinical and pathological characteristics of the tumors were investigated. Furthermore, to test whether the reported correlation between somatostatin receptor expression and neuroendocrine differentiation was maintained in this population, 43 of these tumors, 30 somatostatin receptor-positive and 13 somatostatin receptor-negative, were also examined for morphological and immunohistochemical markers of neuroendocrine differentiation. Three somatostatin receptor-positive tumors were also positive for two or more other markers of neuroendocrine differentiation, suggesting that neuroendocrine breast tumors and somatostatin receptor-positive breast tumors are overlapping, but independent, subgroups of tumors.

To test whether specific genetic alterations are associated with somatostatin receptor-positive or somatostatin receptor-negative breast tumors, we examined in a selected series of 47 somatostatin receptor-positive and 32 somatostatin receptor-negative breast tumors a number of known genetic markers by Southern blotting. Deletions or rearrangements of the retinoblastoma (RB) tumor-suppressor gene were observed in five somatostatin receptor-positive and five somatostatin receptor-negative tumors. In four somatostatin receptor-positive and also in four somatostatin receptor-negative tumors an amplification of the *neu* oncogene was observed. Amplifications of the *int*-2 oncogene were found in two somatostatin receptor-positive and one somatostatin receptor-negative breast tumor. In one somatostatin receptor-positive tumor an amplification of the c-*myc* oncogene was observed, and in another somatostatin receptor-positive tumor a rearrangement of the L-*myc* oncogene was found. These results indicated that no correlation exists between somatostatin receptor expression and alterations of the RB gene or amplification of one of the investigated proto-oncogenes.

II.   CHARACTERISTICS OF THE RADIOPHARMACEUTICAL

A.   Chemistry of [DTPA⁰]octreotide

The N^α-diethyleletriamepenta-acetic acid (DTPA, Fluka) derivative of octreotide was synthesized by Novartis (Basel, Switzerland) using the protected [ε-t-butyloxy-carbonyl-Lys⁵]octreotide as starting material which was available by the reaction of octreotide with di-t-butyl-dicarbonate [$(Boc)_2O$, Fluka] in dimethylformamide. DTPA was coupled to the selectively protected octreotide in form of its dianhydride. Purification of the product was achieved by silica gel chromatography in order to separate the wanted [DTPA⁰-ε-Boc-Lys⁵]octreotide from the contaminating double-substituted DTPA-derivative and unreacted starting material. Deprotecting with trifluoracetic acid and subsequent sequential purification yielded homogeneous [DTPA^0]octreotide (also called [DTPA-D-Phe^1]octreotide) as lyophilisate. The purity was checked by reverse-phase HPLC. Structure and amino acid composition were proven by means of nuclear magnetic resonance, fast atom bombardment mass spectrometry, and amino acid analysis [49].

B. Dosimetry

The effective dose equivalent of 222 MBq [^{111}In-DTPA^0]octreotide (about 16 mSv) is comparable to values for other ^{111}In-labeled radiopharmaceuticals and is acceptable in view of the clinical indications. Furthermore, these radiation doses have to be compared with the values of commonly used imaging techniques for these clinical indications, e.g., CT (chest: 7–11 mSv) [50,51].

C. Radiolabeling

[DTPA^0]octreotide and ^{111}InCl$_3$ (DRN 4901, 370 MBq/ml in HCl, pH 1.5–1.9) are from Mallinckrodt Medical (Petten, The Netherlands). The kit preparation of a patient dose is performed by addition of 222 MBq (6 mCi) ^{111}InCl$_3$ to freeze-dried [DTPA^0]octreotide.

D. Quality Control

Thirty minutes after the start of this procedure quality control is performed by instant thin-layer chromatography with silica gel and 0.1 M sodium citrate, pH 5, as eluent. Under these conditions indium citrate and indium chloride migrate along with the solvent front, whereas peptide-bound ^{111}In stays near the origin.

E. Preclinical Experience

1. [^{111}In-DTPA^0]octreotide, Biodistribution, and (Intracellular) Metabolism

The inhibitory effect of somatostatin on hormone secretion of various glands led to the concept of beneficial effects of somatostatin in the treatment of diseases, based on gland hyperfunction or overproduction of hormones by endocrine-active tumors. However, the tetradecapeptide SS-14 itself is unsuitable for routine treatment, because of its very short half-life of about 3 min in man after intravenous injection due to rapid enzymatic degradation and because of its diversity of action, such as lowering insulin levels. Successful efforts have been undertaken to synthesize somatostatin analogs that are more resistant to enzymatic degradation. Introduction of D-amino acids and shortening of the molecule to the bioactive core sequence resulted in the eight amino acids containing somatostatin analog octreotide (Fig. 1). Nowadays octreotide is widely used with success in the treat-

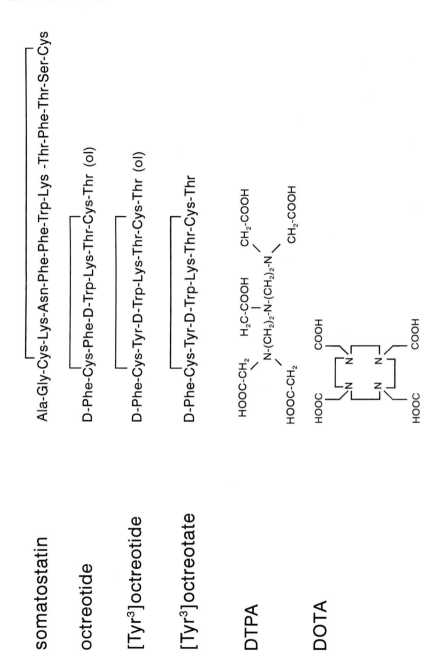

somatostatin

Ala-Gly-Cys-Lys-Asn-Phe-Phe-Trp-Lys -Thr-Phe-Thr-Ser-Cys

octreotide

D-Phe-Cys-Phe-D-Trp-Lys-Thr-Cys-Thr (ol)

[Tyr³]octreotide

D-Phe-Cys-Tyr-D-Trp-Lys-Thr-Cys-Thr (ol)

[Tyr³]octreotate

D-Phe-Cys-Tyr-D-Trp-Lys-Thr-Cys-Thr

DTPA

DOTA

FIGURE 1   Structures of somatostatin, octreotide, [Tyr³]-octreotide, [Tyr³]-octreotate, DTPA, and DOTA.

ment of symptoms of neuroendocrine-active tumors, such as growth hormone-producing pituitary adenomas and gastroenteropancreatic tumors [52–54]. Somatostatin receptors are structurally related, integral membrane glycoproteins. Five different human somatostatin receptor types have been cloned. All subtypes bind SS-14 and SS-28 (a polypeptide of 28 amino acids with SS-14 making up the C-terminus) with high affinity, while the affinity of numerous somatostatin analogs for the five different subtypes differ considerably [31–33]. Octreotide binds with high affinity to the sst_2 (human somatostatin receptor subtype 2), while this analog has a relatively low affinity for sst_3 and sst_5 and shows no binding to sst_1 and sst_4 [31–33,55]. Octreotide scintigraphy is therefore based on the visualization of (an) octreotide-binding somatostatin receptor(s), most probably the sst_2 and sst_5. Somatostatin receptor scintigraphy has been performed at the University Hospital Dijkzigt in Rotterdam since 1987. At first with [^{123}I-Tyr^3]octreotide and since 1989 with [^{111}In-DTPA^0]octreotide as described earlier [51,56].

For preclinical in vivo experiments, male Lewis rats, bearing the CA20948 pancreatic tumor, or Wistar male rats were used. Rats were injected intravenously under ether anesthesia with 3 MBq (0.5 µg of the peptide) radiolabeled peptide. In order to determine nonspecific binding of the radiopharmaceutical, a separate group of rats was injected subcutaneously with 0.5 mg octreotide 30 min before injection of the radiolabeled peptide.

In vivo investigations both in rats and men comparing [^{123}I-Tyr^3]octreotide and [^{111}In-DTPA^0]octreotide showed that the residence time of the two radiopharmaceuticals in somatostatin receptor-positive tissues and tumors was completely different. Twenty-four hours after the injection of the radiopharmaceutical release of radioactivity from somatostatin receptor-positive tissues and tumors was much slower with [^{111}In-DTPA^0]octreotide than with [^{123}I-Tyr^3]octreotide [51], due to differences in metabolism and retention time of the metabolites in the cell [57]. Furthermore, isolated rat liver perfusion experiments with [^{123}I-Tyr^3]octreotide showed that disposal of this compound occurred predominantly by rapid uptake into the liver and excretion via the bile into the intestines, whereas the addition of the relatively large and very hydrophilic DTPA group to the octapeptide molecule [DTPA^0]octreotide favored renal excretion of the latter [57]. The results of our study in perfused rat livers and the rat and human in vivo investigations with [^{123}I-Tyr^3]octreotide and [^{111}In-DTPA^0]octreotide were in very good agreement.

In general, receptor-mediated endocytosis systems have been described [58,59], where cell surface receptors capture their ligands from the extracellular milieu. The receptor-ligand complex is internalized via invagination of the plasma membrane. The resulting intracellular vesicles, termed endosomes, rapidly acidify, which causes the ligand to dissociate from the receptor. The ligand is delivered to the lysosome [60], and the receptor may recycle back to plasma membrane. The whole process takes approximately 15 min [58], and a single receptor can deliver numerous ligand molecules to the lysosomes. We have studied internalization and degradation of radiolabeled [DTPA⁰]octreotide in the somatostatin receptor-positive rat pancreatic tumor cell lines CA20948 and AR42J and in the somatostatin receptor-negative human anaplastic thyroid tumor cell line ARO and detected internalization of the radiopharmaceutical in vitro, in accordance with the findings of Andersson et al. [61], and found that this process was receptor-specific and temperature-dependent [62]. Earlier, we reported in vitro studies using AtT20 mouse pituitary tumor cells for detection of internalization of [^{125}I-Tyr^3]octreotide [63].

Receptor-mediated internalization of [^{111}In-DTPA⁰]octreotide results in degradation to ^{111}In-DTPA-D-Phe in the lysosomes, and this metabolite is not capable passing the lysosomal and/or other cell membrane(s) [64].

2. [DTPA⁰]octreotide, Radionuclide Therapy

A new perspective for patients with somatostatin-positive tumors is peptide receptor radionuclide therapy (PRRT) with [^{111}In-DTPA⁰]octreotide. After internalization of the radiopharmaceutical in the tumor cells, the radioactive ligand is close to the nucleus. Since ^{111}In emits not only gamma rays, which are visualized with somatostatin receptor scintigraphy, but also short-ranged Auger electrons, an effect on tumor cell proliferation could be expected. The radiotoxicity of Auger electrons is very high if their target, the DNA of the cell, is in high nanometer distance [65–67].

We studied the effect of radionuclide therapy in animals inoculated with the somatostatin receptor-positive CA20948 tumor cells and the somatostatin receptor-negative CC-531 tumor cells, respectively. Radionuclide therapy was performed with [^{111}In-DTPA⁰]octreotide. Rats in the experimental groups were injected with 370 MBq (0.5 µg) [^{111}In-DTPA⁰]octreotide IV on days 1 and 8. Rats in the control groups were injected with 0.5 µg [DTPA⁰]octreotide IV according to the same schedule. Another six rats were injected with 1 mg octreotide only, in order to investigate the effect of the blocking itself. All rats were sacrificed 21 days after inoculation of tumor cells, and tumor growth was determined by counting the number of metastases on the surface of the liver lobes.

PRRT with administrations of 370 MBq (0.5 µg) [^{111}In-DTPA⁰]octreotide on day 1 and day 8 induced a significant ($P < .01$) decrease in the number of hepatic metastases 21 days after intraportal injection of CA20948 pancreatic somatostatin receptor-positive tumor cells. PRRT in rats with somatostatin receptor-negative liver metastases did not induce a difference in the number of liver tumor colonies found between the experimental group and the control group. Furthermore, pretreatment with 1 mg octreotide, resulting in a saturation of somatostatin receptors, led to a diminished therapeutic effect of PRRT. The results of these experiments suggest that the effect on tumor growth was due to specific binding of the radioligand to somatostatin receptors [68].

A problem during radionuclide therapy may be caused by the high uptake of radioactivity in the kidneys; small peptides in the blood plasma are filtered through the glomerular capillaries in the kidneys and subsequently reabsorbed almost completely (about 90%) by the proximal tubular cells by carrier-mediated endocytosis. This is also the case for the radiolabeled octapeptide [^{111}In-DTPA[0]]octreotide. After the subsequent degradation process that takes place in the lysosomes of the tubular cells, their labeled degradation products are "trapped" in the lysosomes [64], causing a high dose of radioactivity in the kidneys, thereby reducing the scintigraphic sensitivity for detection of small tumors in the perirenal region and the possibilities for radionuclide therapy. We showed that the renal uptake of [^{111}In-DTPA[0]]octreotide in rats could be reduced about 50% by single intravenous administration of 400 mg/kg L- or D-lysine [69,70], in agreement with other reports [71]. The membranes of renal tubular cells contain negatively charged sites, to which positively charged residues of peptides or proteins are thought to bind [72]. An inhibition of this binding process may explain the effects by administration of the positively charged amino acid lysine (both D- and L-lysine [70]) on [^{111}In-DTPA[0]]octreotide re-uptake.

3. New ^{111}In-Labeled sst$_2$-Binding Analogs for Tumor Scintigraphy and Radionuclide Therapy

We have recently evaluated and compared different (new) ^{111}In-chelator-peptide constructs with regard to binding to octreotide receptors on mouse pituitary tumor cell membranes and internalization in rat pancreatic tumor cells. Furthermore, biodistribution in tumor-bearing rats was investigated in vivo. The analogs tested were [DTPA[0]]octreotide, [DTPA[0],Tyr[3]]octreotide, and [DTPA[0],Tyr[3]]octreotate (structures shown in Fig. 1; in octreotate the C-terminal threoninol has been replaced with the native amino acid threonine; [DTPA[0],Tyr[3]]octreotide and [DTPA[0],Tyr[3]]octreotate were synthesized at Mallinckrodt Medical, St. Louis, Mo). Phe residues were replaced with Tyr to increase the hydrophylicity of the peptides. Furthermore, [DTPA[0],Tyr[3]]octreotate, with the C-terminal threonine, was synthesized to investigate the effects of an additional negative charge on clearance and cellular uptake. In addition, [DOTA[0],Tyr[3]]octreotide was synthesized (by Novartis and H. Mäcke, Basel, Switzerland) and tested, as this compound enables stable radiolabeling with both ^{111}In and the β-particle-emitting radionuclide [90]Y (DOTA = tetraazacyclododecanetetraacetic acid). Radiolabeling with ^{111}In and quality control procedures were mostly as described for [DTPA[0]]octreotide; for radiolabeling of [DOTA[0],Tyr[3]]octreotide, the mixture was heated for 25 min at 100°C.

In in vitro receptor-binding studies, all unlabeled compounds showed high and specific binding for the somatostatin receptors, with IC$_{50}$ values in the low nanomolar range. [DOTA[0],Tyr[3]]octreotide showed the highest affinity of the compounds tested [73]. Comparison of specific internalization of the ^{111}In-labeled compounds in two somatostatin receptor-positive cell lines showed that internalized radioactivity was by far the highest after incubation with [^{111}In-DTPA[0],Tyr[3]]octreotate [73]. Also in biodistribution experiments in sst$_2$-positive CA20948 tumor-bearing rats, uptake in the sst$_2$-expressing organs and tumor of ^{111}In-labeled [DTPA[0],Tyr[3]]octreotide, [DOTA[0],Tyr[3]]octreotide, and [DTPA[0],Tyr[3]]octreotate was significantly higher than that of [^{111}In-DTPA[0]]octreotide at the time points tested. [^{111}In-DTPA[0],Tyr[3]]octreotate showed the highest uptake in the sst$_2$-positive organs of the ^{111}In-labeled peptides tested, also in accordance with the in vitro internalization studies. Uptake of this ^{111}In-labeled peptide in the sst$_2$-positive target organs represented mostly specific binding to the octreotide receptors, as uptake was decreased to <7% of control by pretreatment of the rats with 0.5 mg unlabeled octreotide. Clearance from the blood was rapid. Furthermore, the low uptake of [^{111}In-DTPA[0],Tyr[3]]octreotate in the liver is worth mentioning, which is favorable especially in combination with the rapid blood clearance and high uptake of this compound in the target organs. We concluded that ^{111}In-labeled [DTPA[0],Tyr[3]]octreotide, but especially [DTPA[0],Tyr[3]]octreotate and their DOTA-coupled counterparts, are most promising for scintigraphy and, after coupling to therapeutic radionuclides, for radionuclide therapy of octreotide receptor-positive tumors in humans [73].

III. IMAGE ACQUISITION WITH [[111]IN-DTPA[0]]OCTREOTIDE [56]

The preferred dose of ^{111}In-labeled octreotide, at least 10 µg of the peptide, is about 200 MBq. With such a dose it is possible to perform SPECT, which may increase the sensitivity to detect octreotide receptor-expressing tissues and gives a better anatomical delineation than planar views. Planar and SPECT images are obtained with a large field of view gamma camera, equipped with a medium-energy parallel-hole collimator. The pulse height analyzer windows are centered over both ^{111}In photon peaks (172 keV and 245 keV) with a window width of 20%. Data from both windows are added to the acquisition frames. The acquisition parameters are for planar images (spot views) (anterior and posterior views are necessary!) with a single head camera with analog imaging:

1. Images of head/neck (also from lateral): 300,000 preset counts or 15 min per view at 24 hours and 15 min preset time (about 200,000 counts) at 48 hours after injection.

2. The remainder of the body with separate images of the chest (including as little as possible of the liver and spleen), the shoulders and axillae with upraised arms to detect metastases in the armpits), the upper abdomen (including liver/spleen and kidneys) and lower abdomen:

500,000 counts (or 15 min); with single and dual head cameras with digital imaging: (a) 256 × 256 word matrix; (b) 15 min preset time images; and (c) digital images of upper and lower abdomen are viewed at both low and high intensity settings; those of other parts of the body are viewed at a level optimized for low-radioactivity structures.

For SPECT images the acquisition parameters are: (1) single-head camera (a) 60 projections; (b) 64 × 64 word matrix; (c) *at least* 45 to 60 sec acquisition time per projection, or (2) dual-head camera (a) 60 steps of 6° each; (b) 64 × 64 matrix; (c) *at least* 30 sec acquisition time per step; and (3) triple-head camera (a) 40 steps of 3° each; (b) 64 × 64 word matrix; (c) *at least* 30 sec acquisition time per step (45 sec for SPECT of the head).

SPECT analysis is performed with a Wiener or Metz filter on original data. The filtered data are reconstructed with a Ramp filter. In case the counting time to obtain these "preset" counts for the planar views is short, especially when tissues with relatively high accumulation (e.g., abdominal organs) are included in the field of view or tumor types are being scanned of which it is known that the receptor density is low (as is the case for both breast cancer and lymphomas), additional images with a longer counting time (15 min per planar view) are necessary in order to also visualize small lesions or lesions with low somatostatin receptor density. The above-mentioned counting times per projection for planar imaging with a single-head camera also imply an appropriate (long) duration of whole-body planar scintigraphy with a dual-head camera, e.g., at least about 40 min from head to pelvis or a maximum speed of 3 cm/min. In general, the more counts collected, the better the results in detecting or localizing ligand-receptor-expressing tissue(s).

The importance of SPECT of the chest for breast cancer (primary and metastases) versus planar imaging is not really known at the moment, if the above-mentioned considerations of counting time are taken into account. For instance, Chiti et al. did compare planar imaging with SPECT in patients with breast cancer [74]. In our view, however, the acquisition times they used, of 5 and 10 min at 4 and 24 hours after injection, are too short for planar imaging of breast cancer. Our below-mentioned results have been obtained with planar imaging only. However, our impression is that SPECT of the chest, including iterative reconstruction nowadays, might improve the sensitivity for breast cancer detection. Iterative reconstruction improves the quality of the images by showing less background noise and reconstruction artifacts.

Planar and SPECT studies are preferably performed 24 hours after injection of the radiopharmaceutical. Planar studies after 24 and 48 hours can be carried out with the same protocol. Repeat scintigraphy after 48 hours is especially indicated when 24-hour scintigraphy shows accumulation in the abdomen, which may also represent radioactive bowel content.

A special remark has to be made with respect to the observation of bilateral and diffuse, physiological breast uptake in normal females [75]. This faint uptake occurs at 4 hours after the administration of [^{111}In-DTPA^0]octreotide in nearly 50% of females and decreases at 24 hours to about 15% and is clearly different from the more localized accumulation at the site of breast cancer. At the moment the basis for this finding is unknown.

IV.   CLINICAL APPLICATIONS: [^{111}IN-DTPA^0]OCTREOTIDE AND OTHER PEPTIDES IN BREAST CANCER

A.   Personal Experience

The somatostatin receptor imaging technique ([^{111}In-DTPA^0]octreotide, Octreoscan), has been shown to be successful in the visualization of the primary as well as metastatic tumor sites of a variety of neuroendocrine tumors like carcinoids, islet cell tumors, and paragangliomas [49–51,56]. Validation of this technique was reached by the in vitro demonstration of high-affinity binding sites for somatostatin on those tumors, which had been visualized in vivo [49]. In parallel, a positive somatostatin receptor scan closely predicted a beneficial effect of chronic octreotide therapy on hormonal hypersecretion by these tumors [76].

In a recent study we visualized 39 of 52 primary breast cancers (75%) with somatostatin receptor. There was a close correlation between the in vivo somatostatin receptor scan and subsequent in vitro findings at autoradiography with (^{125}I-Tyr^3) octreotide, also confirming and validating the concept of receptor imaging in this type of tumor [77]. There was considerable variability in the accumulation of radioactivity at somatostatin receptor scintigraphy. A higher density in vivo turned out to correlate in most instances with a homogeneous and dense distribution of somatostatin receptor throughout the tumor at autoradiography, while a lower density of radioactivity over the tumor area in vivo in most instances corresponded with a nonhomogeneous and often sparse distribution of these receptors. Interestingly, the low density of receptors in vivo and in vitro seemed to be due to the occurrence of a noninvasive carcinoma component, mainly being ductal carcinoma in situ.

The high incidence of somatostatin receptor in these 52 carcinomas (as observed with the in vivo technique) might be related to several causes: first, it is hypothesized that in vivo somatostatin receptor visualization of the primary breast cancer is more sensitive than in vitro autoradiography using sections of parts of the tumor only, as this nuclear medical technique investigates in fact the presence of receptors three-dimensionally in the entire tumor; in accordance with this, statistically significantly more T_2 tumors than T_1 tumors were visualized in vivo. Second, our patients might represent a "selected" group in comparison with those found in other countries, as the incidence of ductal carcinomas among the patients with newly diagnosed breast cancers has increased over the last years in the Netherlands after the introduction of routine and especially repeated screening of the population [78]. Significantly more (locally) invasive ductal carcinomas were visualized with this technique.

B.   Comparison with Tumor Markers

CA 15-3 and CEA are the most commonly used tumor markers to monitor patients with recurrent breast cancer. Both markers are elevated in only 5% to 20% of women with primary breast cancer, but elevations between 61% and 84% have been recorded for women with extensive metastatic disease. CA 15-3 seems to be related to the extent of the metastases, the number of metastatic sites, and survival, whereas CEA is only correlated with the extent of disease [79,80].

In this study we showed a higher sensitivity of somatostatin receptor scintigraphy compared with these tumor markers to detect the development of recurrent breast cancer in patients with somatostatin receptor-positive primary breast cancer. Somatostatin receptor scintigraphy demonstrated recurrent disseminated breast cancer in six (only one of whom was symptomatic for recurrence) of 28 patients with somatostatin receptor-positive primary tumors. All six patients had normal CA 15-3 and CEA serum values. Another three of these 28 patients had abnormal serum tumor markers, two of whom had an abnormal somatostatin receptor scintigram. The third patient, who only showed marginally elevated CA 15-3 serum levels both at first presentation and at follow-up, is clinically in complete remission 3.2 years after operation. Possibly the CA 15-3 in this patient is false-positive for breast cancer.

C.   Biological Behavior

Very little is known concerning the biological behavior of somatostatin receptor-positive human breast cancer. In a retrospective study involving 110 patients Foekens et al. [40] suggested that the presence of somatostatin receptor might predict a longer disease-free survival. Also in vitro studies in more than 300 breast cancer samples showed an inverse relationship between somatostatin and EGF-receptor expression [16,48]. These observations suggest that patients with somatostatin receptor-positive cancers might have a relatively good prognosis. This, however, seems not to be substantiated by our observations. In the follow-up after 50 to 65 months we found that, from the 37 patients with a somatostatin receptor-positive primary tumor, at least 19 (55%) had extensive metastases (four had died), including six of 26 symptom-free patients who had (multiple) histologically proven metastases, as initially visualized at follow-up somatostatin receptor scintigraphy. In two patients (15%) recurrent disease was found at follow-up in patients with somatostatin receptor-negative primary tumors.

D.   Review of Somatostatin Receptor Scintigraphy of Breast Cancer in Medical Literature

Only a few studies report the use of somatostatin receptor scintigraphy in breast cancer [74,77,81–83]. Chiti et al. show a positivity of somatostatin receptor scintigraphy in 15 out of 16 primary tumors (size range 5 to 36 mm, mean 29 mm) and five of the six cases of metastatic axillary node involvement [74]. No difference in sensitivity between somatostatin receptor scintigraphy and ^{99m}Tc-MIBI scintigraphy in these same patients was observed. The sizes of negative primary tumors were 7 mm (somatostatin receptor scintigraphy) and 5 mm (^{99m}Tc-MIBI scintigraphy). These authors emphasize the use of SPECT for both radioligands (see remarks in Section III).

Other reported studies used only about 3 mCi of the ^{111}In-labeled [DTPA[0]]octreotide [81–83]. In our view, this is too low a dose for detecting tumors with a rather low density of somatostatin receptors, e.g., breast cancer. Nevertheless, the observed sensitivities to detect primary tumors were as follows: 18/24 patients, 16/17 cancers, and 9/9 patients, respectively. Axillary lymph node metastases were found in 5/6 patients [82] and 4/4 and 0/3 patients with palpable and nonpalpable lymph nodes [83], respectively.

No studies have been reported to day in which somatostatin receptor scintigraphy has served as a possible predictor (in a subgroup of patients) for the efficacy of somatostatin analogs in combination with tamoxifen.

E.   Case Illustrations

1.   Case 1

A 77-year-old female who had a breast amputation at the right side 5 years before she presented with a palpable mass on the left. The ^{111}In-labeled [DTPA[0]] octreotide scintigram (left anterior view of the chest) showed a hot spot and diffuse distribution of tracer accumulation in a larger area (Fig. 2). Histopathology showed a small infiltrating tumor with a large extensive ductal carcinoma in situ component.

2.   Case 2

A 49-year-old female with a 3.5-cm infiltrating ductal carcinoma. Two axillary lymph nodes were found to be positive at histology. The ^{111}In-labeled [DTPA[0]]octreotide scintigram showed only the hotspot at the site of the primary tumor (Fig. 3A,B, left anterior and left lateral views of the chest). Adjuvant treatment consisted of chemotherapy and radiation of the thoracic wall. The [111]In-

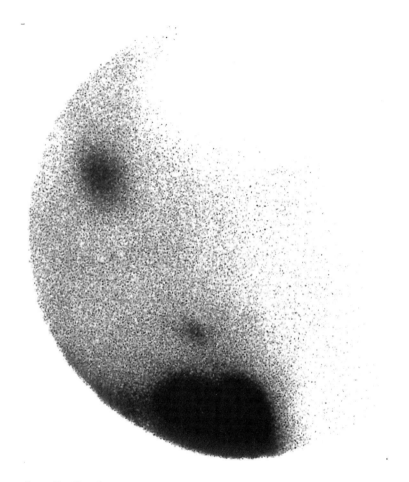

FIGURE 2   Case 1.

labeled [DTPA^0]octreotide scintigram at the follow-up shows typical pulmonary postradiation effects (Fig. 4A,B, anterior and posterior views of the chest).

3.   Case 3

A 42-year-old female presenting with a T_2N_1 (four positive axillary lymph nodes) infiltrating ductal carcinoma for which a modified radical mastectomy was performed (Fig. 5, left anterior view of chest and axilla). Adjuvant therapy consisted of chemotherapy (six times CMF). After 16 months, as part of our study, an ^{111}In-labeled [DTPA^0]octreotide scintigram was performed which showed tracer distri-

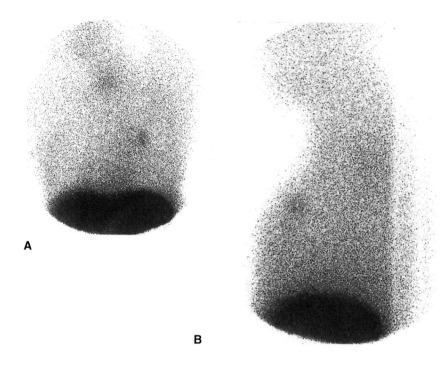

A

B

Figure 3   Case 2.

bution compatible with pleural carcinomatosis (Fig. 6A,B, anterior and posterior views of the chest), which was confirmed by cytological smear analysis of pleural fluid from the left thorax.

4.   Case 4

A 54-year-old patient presenting with a right-sided homonymous hemianopsia and hypocortisolism. CT scanning demonstrated a pituitary tumor (Fig. 7A, coronal view of the pituitary). The patient underwent an ^{111}In-labeled [DTPA^0]-octreotide scintigram because of a suspected nonsecreting pituitary adenoma. The ^{111}In-labeled [DTPA^0]octreotide scintigram demonstrated not only an enlarged pituitary area of tracer accumulation of normal intensity (Fig. 7B,C, right lateral view of the head; and coronal view of SPECT), but also definite abnormalities in the chest area (Fig. 8A,B, anterior and posterior views of the chest). The combination of pituitary and chest accumulation points to pathology other than the suspected nonsecreting pituitary adenoma. After informing the referring physician about the results, we learned about a history of breast cancer. The pituitary lesion proved to be metastatic breast cancer.

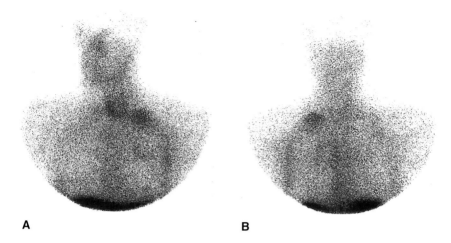

A   **B**

FIGURE 4   Case 2.

5. Case 5

A 47-year-old female who was operated in March 1990 for a large carcinoid of the appendix. At the end of April 1990 she had an ^{111}In-labeled [DTPA⁰]octreotide scintigram to see whether any metastatic disease of the carcinoid was present. The ^{111}In-labeled [DTPA⁰]octreotide scintigram showed no abnormalities pointing to the absence of carcinoid metastases, although faint and diffuse tracer uptake can be seen in the region of the left breast (Fig. 9, anterior view of the chest). In November 1990 (thus only 6 months later) she presented with a palpable breast tumor on the right side, with no clinically suspected lymph nodes. A mammography detected a suspected lesion on the right side and a large area of microcalcifications on the left. Another ^{111}In-labeled [DTPA⁰]octreotide scintigram was performed which showed a hotspot in both breasts as well as a hot spot in the right armpit (Fig. 10a,b, anterior and left anterior oblique views of the chest). A modified radical mastectomy on the right side and an incision biopsy of the area with the microcalcifications on the left side were performed. Histopathology showed a T_2N_1 (two positive axillary lymph nodes) infiltrating ductal carcinoma on the right side and a ductal carcinoma in situ without any infiltration in the biopsy specimen of the left breast. Adjuvant chemotherapy (six times CMF) was started, and an ablation of the left breast was planned after finishing the adjuvant treatment. However, before the operation in July 1991 it was obvious from the mammography that an infiltrating tumor was present. Therefore a modified radical

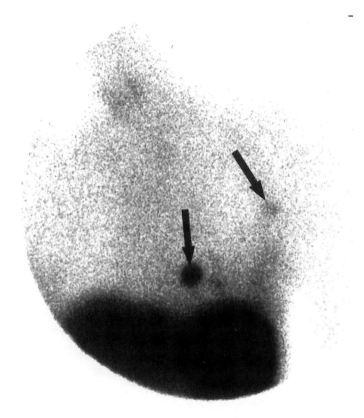

FIGURE 5   Case 3.

mastectomy was again done. A small infiltrating ductal carcinoma was found with an extensive ductal carcinoma in situ component and again two axillary lymph nodes were positive.

F. Possible Impact of Radiolabeled Somatostatin Analogs in the Treatment of Patients with Breast Cancer

I. Introduction

In vitro studies with breast cancer cell lines indicate a direct receptor mediated inhibitory effect of unlabeled (= nonradioactive) somatostatin analogs on cell proliferation [84]. The results of prospective, controlled studies on the use of unlabeled somatostatin analogs in patients with breast cancer have not been published

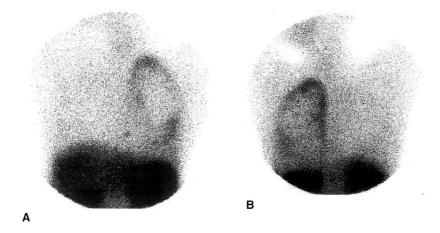

A   B

FIGURE 6   Case 3.

yet. Interesting animal data have been reported showing the additive effect of unlabeled somatostatin analogs on the antiproliferative effect of tamoxifen treatment on breast cancer [85]. The precise role of somatostatin receptors and/or their density at the plasma membrane of breast cancer cells in this additive effect of somatostatin analogs, if any, has yet to be determined. The mechanism of action of unlabeled somatostatin and its analogs is twofold, via a direct (somatostatin receptors) and indirect effect (e.g., influence on production of growth factors such as PRL, GH, and IGF-I). Their possible effect on angiogenesis might in theory be related to both direct and indirect influences.

2. Radiolabeled Somatostatin Analogs

In vitro studies underestimate the presence of somatostatin receptors, because often only small tissue samples from breast cancer with frequently heterogeneous distribution of somatostatin receptors are investigated. Peptide receptor scintigraphy is able to detect the presence of these receptors in the whole tumor and has therefore shown to have a higher sensitivity for peptide receptor detection in breast cancer than in vitro studies so far reported. It would be very interesting to see what the possible effect of unlabeled somatostatin analog treatment is in the subgroup of patients with breast cancer having a positive somatostatin receptor scintigraphy as opposed to the subgroup with a negative somatostatin receptor scintigraphy. The positivity of somatostatin receptor scintigraphy can also be expressed in grades to give an impression of the density of the receptors, thereby enabling study of the possible impact of the density on the effect of unlabeled

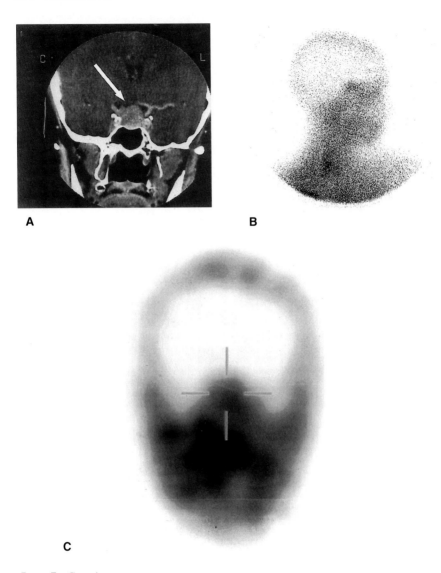

A   B

C

Figure 7   Case 4.

somatostatin analog treatment for breast cancer. Unfortunately, human studies on the effect on unlabeled somatostatin analogs do not include somatostatin receptor scintigraphy, but often rely on in vitro analyses.

The grading of somatostatin receptor density might also be of importance for the future use of somatostatin analogs labeled with radionuclides emitting β-particles (e.g., ^{90}Y) showing a crossfire with acceptable tissue penetration in order

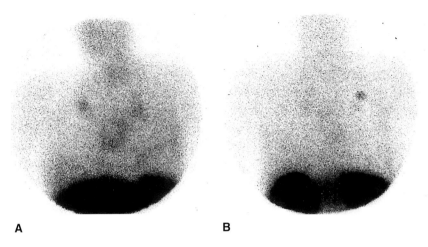

A   B

FIGURE 8   Case 4.

to overcome the problem of the heterogenetic distribution of breast cancer cells expressing somatostatin receptors. The first promising results with peptide receptor radionuclide therapy with multiple administrations of high doses of ^{111}In-labeled [DTPA^0]octreotide in patients with gastroenteropancreatic neuroendocrine tumors have been reported [86,87]. The tissue penetration of Auger electrons emitted by ^{111}In is probably too short to get an antiproliferative effect with this radionuclide in breast cancer. Since the distribution and density of somatostatin receptors in gastroenteropancreatic neuroendocrine tumors is more favorable, these tumors are better candidates for peptide receptor radionuclide therapy with multiple administrations of high doses of ^{111}In-labeled [DTPA^0]octreotide.

3. Potential of Peptide Receptor Scintigraphy of Breast Cancer with Other Somatostatin Analogs

Five subtypes of human somatostatin receptors have been cloned. The somatostatin analog octreotide competes with somatostatin binding to the somatostatin receptor subtype 2 (sst_2) in the low nanomolar range (0.1 to 1 nM), in contrast to higher values (lower affinity) for types sst_3 and sst_5 (10 to 100 nM), and sst_1 and sst_4 (>1000 nM). The somatostatin receptor subtype expression (sst_{1-5}) in somatostatin receptor positive breast cancer has been studied by mRNA analysis and receptor autoradiography [88,89]. Although all five somatostatin receptor subtypes in breast cancer are expressed, the majority of breast cancers show a preference for sst_2. Thus, radiolabeled octreotide and any somatostatin analog with a preferential binding to sst_2 are the appropriate radioligands for scintigraphy and future radionuclide therapy of somatostatin receptor-positive breast cancers.

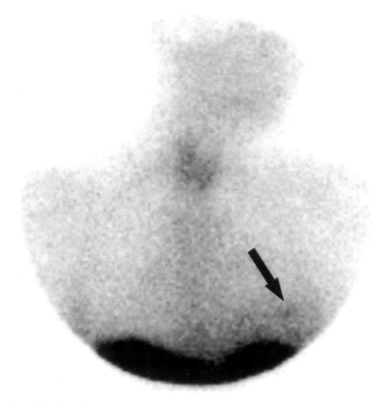

FIGURE 9   Case 5.

G.   Peptide Receptor Scintigraphy of Breast Cancer with Other Peptides

After the introduction of somatostatin receptor scintigraphy with radiolabeled octreotide for various cancers, other radiolabeled peptides derived from hormones, growth factors, and antitumor antibodies were considered candidates for peptide receptor scintigraphy and radionuclide therapy [50,56]. At the moment, the available information of these candidates is scarce and mainly based on in vitro studies using breast cancer tissue samples. In vivo scintigraphy in patients with breast cancer with these other peptides has hardly been reported. The following examples of receptors have been identified in vitro in human breast cancers.

Vasoactive intestinal peptide (VIP), a 28-amino-acid neuroendocrine mediator, has been found in 100% of both the primary tumors (n = 24) and metastases

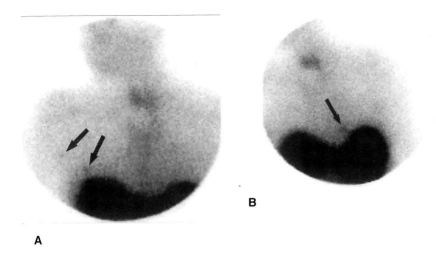

FIGURE 10   Case 5.

(n = 15), apparently with a homogeneous distribution over the whole tumor [90]. Both ductal and lobular breast cancers are VIP receptor-positive. On the basis of these interesting data, VIP receptor scintigraphy might become a sensitive tool for both the detection of the primary tumor and its metastases of breast cancer. VIP receptor scintigraphy with ^{123}I-VIP has been reported, but not in patients with breast cancer [91].

The theoretical application of VIP receptor scintigraphy on the basis of results of autoradiography studies is very broad. However, some reservation with regard to its possible use for peptide receptor scintigraphy in breast cancer is the in-house labeling with [123]I (costs, logistics, manpower) and the intense accumulation of ^{123}I-VIP in the lung for the first hours after injection. Furthermore, as long as there is no chelated VIP analog available that enables easier labeling with a radionuclide and that might be used in the future for peptide receptor radionuclide therapy, if ever possible because of the high accumulation in the lung, the available alternatives in nuclear medicine, e.g., MIBI and FDG, will in our view prevail for the near future.

Substance P receptor scintigraphy with ^{111}In-labeled DTPA-chelated substance P has also been performed in patients with autoimmune diseases but not in patients with breast cancer [92]. Substance P, an undecapeptide, belongs to the family of tachykinins. This peptide acts as a neurotransmitter in the central nervous system, has vasodilator potency, and increases vascular permeability. Furthermore, it affects the immune response and angiogenesis. Receptor autoradiography studies with radiolabeled substance P have shown a 50% positivity for the presence of substance P receptors in breast cancer tumor samples (n = 16), whereas all samples showed the presence of substance P receptors in the vessels of the tumoral stroma [93]. In most of the tumors the distribution of substance P receptors was nonhomogeneous. The role of substance P receptors in breast cancer and the application of radiolabeled substance P ligands have to be established in the future.

With several in vitro assay techniques EGF receptors have been found in nearly 50% of breast cancer tumors [see review, 94]. This 53-amino-acid polypeptide can affect proliferation and differentiation of many cells. Both EGF and transforming growth factor-α (TGFα) can activate the EGF receptor. For breast cancer there may exist a negative relation between the expression of EGF receptor and estrogen and somatostatin receptors. Also the level of expression of EGF receptor on tumor cells might represent a useful prognostic factor in breast cancer. It has been associated with a poor response to endocrine therapy and a decreased overall survival.

The use of radiolabeled EGF is of course a very attractive idea for nuclear oncology and already reported for a ^{111}In-chelated human EGF [95], whereas a radioiodinated EGF has been investigated in one of our patients (unpublished data). The very rapid and high hepatic degradation of this large molecule after its intravenous administration is a real obstacle for in vivo scintigraphy. Hopefully, other derivatives of EGF, e.g., chelated fragments, may overcome this problem.

A lower percentage (about 30%) of breast cancer membranes from 100 tumor samples expressed receptors of bombesin (or for its mammalian counterpart, gastrin-releasing peptide [GRP]), a tetradecapeptide [96]. Also these receptors might be involved in the growth of breast cancer. The development of chelated bombesin/GRP analogs for their use in nuclear medicine is in progress.

Another interesting peptide receptor for nuclear medicine is that of cholecystokinin-B (CCK-B) or gastrin, especially for medullary thyroid cancer and small-cell lung cancer [97]. Unfortunately, according to in vitro studies, only 8% of the breast cancer seem to express these receptors. Thus the use of radiolabeled radioligands for binding to the CCK-B/gastrin receptor in breast cancer might be of minor importance.

The above-mentioned peptides are derived from native hormones. Also peptides constituting part of monoclonal antibodies, the so-called amino acid sequences in the complementarity-determining regions (CDRs) of the variable domains, have been reported as candidates for their use in radiolabeled form for scintigraphy after binding to tumor-associated antigens [98]. One example is a synthetic pentadecapeptide αM2, radiolabeled with ^{99m}Tc, derived from the idiotype of a murine antitumor monoclonal antibody (ASM2) directed against polymorphic epithelial mucin. It has been reported that 14 out of 15 primary breast cancer tumors were positive with scintigraphy, as well as 16 out of 26 lymph node metastases and 14 out of 19 other sites.

V. SUMMARY

It is clear from the above-mentioned information that radiolabeled peptides are new radioligands for scintigraphy of breast cancer. In the opinion of the authors, their future application in breast cancer scintigraphy has to be aimed at their in vivo use as prognostic predictors and not necessarily for localization per se, since other powerful alternatives are already available in nuclear medicine. An exception might be the demonstration or localization of the presence of recurrence of breast cancer, since up to now it is questionable whether sensitive technique(s) exist(s) to show the recurrence of disease in an early phase [99,100]. Somatostatin receptor scintigraphy might be an exception for this objective [77; see above]. Also, peptide receptor radionuclide therapy using radionuclides with appropriate particle ranges may become an new treatment modality. One might consider the use of radiolabeled somatostatin analogs first in an adjuvant setting after surgery of somatostatin receptor-positive primary breast cancer to eradicate occult metastases and, second, for breast cancer recurrence at a later stage. Studies with the aim to find compounds which upregulate in vivo the density of somatostatin receptors on tumors were not successful up to now. Thus, the only way to obtain the highest accumulation of a radiolabeled somatostatin analog in a tumor is by selecting an analog showing the highest binding and a concomitant appropriate biodistribution. New developments in this area, especially for somatostatin analogs, have been mentioned here. Also, the use of radiosensitizers may enhance the radiobiologic effect of peptide receptor radionuclide therapy.

Peptide receptor scintigraphy for breast cancer in general might also flourish in the future if these peptides are related to peptide compounds which might be introduced for treatment of breast cancer in a nonradioactive form (e.g., analogs and/or antagonists of somatostatin [84,85], EGF, VIP, and bombesin). After all, peptide receptor scintigraphy is a simple, sensitive, noninvasive tool to show the presence or absence of specific receptors on tumor in vivo.

REFERENCES

1. Schönbrunn A, Tashjian A. Characterization of functional receptors for somatostatin in rat pituitary cells in culture. J Biol Chem 253:6473–6483, 1978.
2. Reubi JC, Kvols LK, Krenning EP, Lamberts SWJ. Distribution of somatostatin receptors in normal and tumor tissue. Metabolism 39(9 suppl 2):78–81, 1990.
3. Reubi JC, Krenning EP, Lamberts SWJ, Kvols LK. Somatostatin receptors in malignant tissues. J Steroid Biochem Mol Biol 37:1073–1077, 1990.
4. Reubi JC, Kvols LK, Waser B, et al. Detection of somatostatin receptors in surgical and percutaneous needle biopsy samples of carcinoids and islet cell carcinomas. Cancer Res 50:5969–5977, 1990.

5. Reubi JC, Modigliani E, Calmettes C, Kvols LK, Krenning EP, Lamberts SWJ. In vitro and in vivo identification of somatostatin receptors in medullary thyroid carcinomas, pheochromocytomas and paragangliomas. In: Calmettes C, Guliana JM, eds. Medullary Thyroid Carcinomas. London: John Libbey Eurotext, 1991;211:85–87.

6. Warren WH, Lee I, Gould VE, Memoli VA, Jao W. Paragangliomas of the head and neck: ultrastructural and immunohistochemical analysis. Ultrastruct Pathol 8:333–343, 1985.

7. Hamid QA, Bishop AE, Rode J et al. Duodenal gangliocytic paragangliomas: a study of 10 cases with immunocytochemical neuroendocrine markers. Hum Pathol 17:1151–1157, 1986.

8. Lundberg JM, Hamberger B, Schultzberg M, et al. Enkephalin- and somatostatin-like immuno-reactivities in human adrenal medulla and pheochromocytoma. Proc Natl Acad Sci USA 76:4079–4083, 1979.

9. Reubi JC, Chayvialle JA, Franc B, Cohen R, Calmettes C, Modigliani E. Somatostatin receptors and somatostatin content in medullary thyroid carcinomas. Lab Invest 64:567–573, 1991.

10. McKinney M, Barrett RW: Biochemical evidence for somatostatin receptors in murine neuroblastoma clone N1E-115. Eur J Pharmacol 162:397–405, 1989.

11. Reubi JC, Cortes R, Maurer R, Probst A, Palacios JM. Distribution of somatostatin receptors in the human brain: an autoradiographic study. Neuroscience 18:329–346, 1986.

12. Reubi JC, Lang W, Maurer R, Koper JW, Lamberts SWJ. Distribution and biochemical characterization of somatostatin receptors in tumors of the human central nervous system. Cancer Res 47:5758–5764, 1987.

13. Reubi JC, Maurer R, von Werder K, Torhorst J, Klijn JGM, Lamberts SWJ. Somatostatin receptors in human endocrine tumors. Cancer Res 47:551–558, 1987.

14. Reubi JC, Maurer R, Klijn JGM, et al. High incidence of somatostatin receptors in human meningiomas: biochemical characterization. J Clin Endocrinol Metab 63:433–438, 1986.

15. Reubi JC, Horisberger U, Lang W, Koper JW, Braakman R, Lamberts SWJ. Coincidence of EGF receptors and somatostatin receptors in meningiomas but inverse, differentiation-dependent relationship in glial tumors. Am J Pathol 134:337–344, 1989.

16. Reubi JC, Waser B, Foekens JA, Klijn JGM, Lamberts SWJ, Laissue J. Somatostatin receptor incidence and distribution in breast cancer using receptor autoradiography: relationship to EGF receptors. Int J Cancer 46:416–420, 1990.

17. Fekete M, Wittliff JL, Schally AV. Characteristics and distribution of receptor for [D-Trp^6]-luteinizing-hormone-releasing hormone, somatostatin, epidermal growth factor and sex steroids in 500 biopsy samples of human breast cancer. J Clin Lab Anal 3:137–141, 1989.

18. Papotti M, Macri L, Bussolati G, Reubi JC. Correlative study on neuroendocrine differentiation and presence of somatostatin receptors in breast carcinomas. Int J Cancer 43:365–369, 1989.

19. Reubi JC, Waser B, Sheppard M, Macaulay V. Somatostatin receptors are present in small-cell but not in non-small-cell primary lung carcinomas. Int J Cancer 45:269–274, 1990.

20. Sagman U, Mullen JB, Kovacs K, Kerbel R, Ginsberg R, Reubi JC. Identification of

somatostatin receptors in human small cell lung carcinoma. Cancer 66:2129–2133, 1990.

21. Thermos K, Reisine T. Somatostatin receptor subtypes in clonal anterior pituitary cell lines AtT-20 and GH₃. Mol Pharmacol 33:370–377, 1988.

22. Srikant CB, Heisler S. Relationship between binding and biopotency of somatostatin-14 and somatostatin-28 in mouse pituitary tumor cells. Endocrinology 117:271–278, 1985.

23. Murthy KK, Srikant CB, Patel YC. Evidence for multiple protein constituents of the somatostatin receptor in pituitary tumor cells: affinity cross-linking and molecular characterization. Endocrinology 125:948–956, 1989.

24. Schönbrunn A, Rorstad OP, Westendorf JM, Martin JB. Somatostatin analogs: correlation between receptor binding affinity and biological potency in GH pituitary cells. Endocrinology 113:1559–1567, 1983.

25. Wang HL, Bogen C, Reisine T, Dichter M. Somatostatin-14 and somatostatin-28 induce opposite effects on potassium currents in rat neocortical neurons. Proc Natl Acad Sci USA 86:9616–9620, 1989.

26. Dichter M, Wang HL, Reisine T. Electrophysiological effects of somatostatin-14 and somatostatin-28 on mammalian central nervous system neurons. Metabolism 39(suppl 1):86-90, 1990.

27. Reubi JC. Evidence of two somatostatin-14 receptor types in rat brain cortex. Neurosci Lett 49:259–263, 1984.

28. Reubi JC, Probst A, Cortes R, Palacios JM. Distinct topographical localization of two somatostatin receptor subpopulations in the human cortex. Brain Res 406:391–396, 1987.

29. Reubi JC, Krenning E, Lamberts SWJ, Kvols LK. In vitro detection of somatostatin receptors in human tumors. Metabolism 41(suppl 2):104–110, 1992.

30. Bell GI, Reisine T. Molecular biology of somatostatin receptors. Trends Neurosci 16(1):34–38, 1993.

31. Yamada Y, Kagimoto S, Kubota A, et al. Cloning, functional expression and pharmacological characterization of a fourth (hSSTR4) and a fifth (hSSTR5) human somatostatin subtype. Biochem Biophys Res Commun 195(2):844–852, 1993.

32. Bruno JF, Berelowitz M. Somatostatin receptors: orphan that found family and function. Mol Cell Neurosci 4:307–309, 1993.

33. Rohrer L, Raulf F, Bruns C, Buettner R, Hofstaedter F, Schüle R. Cloning and characterization of a fourth human somatostatin receptor. Proc Natl Acad Sci USA 90:4196–4200, 1993.

34. Vogler E. Über das basilare Helle-Zellen-Organ der menschlichen Brustdrüse. Klin Med 2:159–168, 1947.

35. Freyter F, Hartmann G. Über die carcinoide wuchsform des carcinoma mammae, insbesondere das carcinoma solidum (gelatinosum) mammae. Frankfurter Z Pathol 73:24–39, 1963.

36. Gould VE, Chejfec G. Case 13: lobular carcinoma of the breast with secretory features. Ultrastruct Pathol 1:151–156, 1980.

37. Gould VE, Jao W, Battifora H. Ultrastructural analysis in the differential diagnosis of breast tumors. Pathol Res Pract 167:45–70, 1980.

38. Bussolati G, Gugliotta P, Sapino A, Eusebi V, Lloyd R. Chromogranin-reactive

endocrine cells in argyrophilic carcinomas (carcinoids) and normal tissue of the breast. Am J Surg Pathol 120:186–192, 1985.

39. Nobels FRE, Kwekkeboom DJ, Coopmans W, et al. Chromogranin A as serum marker for neuroendocrine neoplasia: comparison with neuron-specific enolase and the α-subunit of glycoprotein hormones. J Clin Endocrinol Metab 82:2622–2628, 1997.

40. Foekens JA, Portengen H, van Putten WLJ, et al. Prognostic value of receptors for insulin-like growth factor 1, somatostatin, and epidermal growth factor in human breast cancer. Cancer Res 49:7002–7009, 1989.

41. Bootsma A, van Eijck CHJ, Schouten KK, et al. Somatostatin receptor-positive primary breast tumors: genetic, patient and tumor characteristics. Int J Cancer 54(3): 357–362, 1993.

42. Callahan R. Genetic alterations in primary breast cancer. Breast Cancer Res Treat 13:191–203, 1989.

43. Varley JM, Armour J, Swallow JE, et al. The retinoblastoma gene is frequently altered leading to loss of expression in primary breast tumors. Oncogene 4:725–729, 1989.

44. Adnane J, Gaudray P, Simon MP, Simony-Lafontaine J, Jeanteur P, Theillet C. Proto-oncogene amplification and human breast tumor phenotype. Oncogene 4:1389–1395, 1989.

45. vande Vijver MJ, Peterse JL, Mooi WJ, et al. NEU-protein overexpression in breast cancer. Association with comedo-type ductal carcinoma in situ and limited prognostic value in stage II breast cancer. N Engl J Med 319:1239–1245, 1988.

46. Harbour JW, Lai SL, Whang-Peng J, Gazdar AF, Minna JD, Kaye FJ. Abnormalities in structure and expression of the human retinoblastoma gene in SCLC. Science (Wash. DC) 241:353–356, 1988.

47. Wong AJ, Ruppert JM, Eggleston J, Hamilton SR, Baylin SB, Vogelstein B. Gene amplification of c-myc and N-myc in small cell carcinoma of the lung. Science (Wash. DC) 233:461–464, 1986.

48. Reubi JC, Torhorst J. Relationship between somatostatin, epidermal growth factor and steroid hormone receptors in breast cancer. Cancer 64:1254–1260, 1989.

49. Bakker WH, Albert R, Bruns C, et al. [^{111}In-DTPA-D-Phe^1]-octreotide, a potential radiopharmaceutical for imaging of somatostatin receptor-positive tumors: synthesis, radiolabeling and in vitro validation. Life Sci 49:1583–1591, 1991.

50. Krenning EP, Kwekkeboom DJ, Bakker WH, et al. Somatostatin receptor scintigraphy with [^{111}In-DTPA-D-Phe^1] and [^{123}I-Tyr^3]-octreotide; the Rotterdam experience with more than 1000 patients. Eur J Nucl Med 20:716–731, 1993.

51. Krenning EP, Bakker WH, Kooij PPM, et al. Somatostatin receptor scintigraphy with [^{111}In-DTPA-d-Phe^1]-octreotide in man: metabolism, dosimetry, and comparison with [^{123}I-Tyr^3]-octreotide. J Nucl Med 33:652–658, 1992.

52. Lamberts SWJ, Uitterlinden P, Verschoor L, van Dongen KJ, del Pozo E. Long-term treatment of acromegaly with the somatostatin analogue SMS 201-995. N Engl J Med 313:1576–1580, 1985.

53. Lamberts SWJ. The role of somatostatin in the regulation of anterior pituitary hormone secretion and the use of its analogs in the treatment of human pituitary tumors. Endocrin Rev 9:417–436, 1988.

54. Lamberts SWJ, Krenning EP, Reubi JC. The role of somatostatin and its analogues in the diagnosis and treatment of tumors. Endocrin Rev 12:450–482, 1991.

55. Kubota A, Yamada Y, Kagimoto S, et al. Identification of somatostatin receptor sub-types and an implication for the efficacy of somatostatin analogue SMS 201-995 in treatment of human endocrine tumors. J Clin Invest 93:1321–1325, 1994.

56. Krenning EP, Kwekkeboom DJ, Pauwels S, Kvols LK, Reubi JC. Somatostatin receptor scintigraphy. In: Freeman LM, ed. Nuclear Medicine Annual. New York: Raven Press, 1995:1–50.

57. de Jong M, Bakker WH, Breeman WAP, et al. Hepatobiliary handling of iodine-125-Tyr3-octreotide and indium-111-DTPA-D-Phe1-octreotide by isolated perfused rat liver. J Nucl Med 4:2025–2030, 1993.

58. Schwarz AL, Fridovich SE, Lodisch HF. Kinetics of internalization and recycling of the asialoglycoprotein receptor in hepatoma cell line. J Biol Chem 257:4230–4237, 1982.

59. Weigel PH. Mechanisms of cellular processing and degradation of internalized soluble glycoproteins. In: Allen HJ, Kisaulis EC, eds. Glycoconjugates, Composition, Structure and Function. New York: Marcel Dekker, 1992.

60. Duncan JR, Welch MJ. Intracellular metabolism of indium-111-DTPA-labeled receptor targeted proteins. J Nucl Med 34:1728–1738, 1993.

61. Andersson P, Forssel-Aronsson E, Johanson V, et al. Internalization of In-111 into human neuroendocrine tumor cells after incubation with indium-111-DTPA-D-Phe[1] octreotide. J Nucl Med 37:2002–2006, 1996.

62. de Jong M, Bernard HF, de Bruin E, et al. Internalization of radiolabeled [DTPA[0]]octreotide and [DOTA[0],Tyr[3]]octreotide: peptides for somatostatin receptor-targeted scintigraphy and radionuclide therapy. Nucl Med Commun. In Press.

63. Hofland LJ, van Koetsveld PM, Waaijers M, Zuyderwijk J, Breeman WAP, Lamberts SWJ. Internalization of the radioiodinated somatostatin analogue, [^{125}I-Tyr[3]]octreotide by mouse and human pituitary tumor cells: increase by unlabeled octreotide. Endocrinology 136:3698–3706, 1995.

64. Duncan JR, Stephenson MT, Wu HP, Anderson CJ. Indium-111-diethylenetriaminepentaacetic acid-octreotide is delivered in vivo to pancreatic, tumor cell, renal, and hepatocyte lysosomes. Cancer Res 57:659–671, 1997.

65. Bambyrek W, Craseman B, Fink WR. X-ray fluorescence yields, Auger, and Coster-Kronig transition probabilities. Rev Phys 44:716–813, 1972.

66. Howell RW. Radiation spectra for Auger electron emitting radionuclides. Report No. 2 of AAPM Nuclear Medicine Task Group. Med Phys 19:1371–1383, 1992.

67. Adelstein SJ. The Auger process: a therapeutic promise? AJR 160:707–713, 1993.

68. Breeman WAP, Slooter GD, Marquet R, van Eijck CHJ, Krenning EP. Peptide receptor radionuclide therapy (PRRT) with [^{111}In-DTPA[0]]octreotide in rats bearing the pancreatic somatostatin receptor (SSR) positive tumor CA20948. J Nucl Med 38(5):59P, 1997. Abstract.

69. De Jong M, Rolleman EJ, Bernard BF, et al. Inhibition of renal uptake of indium-111-DTPA-octreotide in vivo. J Nucl Med 37:1388–1392, 1996.

70. Bernard HF, Krenning EP, Breeman WAP, et al. D-Lysine for reduction of renal [^{111}In-DTPA[0],D-Phe[1]]octreotide and [^{90}Y-DTPA[0],D-Phe[1],Tyr[3]]octreotide uptake. J Nucl Med 38:1929–1933, 1997.

71. Hammond PJ, Wade AF, Gwilliam ME, et al. Amino acid infusion blocks renal tubu-

lar uptake of an indium-labelled somatostatin analogue. Br J Cancer 67:1437–1439, 1993.

72. Mogensen CE, Solling K. Studies on renal tubular protein reabsorption: partial and near complete inhibition by certain amino acids. Scand J Clin Lab Invest 37:477–486, 1977.

73. De Jong M, Breeman WAP, Bakker WH, et al. Comparison of ^{111}In-labeled somatostatin-analogs for tumor scintigraphy and radionuclide therapy. Cancer Res. 58:437–441, 1998.

74. Chiti A, Agresti R, Maffioli L, et al. Breast cancer staging using technetium-99m sestamibi and indium-111 pentetreotide single-photon emission tomography. Eur J Nucl Med 24:192–196, 1997.

75. Leners N, Jamar F, Fiasse R, Ferrant A, Pauwels S. In-111-pentetreotide uptake in endocrine tumors and lymphoma. J Nucl Med 37(6):916–922, 1996.

76. Lamberts SWJ, Hofland LJ, van Koetsveld PH, et al. Parallel in vivo and in vitro detection of functional somatostatin receptors in human endocrine pancreatic tumors: consequences with regards to diagnosis, localization and therapy. J Clin Endocrinol Metab 71(3):566–574, 1990.

77. van Eijck CHJ, Krenning EP, Bootsma A, et al. Somatostatin receptor scintigraphy in primary breast cancer. Lancet 343(8898):640–643, 1994.

78. van Bon-Martens MJH, Verbeek ALM, Peters PHM, Luning P, Werre JM. Een overzicht van de epidemiologie van borstkanker in Nederland. Ned Tijdschr Geneeskd 134(6):287–291, 1992.

79. Hayes DF, Zurawski VR Jr, Jufe DW. Comparison of circulating CA 15-3 and carcino-embryonic antigen levels in patients with breast cancer. J Clin Oncol 4:1542–1550, 1986.

80. Colomer R, Ruibal A, Salvador L. Circulating tumor marker levels in advanced breast carcinoma correlate with the extent of metastatic disease. Cancer 64:1674–1681, 1989.

81. Bajc M, Ingvar C, Palmer J. Dynamic indium-111-pentetreotide scintigraphy in breast cancer. J Nucl Med 37(4):622–626, 1996.

82. Vural G, Unlu M, Atasever T, Ozur I, Ozdemir A, Gokcora N. Comparison of indium-111 octreotide and thallium-201 scintigraphy in patients mammographically suspected of having breast cancer: preliminary results. Eur J Nucl Med 24(3):312–315, 1997.

83. Limouris GS, Rassidakis A, Kondi-Paphitti A, et al. Receptor scintigraphy of non-neuroendocrine cancers with In-111 pentetreotide. Hybridoma 16:133–137, 1997.

84. Weckbecker G, Raulf F, Stolz B, Bruns C. Somatostatin analogs for diagnosis and treatment of cancer. Pharmacol Ther 60:245–264, 1993.

85. Weckbecker G, Tolcsvai L, Stolz B, Pollak M, Bruns C. Somatostatin analogue octreotide enhances the antineoplastic effects of tamoxifen and ovariectomy on 7,12-dimethylbenz(a)anthracene-induced rat mammary carcinomas. Cancer Res 54:6334–6337, 1994.

86. Krenning EP, Kooij PPM, Bakker WH, et al. Radiotherapy with a radiolabeled somatostatin analogue [^{111}In-DTPA-D-Phe[1]]-octreotide: A case history. Ann NY Acad Sci 733:496–506, 1994.

87. Krenning EP, Kooij PPM, Pauwels S, et al. Somatostatin receptor: scintigraphy and radionuclide therapy. Digestion 57:57–61, 1996.

88. Schaer JC, Waser B, Mengod G, Reubi JC. Somatostatin receptor subtypes sst1, sst2, sst3, and sst5 expression in human pituitary, gastroentero-pancreatic and mammary tumors: comparison of mRNA analysis with receptor autoradiography. Int J Cancer 70:530–537, 1997.

89. Evans AA, Crook T, Laws SAM, Gough A, Royle GT, Primrose JN. Analysis of somatostatin receptor subtype mRNA expression in human breast cancer. Br J Cancer 75:798–803, 1997.

90. Reubi JC. In vitro identification of VIP receptors in human tumors: potential clinical implications. Ann NY Acad Sc 805:753–759, 1996.

91. Virgolini I, Raderer M, Kurtaran A, et al. Vasoactive intestinal peptide-receptor imaging for the localization of intestinal adenocarcinomas and endocrine tumors. N Engl J Med 331:1116–1121, 1994.

92. van Hagen PM, Breeman WA, Reubi JC, et al. Visualization of the thymus by substance P receptor scintigraphy in man. Eur J Nucl Med 23(11):1508–1513, 1996.

93. Hennig IM, Laissue JA, Horisberger U, Reubi JC. Substance-P receptors in human primary neoplasms: tumoral and vascular localization. Int J Cancer 61:786–792, 1995.

94. Klijn JGM, Berns PMJJ, Schmitz PIM, Foekens JA. Epidermal growth factor receptor (EGF-R) in clinical breast cancer: update 1993. Endocrin Rev 1(1):171–174, 1993.

95. Remy S, Reilly RM, Sheldon K, Gariepy J. A new radioligand for the epidermal growth factor receptor: [111]In labeled human epidermal growth factor derivatized with a bifunctional metal-chelating peptide. Bioconjugate Chem (6):683–690, 1995.

96. Halmos G, Wittliff JL, Schally AV. Characterization of bombesin/gastrin-releasing peptide receptors in human breast cancer and their relationship to steroid receptor expression. Cancer Res 55:280–287, 1995.

97. Reubi JC, Schaer JC, Waser B. Cholecystokinin (CCK)-A and CCK-B/gastrin receptors in human tumors. Cancer Res 57:1377–1386, 1997.

98. Sivolapenko GB, Douli V, Pectasides D, et al. Breast cancer imaging with radiolabeled peptide from complementarity-determining region of antitumor antibody. Lancet 346:1662–1666, 1995.

99. Investigators GIVIO. Impact of follow-up testing on survival and health-related quality of life in breast cancer patients. JAMA 271(20):1587–1592, 1994.

100. Rosselli Del Turco M, Palli D, Cariddi A, Ciatto S, Pacini P, Distante V. Intensive diagnostic follow-up after treatment of primary breast cancer. JAMA

7
Breast Imaging with Radiolabeled Estrogen Receptor Ligands

Klemens Maria Scheidhauer and Anton Scharl
University Hospital, Cologne, Germany

I. INTRODUCTION

Estrogens enter tumor cells by passive diffusion and bind with high affinity and specificity to estrogen receptors (ER) [1]. Estrogen receptors are ligand-activated (transcription regulators); the interaction of the ligand-receptor complexes with DNA occurs at special transcription-activating nucleotide sequences, referred to as estrogen-responsive elements (EREs) that lie within the respective promoter regions. The metabolic effect of estrogens takes place through an activation of genes whose gene products control the cell cycle. Those changes occur in DNA transcription that in turn affect cellular protein synthesis [2,3].

The expression of estrogen receptors in mammary carcinomas indicates advanced functional differentiation within the tumor accompanied by a high degree of morphological differentiation [4,5]. The expected correlation between mammographically revealed parenchymal alterations and estrogen receptor concentrations in tumor cells has not, however, been found [6]. Furthermore, patients with receptor-positive carcinomas tend to have a more favorable prognosis [4,7–9].

The measurement of estrogen receptor status of primary tumors is one of the basic diagnostic methods used in assessing mammary carcinomas. For biochemical or histochemical measurement of receptor status adequate amounts of tumor tissue must be obtained through surgery or biopsy. These methods are therefore usually performed on primary tumors and only rarely on a recurrent tumor or metastases [10]. The latter approach often fails due to insufficient sample tissue. It is possible to perform qualitative and quantitative receptor analysis on cryo-conserved tissue and even on formalin-fixed tissue, by immunohistochemistry or enzyme immunoassay and use of monoclonal antibodies [4,11]. The results of these various approaches are somewhat divergent [12,13]. The receptor distribution in the tumor is often inhomogeneous and can also vary between primary tumors and metastases [13–15].

Positive ER status is a determining factor for the success of hormone therapy and for prognostication. The mammary gland normally contains hormone receptors; the concentration is markedly raised in more than 50% of mammary carcinomas [16,17]. The pattern of growth of mammary carcinomas can be influenced by changes in the hormonal milieu. Endocrine therapy is effective against receptor-negative tumors in only 10% of patients, while for receptor-positive carcinomas, a successful outcome can be expected in 40% to 70% of cases [18–20]. The receptor content of the cells decreases with increasing dedifferentiation, and can also be influenced by endocrine, chemo-, or radiation therapy [21,22]. Detection of endocrine receptors and receptor-oriented endocrine therapy have now become standard methods for diagnosis and treatment of breast cancer patients [20].

A noninvasive receptor diagnosis by scintigraphic imaging of receptors would allow simultaneous assessment of receptor status in several tumor locations at once—for instance, in metastases in different organs as well as in the primary tumor. It would also be possible to take sequential receptor measurements throughout the course of the disease. Last, but not least, the technique would open up new possibilities for scientific studies into, for instance, the kinetics of ligands and ligand-receptor binding. So far, our knowledge of hormone receptors has rested on measurements taken at the moment of tissue extraction. It has therefore been impossible up to now to investigate the dynamics of the expression of estrogen receptors. A scintigraphic method for diagnosing receptor levels might enable us to detect pathological alteration at a cellular level in vivo.

The search for radiolabeled receptor-specific derivatives for in vivo scintigraphic detection of receptors began back in the 1940s and '50s [23,24]. A small number of studies have since investigated how suitable scintigraphic imaging with labeled estrogen derivatives is as a noninvasive technique for in vivo scanning of tissues with high concentrations of estrogen receptors [25–29]. A number of research groups have developed their own series of radiolabeled estrogen derivatives but few of these have been tested in vivo [30–32]. The first trials of in vivo receptor scintigraphic imaging in humans were performed using the positron emitter ^{18}F published as 16-α-[^{18}F] fluoro-17-β-estradiol [26], later followed by derivatives labeled with gamma and Auger electron emitters.

II. CHARACTERISTICS OF RADIOLABELED ESTROGEN RECEPTOR LIGANDS

In 1979 Hochberg developed the biologically active, radiolabeled steroid hormone (iodine-125)-16-α-iodo-estradiol, that fulfilled the necessary criteria for a radiotracer to detect hormone receptors: that is, it combined high receptor affinity with a low degree of unspecific binding, and also exhibited good chemical and metabolic stability [33]. This compound was synthesized by exchanging iodine for bromine in the 16-β position. The fundamental disadvantage of this synthesis was that the long reaction time, which lasted about 2 days, limited the choice of isotope to iodine-125 on account of its long half-life (60 days). However, this isotope's low-energy gamma radiation renders it unsuitable for in vivo scintigraphy. By inserting a Kronenester (benzo-15-Krone-5) as a catalyst for the nucleophile halogen exchange reaction, the reaction time for the labeling was reduced to 20 min, thus allowing use of iodine-123 (half-life: 13 hours) [34,35]. The exact chemical name of this compound is: 16-α-iodo-estradiol-1,3,5-(10)triene-3,17-β-diol or E_2 for estradiol and ^{123}I-E_2 for the labeled form. This estradiol was introduced in the United States and in a multicenter study in Germany [25,27,29]. In addition, further estrogen derivatives such as 11-β-methoxy-E_2 and 16-α-iodovinyl-11-β-methoxy estradiol were applied clinically. These performed better than 16-α-E_2, at equivalent or even higher receptor specificity [36–38]. Recently, a Dutch research group published their findings from animal experiments with other ^{123}I-labeled estradiol derivatives [39] and the results of preliminary clinical trials of 11-β-methoxy-17-α[I-123] iodovinyl estradiol or Z-[I-123]MIVE for short [28,40,41].

The two clinically tested ^{123}I-labeled substances mentioned are rapidly eliminated from the blood. They are also rapidly washed-out of receptor-negative tissue. Transhepatic elimination leads to a rapid, intensive accumulation of the tracer in the liver and subsequent excretion through the intestines. These findings correspond with the results of animal trials [42–44]. The binding of the tracer to receptors leads to steady accumulation over a period of several hours in receptor-rich tissues. This provides very early imaging in the thoracic region which is of primary importance for mammary carcinomas. Z-17-α-iodovinyl-11-β-chloromethyl estradiol was further modified by blocking the metabolic reaction at the 3-0 position that takes place in the liver. This raised the concentration of the tracer in tumors and lowered accumulation in the liver; it reduced irradiation of the intestines and raised the tumor-blood quotient [45]. There are not yet any reports of clinical trials using this tracer.

III.   TECHNICAL ASPECTS

For PET tracers (^{18}F-labeling, half-life: 110 min) the new generation of scanners with the widest field of view should be used, in order to scan and take measurements over the greatest possible area within the time available. It is particularly important to include the axillary lymph nodes in the examination. There have been no accounts so far of whole-body scanning techniques with this tracer in clinical practice. The reported acquisition time of 90 to 110 min after injection (PI) is favorable, though, from experience with FDG-PET and the fast elimination of the tracer from the blood, earlier measurements, within about 30 min PI should also be feasible. Wherever possible, the tracer should not be applied to the affected side, since this can produce false-positive focal results owing to retention of radioactivity in the region where the veins branch.

Gamma camera scintigraphy with ^{123}I-labeled estrogen derivatives can be taken about 20 min PI but is optimal at about 1 to 3 hours PI, by which time accumulation of activity in the liver has been reduced. Intravenously applied ^{123}I-E$_2$ is rapidly eliminated from the blood, so that, after only 10 min, whole-body images show no significant traces of the marker anywhere in the blood pool (Fig. 1). In images taken at a much later point (up to 24 hours PI), the tumor/background quotients are higher but the count rates lower, so that extremely long measuring times are needed to obtain images of satisfactory quality. Data are recorded using conventional large field gamma cameras or SPECT cameras. The collimator should be a low-energy, high-resolution model. In addition to planar views of the thorax and whole-body scintigraphs, SPECT tomographs of the thorax should also be taken. Special positioning techniques, such as the abdominal position, combined with the use of recesses in the examination couch for lateral views of the breasts can be helpful. The exposure time for single planar images should generally not exceed 10 min per image as it is unreasonable to expect patients to undergo SPECT for longer than 30 to 40 min. The thyroid glands should be blocked at regular intervals, for instance with perchlorate; otherwise, a concentration of activity of free iodine in the thyroids and salivary glands will be seen in late acquisitions due to radiolysis (Fig. 2).

Owing to the excess emission from the caudal thoracic segments, arising from accumulated radioactivity in the liver, intense amplification is often necessary before these pictures can be evaluated. Covering the areas of maximum activity around the liver with a protective lead apron, normally used for X-ray examinations, can be helpful here. Tomographic techniques have to be used to establish the exact spatial arrangement of the overlapping structures. Even if the tumor uptake is completely overlayed by high background activity, SPECT proved to provide correct localization of specific uptake of estradiol even in small lesions (Figure 3a–d). Very high activity peaks may, however, produce reconstruction artifacts and thereby diminish the representational value of the images, especially around the liver. The regional lymph outflow areas (mediastinum, axillae, and supraclavicular fossae) and the contralateral breast can usually be covered completely by SPECT, as long as all the regions to be investigated lie within the field of view of the gamma camera. Large-field cameras are usually needed to achieve this [29].

IV. CLINICAL APPLICATIONS

Altogether, radiolabeled estrogen derivatives are used relatively seldom in clinical practice, owing to difficulties inherent in the labeling technique and the very small

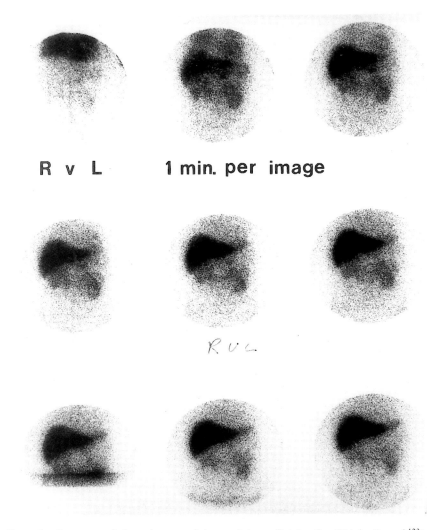

FIGURE 1   Sequence of planar images of the trunk immediately after IV-injection of ^{123}I-labeled estradiol (1 min/image): fast clearing of blood pool to liver and kidneys activity. From Ref. 29.

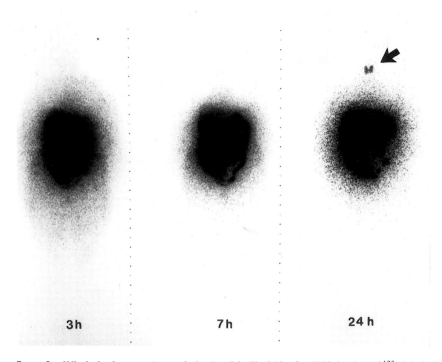

3 h   **7 h**   **24 h**

FIGURE 2   Whole-body scans (ventral view) at 3 h, 7h, 24 h after IV injection of ^{123}I-labeled estradiol showing hepatobiliary excretion of the tracer; thyroid uptake (arrow) in the 24-h image is due to in vivo radiolysis. From Ref. 29.

amount of tracer substances available. Furthermore, patenting procedures prevented more frequent, commercial application of this promising diagnostic technique. The clinical studies published to date have included a disproportional number of patients with confirmed primary mammary carcinomas or established metastases and fewer patients with only suspected mammary carcinomas. The PET tracer 16-α-[18F]fluoro-17-β-estradiol has been used only in relatively small groups of patients, for logistic reasons and owing to the limited capacity of the PET scanner [26,46]: Mintun's findings are taken from a group of 12 patients with primary mammary carcinomas with tumors ranging from 1.6 to 6 cm and one patient with a benign tumor in which the tracer failed to accumulate at all. All carcinomas, however, showed an accumulation of 16-α-[18F]fluoro-17-β-estradiol, which was described as marked in some cases but slight or only questionable in others. Quantitative measurement of tracer uptakes revealed a high correlation ($r = .96$) with estrogen receptor concentration, measured postoperatively in vitro.

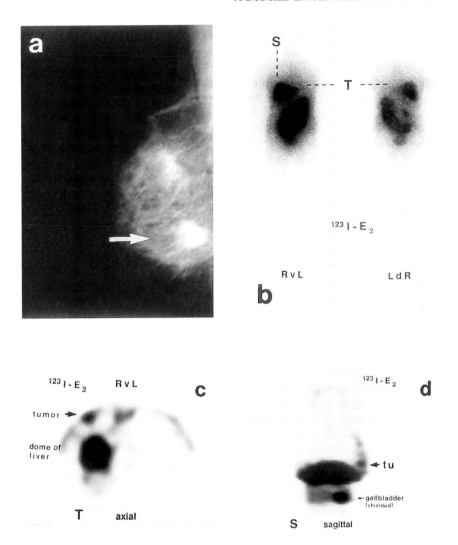

FIGURE 3 Primary carcinoma (pT1) located in the lower lateral quadrant of the right breast. (a) Lateral mammography (white arrow: tumor); (b–d) ^{123}I-estradiol scintigraphy as a 2-h whole-body scan (b) with spotted marks of the SPECT slices (c,d): transverse, resp. sagittal SPECT slices of the thorax unmask and depict the focal uptake in the tumor not detectable in the whole-body scan. From Ref. 29.

However, both false-positive and false-negative results were obtained in the region of the axillary lymph nodes. The PET scanner used for this study had a field of view of 10 cm, which is relatively narrow, suggesting that the axillary region was incompletely scanned and that possible artifacts may have arisen at the edge of the field. The authors particularly recommend regular scanning throughout hormone therapy to monitor the response to therapy and check for metastases.

The good quantitative correlation between in vitro measurements of estrogen receptor concentration and in vivo PET readings could not be reproduced in McGuire's next study performed by the same research group on patients with metastases of a mammary carcinoma. A number of factors could explain this: for one, the in vitro values were obtained from primary tumors, but the receptor content of primary tumor tissue and metastases differ in 20% to 25% of patients [47]. The sensitivity of receptor scintigraphy was 93% in 57 metastases (n = 16 patients), which is indeed high. However, the presence of a receptor-positive primary tumor was one of the criteria for inclusion in the study. Two false-positive findings were reported (radiation fibrosis and a fatigue fracture), but, in this study, only small axial areas of 10 or 20 cm were scanned. Seven patients were given a further scan after commencement of hormone therapy with antiestrogen (= receptor blockade). In each case this led to a marked reduction of activity—on average by almost two-thirds of the original level. This is evidence of the high specificity of the tracer used for the receptor [46].

Larger groups of patients were examined using ^{123}I-labeled tracers as part of a multicenter study run in Germany, using the then commercially available tracer ^{123}I-E$_2$ [29]. Here research is being focused on technical and tracer-related problems in receptor scintigraphy that have been partly solved by recent technical advances in data processing. Further studies with groups of > 20 patients have been run in the U.S. [25,27]. ^{123}I-E$_2$ is applied intravenously in a volume of 6 to 10 ml, corresponding to less than 20 ng E$_2$ and an activity of about 110 MBq iodine-123. As is to be expected with a substance applied in such low amounts, no side effects were reported in any of the studies. Experiments with a subcutaneous tracer injection as a form of lymph scintigraphy for specific imaging of lymph node metastases were unsuccessful. The accumulation contrast of the detected tumors was relatively low in all studies. Tumor/nontumor quotients in the region of 1.3 to 2.1 were obtained for tumors of up to 4 cm diameter. The sensitivity of ^{123}I-E$_2$-scintigraphy for tumor detection in primary diagnosis is also relatively low, at 67%. Since benign alterations can also show positive receptor status (e.g., mastopathy), this makes it impossible to differentiate between malignant and benign lesions. ^{123}I-E$_2$-scintigraphy cannot therefore be used as a screening method. A differentiation between a focal concentration (= malignant) and a diffuse accumulation (= mastopathy), such as that discussed by Preston (D. Preston, personal communication, 1991), has not yet been described in any other studies.

Four patients had multiple skeletal metastases that had been unequivocally detected by skeletal scintigraphy and by X-ray examinations. In none of these cases was it possible to find all these foci by ^{123}I-E$_2$ scintigraphy. In one patient, it was noticed that on the one hand not all the foci detected by skeletal scintigraphy were visible, especially those in the central portions of the skeleton that overlapped with the high level of radioactivity in the liver. Some individual foci, on the other hand, were visualized much more clearly in a ^{123}I-E$_2$ scintigram than in a skeletal scintigram. This could be interpreted as a sign of bone marrow metastasis. Figure 4 shows a receptor-positive bone metastasis with semiquantitative evaluation by ROI technique: tumor to nontumor ratio exceeds 1.6. Again SPECT only depicted metastases in central location of the trunc as demonstrated in Figure 5a–c: a lung metastasis (Fig. 5a: thorax X-ray) with a faint diffuse uptake in the planar image (Fig. 5b) is clearly shown in the transverse SPECT slice with a tumor to nontumor ratio of 1.6. The sensitivity for detection of distant metastases came to 67%, which is not particularly high [29]. However, for analysis of receptor scintigraphs there is little sense in comparing the results of this functional process with values obtained from routine morphological-anatomical diagnosis. With receptor ligands of sufficiently high specificity, receptor-negative tumors

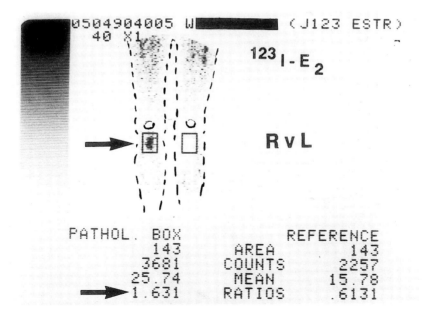

Figure 4   Estrogen receptor-positive bone metastasis of the right tibia head with semi-quantitative ROI evaluation: tumor to nontumor ratio exceeds 1.6 (arrows). From Ref. 29.

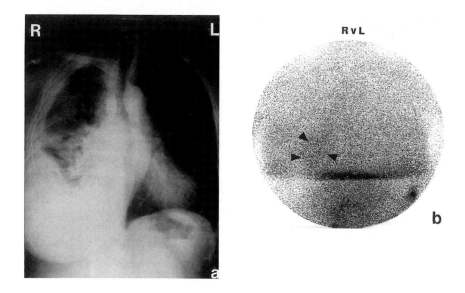

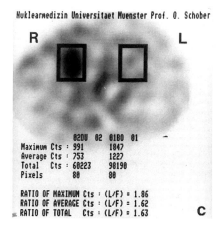

FIGURE 5   Lung metastasis of breast cancer. (a) X-ray of the thorax showing right-sided metastasis with pleural effusion. (b) Planar ^{123}I-estradiol scintigraphy of the thorax with shielded liver: faint diffuse uptake (arrowheads). (c) Transverse SPECT slice of the thorax: focal uptake in the right-sided tumor; uptake ratio: 1.6 (ROI technique). From Ref. 29.

should not be detectable. The detection rate of 67% for primary tumors agrees more or less with the incidence of receptor-positive mammary carcinomas [16]. A comparison of receptor scintigraphy with the results of in vitro receptor measurements is more meaningful. In one group of 20 carcinomas under examination, in vivo scintigraphic findings agreed with in vitro assessment of receptor status in 15 cases (75%) [48]. This matches the degree of overlap observed between the results from different methods of measuring receptor status in vitro—e.g., immunohistochemistry and the dextran charcoal coated ligand binding assay [12,13].

Few patients exhibited an axillary metastasis, although both retrosternal and parasternal foci of activity were revealed by scintigraphic imaging in isolated cases. Since there is no target organ for ER in the mediastinum, and the rapid clearance through blood pool activity excludes the possibility of false diagnosis, the likelihood of lymph node metastases being involved is now under discussion. Preston reported obtaining positive scintigrams long before a carcinoma could be verified histologically [49]. Only the systematic monitoring of clinical course can provide information in such cases. Considering the drastic nature of the most common forms of therapy and the prognostic importance of receptor status, this seems to be an extremely interesting observation and calls for further investigation through scientific studies and monitoring of clinical course.

Kenady et al. [25] achieved a sensitivity and specificity of > 92% in one group of 29 patients. The process of patient selection and tumor characteristics were not, however, clearly described. A series of recurrent tumors was also investigated. The lowest limit for detectable tumor size was given as 1 to 2 cm but no more exact details were provided, making a comparison of this study with other similar investigations difficult [25]. False-positive results could be observed in conditions prevailing after operative exploration. Nevertheless, it should be noted that there was close agreement among the results obtained by different groups.

The most recent results of clinical trials with 11-β-methoxy-17-α-[I-123]iodovinyl estradiol, or [I-123]MIVE for short, have been published by a research group in Amsterdam [40,41]. In one group of 11 patients, all tumors were detected by this tracer. The tumor/background ratio lay between 1.3 and 2.9, which is roughly that achieved with ^{123}I-E$_2$ scintigraphy. Unfortunately, the in vitro measurements of tumor receptor status were not given. In three of the patients, subsequent control scans, run shortly after commencement of antiestrogen therapy with Tamoxifen (= receptor blockade), showed no longer tracer uptake. This suggests that a specific, receptor-induced uptake mechanism operates in the case of Z-[I-123]MIVE. In a second group of patients, with recurrent tumors and metastases, the same substance detected all the lesions known to be present [41]. The highest tumor/background quotients, reaching values of 9.7, were found for bone/bone marrow. This confirms the well-known observation that ^{123}I-E$_2$ accumulates particularly readily in bone and bone marrow.

V. SUMMARY

Radiolabeled estrogen receptor ligands are tracers that can be used for functional receptor diagnosis. Their specificity toward receptors, together with the fact that only 50% to 70% of mammary carcinomas are receptor-positive, renders them unsuitable for detection of primary tumors or metastases, and this means that estrogen receptor scintigraphy can be used neither for tumor screening nor for staging.

However, both ^{18}F-labeled and ^{123}I-labeled estradiol derivatives are suitable for in vivo imaging of estrogen receptors. Their high specificity, established in animal experiments and in vitro studies, has been reproduced in in vivo applications in humans. Tracers with positron radiation emitters are, however, hardly suitable for broad application owing to the short half-life of ^{18}F, which would mean that users would need to be situated close to a cyclotron and a correspondingly equipped radiochemical laboratory. The number of available PET scanners, on the other hand, has increased dramatically over the last few years in Germany, so this, at least, does not present a limiting factor. All the same, ^{123}I-labeled estradiol derivatives will find more widespread application, since the number of gamma cameras incorporating modern multihead systems is several times greater.

The results of studies with ^{123}I-E$_2$ scintigraphy published to date are very promising, even given the initial technical problems mentioned above. As a method of examination, it could be optimized by using improved tracers with a higher tumor contrast and less disturbance from overlapping in diagnostically relevant locations—for instance, by selecting tracers with higher activities whose excretion is more renal than hepatobiliary. The use of modern multihead camera systems can also be expected to improve the photon yield.

A potential area for clinical application of E$_2$ scintigraphy is noninvasive measurement of receptor status in established lesions—for instance, to detect alterations in the receptor population during the course of therapy. It is a technique that could be used to examine several lesions simultaneously, and to run sequential scans to monitor the course of disease. Furthermore, receptor scintigraphy would present an ideal tool for scientific studies of the kinetics of ligands and ligand-receptor bindings as well as the dynamics of expression of estrogen receptors. The software now available for image fusion would allow the combination of morphological diagnostic data (CT, MRT) or unspecific tumor scintigraphy such as FDG-PET with specific functional information obtained by receptor scintigraphy [50].

Perhaps the most important observation, however, is that attachment of the radioisotope-ligand complexes to DNA opens the possibility of performing so-called site directed therapy, employing low-energy radiation emitters with a very limited range (Auger electrons). Localized double-stranded breaks of DNA (molecular surgery) and a selective toxicity for receptor-positive cells [51,52] have been already achieved in vitro.

REFERENCES

1. Wittliff J. Steroid hormone receptor in breast cancer. Cancer 53:630, 1984.
2. Beato M. Gene regulation by steroid hormones. Cell 56:335, 1989.
3. Lippman ME. In: Lippman ME, Lichter AS, Danforth DN, eds. Diagnosis and Management of Breast Cancer. Philadelphia: Saunders, 1988:326.
4. Göhring U-J, Scharl A, Ahr A. Der Stellenwert der immunhistochemischen Bestimmung von Rezeptoren, Gewebsproteasen, Tumorsuppressorproteinen und Proliferationsmarkern als Prognoseindikatoren beim primaeren Mammakarzinom. Geburtsh Frauenheilk 56:177–183, 1996.
5. Tulusan AH, Hamann M, Prestele H, et al. Correlation of the receptor content and ultrastructure of breast cancer cells. Arch Gynec, 231:177, 1982.
6. Ciatto S, Cecchini S, Iossa A. Association of estrogen receptors with parenchymal pattern at mammography. Radiology 170:695–697, 1989.
7. Alexieva-Figusch J, Van Putten WLJ, Blankenstein MA, Blonk–Van der Wijst J, Klijn JGM. The prognostic value and relationship of patient characteristics, estrogen and progestin receptors, and site of relapse in primary breast cancer. Cancer 61:758–768, 1988.
8. Chevallier B, Heintzmann F, Mosseri V, et al. Prognostic value of estrogen and progesterone receptors in operable breast cancer. Cancer 62:2517–2524, 1988.
9. Kaufmann M, Klinga K, Kühn W, Abel U. Proliferations-Index, axillärer Lymphknotenstatus, Hormonrezeptoren und Alter als Prognosefaktoren beim primären Mammakarzinom. Geburtsh Frauenheilk 49:104–108, 1989.
10. Wagner RK, Gassel WD. Hormonrezeptorbestimmung aus gezielten Knochenmarksbiopsien beim Mammakarzinom. Tumor Diagn Ther 10:252–256, 1989.
11. Andersen J, Poulsen HS. Immunohistochemical estrogen receptor determination in paraffin-embedded tissue. Prediction of response to hormonal treatment in advanced breast cancer. Cancer, 64:1901–1908, 1989.
12. Beck T, Pollow K, Grill HJ, Weikel W, Kreienberg R. Hormonrezeptornachweis der Mammakarzinome: Additive Information immunhistochemischer und histologischer Untersuchungen zum biochemischen Rezeptorassay. Tumor Diagn Ther 10:104–108, 1989.
13. Scharl A, Vierbuchen M, Würz H. Immunhistochemischer Nachweis von Östrogen- und Progesteronrezeptoren beim Mammakarzinom mit Hilfe monoklonaler Antikörper: Vergleich mit der biochemischen Rezeptoranalyse. Pathologe, 10:31–38, 1989.
14. Allegra JC, Barlock A, Huff KK, Lippman ME. Changes in multiple or sequential estrogen receptor determinations in breast cancer. Cancer 45:792–794, 1980.
15. Klinga K, Kaufmann M, Runnebaum B, Kubli F. Distribution of estrogen and progesterone receptors on primary tumor and lymph nodes in individual patients with breast cancer. Oncology 39:337–339, 1982.
16. DeSombre ER, Holt JA, Herbst AL. In: Gold JJ, Josimovich JB, eds. *Gynecologic Endocrinology.* New York: Plenum Publishing 1987:511.
17. Osborne CK, Yockmowitz MG, Knicht WA, McGuire WL. The value of estrogen and progesterone receptors in the treatment of breast cancer. Cancer 46:2884–2888, 1980.
18. Osborne CK. In: Harris JR, Hellan S, Henderson IC, Kinne DW, eds *Breast Diseases.* Philadelphia: Lippincott 1987:210.

19. Rausch D, Kiang DT. In: Stoll BA, ed. *Endocrine Management of Cancer. 2. Contemporary Therapy.* London: Karger 1988, vol. 2, p. 102.

20. Schnürch HG, In: Bender H-G, Eds. *Gynäkologische Onkologie.* Stuttgart; Thieme, 1991:376–423.

21. Maysinger D, Marcus CS, Wolf W, Tarle M, Casanova J. Preparation and high-performance liquid chromatography of iodinated diethylstilbestrols and some related steroids. Chromatogr 130:129–138, 1977.

22. Mende T, Hennig K, Wollny G, Gens J. Experimentelle Untersuchungen über die Verteilung von intravenös injiziertem, jodmarkiertem Cytonal (Diäthylstilbestroldiphosphat). Z Urol Nephrol 71:529–534, 1978.

23. Glascock RF, Hoekstra WG. Selective accumulation of tritium-labelled hexoestrol by the reproductive organs of immature female goats and sheep. Biochem J 72:673–682, 1959.

24. Twombly GH, Schoenewaldt EF. The metabolism of radioactive dibromoestrone in man. Cancer 3:601–607, 1950.

25. Kenady DE, Pavlik EJ, Nelson K, et al. Images of estrogen-receptor-positive breast tumors produced by estradiol labeled with iodine I-123 at 16a. Arch Surg 128:1373–1381, 1993.

26. Mintun MA, Welch MJ, Siegel BA, et al. Breast cancer: PET imaging of estrogen receptors. Radiology 169:45–48, 1988.

27. Preston DF, Spicer JA, Baranczuk RA, et al. Clinical results of breast cancer detection by imageable estradiol (I-123 E2). Eur J Nucl Med 16 (suppl):S123, 1990.

28. Rijks LJM, Bakker PJM, van Tienhoven G, et al. Imaging of estrogen receptors in primary and metastatic breast cancer patients with ^{123}I-labelled Z-MIVE. J Clin Oncol 1997. In press.

29. Scheidhauer K, Müller S, Smolarz K, Bräutigam P, Briele B. Tumorszintigraphie mit [123]J-markiertem Östradiol beim Mammakarzinom-Rezeptorszintigraphie. Nuklearmedizin, 30:84–99, 1991.

30. Mathias CJ, Welch MJ, Katzenellenbogen JA, et al. Characterization of the uptake of 16a-((^{18}F)fluoro)-17β-estradiol in DMBA-induced mammary tumors. Nucl Med Biol 14:15–25, 1987.

31. McManaway ME, Jagoda EM. Binding characteristics and biological activity of 17a-(^{125}I)iodovinyl-11β-methoxyestradiol, an estrogen receptor-binding radiopharmaceutical, in human breast cancer cells (MCF-7). Cancer Res 46:2386–2389, 1986.

32. Scharl A, Göhring U-J, Scheidhauer K, Schomäcker K. In: Klapdor R, ed. *Current Tumor Diagnosis: Applications, Clinical Relevance, Trends.* München: W. Zuckschwerdt, 1994: 1–4.

33. Hochberg RB. Iodine-125-labeled estradiol: a gamma emitting analog of estradiol that binds to the estrogen receptor. Science 205:1138–1140, 1979.

34. Baranczuk RJ, Spicer J, Duncan WP, Rotert GA. Bio-Medical Research Laboratories, Kansas.

35. Pavlik EJ, Nelson K, Gallion HH, et al. Characterization of high specific activity (16a-^{123}I)iodo-17β-estradiol as an estrogen receptor-specific radioligand capable of imaging estrogen receptor-positive tumors. Cancer Res 50:7799–7805, 1990.

36. Eckelmann WC, Reba RC, Gibson RE, et al. Receptor-binding radiotracers: a class of potential radiopharmaceuticals. J Nucl Med 20:350–357, 1979.

37. Hanson RN, Seitz DE, Botarro JC. E-17a-(^{125}I)iodovinylestradiol: an estrogen-receptor-seeking radiopharmaceutical. J Nucl Med 23:431–436, 1982.

38. McGuire WL, Clark GM. Progesterone receptors and human breast cancer. Eur J Cancer Clin Oncol 19:1681, 1983.

39. Rijks LJM, Boer GJ, Endert E, et al. The stereoisomers of 17a-(^{123}I)iodovinylestradiol and its 11β-methoxy derivative evaluated for the estrogen receptor binding in human MCF-7 cells and rat uterus, and their distribution in immature rats. Eur J Nucl Med; 23:295–307, 1996.

40. Rijks LJM, van Tienhoven G, Noorduyn LA, de Bruin K, Boer GJ, Janssen AGM. Imaging of primary breast cancer with the estrogen receptor specific radioligand Z-(I-123) MIVE, EANM. Eur J Nucl Med 23:1096, 1996.

41. Rijks LJM, Bakker PJM, Veenhof CHN, Boer GJ, de Bruin K, Janssen AGM. Imaging of recurrent or metastatic breast cancer with the estrogen receptor specific ligand Z-(I-123)MIVE, EANM. Eur J Nucl Med 23:1226, 1996.

42. Scharl A, Beckmann MW, Artwohl JE, Kullander S, Holt JA. Rapid liver metabolism, urinary and biliary excretion, and enterohepatic circulation of 16α-radioiodo-17β-estradiol. Int J Radiat Oncol Biol Phys 21:1235–1240, 1991.

43. Scharl A, Holt JA. Rapid vascular escape of arterially injected 16α-radioiodo, 17β-estradiol. Int J Radiat Oncol Biol Phys 26:285–290, 1993.

44. Scharl A, Beckmann MW, Artwohl JE, Holt JA. Comparisons of dynamic blood tissue exchange of radioiodine after intra-venous or intra-arterial injection of radioiodoestradiol. Int J Radiat Oncol Biol Phys 32:137–146, 1995.

45. Quivy J, Delcorde A, Leclercq G, Frühling J. Blocking the 3-0 position could increase the tumor uptake level of the breast cancer radiopharmaceuticals steroid agent, Z-CMIV, EANM. Eur J Nucl Med 23:1135, 1996.

46. McGuire AH, Dehdashti F, Siegel BA, et al. Positron tomographic assessment of 16a-(^{18}F)fluoro-17β-estradiol uptake in metastatic breast carcinoma. J Nucl Med 32:1526–1531, 1991.

47. Kamby C, Rasmussen B, Kristensen B. Oestrogen receptor status of primary breast carcinomas and their metastases. Relation to pattern of spread and survival after recurrence. Br J Cancer; 60:252–257, 1989.

48. Scheidhauer K, Smolarz K, Jackisch C, et al. In: Klapdor R, eds. *Tumor Associated Antigens, Oncogenes, Receptors, Cytokines in Tumor Diagnosis and Therapy at the Beginning of the Nineties.* München: W. Zuckschwerdt, 1992:588–589.

49. Preston DF. SPECT scan may detect breast lesions sooner. In: Cos A, ed. Radiology. Dallas: National Conference, 1996.

50. Pietrzyk U, Scheidhauer K, Scharl A, Schuster A, Schicha H. Presurgical visualization of primary breast carcinoma with PET emission and transmission imaging. J Nucl Med 36:1882–1884, 1995.

51. Beckmann MW, Scharl A, Rosinski B, Greene GL, Holt JA. Breaks in DNA accompany estrogen receptor-mediated cytotoxicity from 16α(^{125}I)iodo-17β-estradiol ((125I)E). J Cancer Res Clin Oncol 119:207–214, 1993.

52. DeSombre ER, Shafft B, Hanson RN, Kulvanen PC, Hughes A. Estrogen receptor-directed radiotoxicity with Auger electrons: specificity and mean lethal dose. Cancer Res 52:5752–5758, 1992.

8

Thallium Imaging in the Evaluation of Breast Malignancies

Alan D. Waxman

Cedars-Sinai Medical Center and University of Southern California School of Medicine, Los Angeles, California

I. INTRODUCTION

Thallium-201 (Tl-201) has been used for the evaluation of myocardial perfusion as well as myocardial viability. It has been shown to be a safe, nontoxic agent with acceptable radiation burden to the patient [1]. Tl-201 has also been shown to have a clinically relevant role for a variety of oncologic applications.

II. MECHANISM OF UPTAKE

There are several mechanisms which are felt to play a major role in determining the level of Tl-201 uptake by tumor cells. Table 1 lists possible mechanisms thought to be involved in determining Tl-201 concentration in malignancies.

It has been demonstrated that blood flow to malignant tissue appears important for delivery purposes [1–4]. Poorly vascularized tumors, especially if necrotic, appear to take up less than the same tumor type with little or no necrosis. At this time, there have been no reports comparing vascularity of tumors with degree of Tl uptake.

Waxman et al. [5] demonstrated that the degree of thallium uptake in a tumor was more closely related to cell type than any other single factor. This was based on a lymphoma model which demonstrated that highly vascular aggressive

TABLE I   Factors Which Impact Tl-201 Uptake in Tumors

Tumor viability
Tumor histology
Sodium-postassium ATPase pump
Sodium-potassium-chloride cotransport system
Calcium ion channel
Cell membrane permeability
Vascular immaturity
Blood perfusion

tumors such as diffused large-cell lymphomas were shown to have less activity than slower-growing indolent tumors such as cell low-grade lymphomas [5].

Tl is thought to behave similarly to potassium with respect to cellular biochemistry and physiology [6–8]. The sodium potassium ATPase system in the cell membrane is thought to play a key role in thallium entry into tumor cells [4,9,10]. A high potassium concentration within the cell is maintained compared with the extra cellular space in large part due to the sodium potassium pump. Sessler and co-workers [10] studied the cellular uptake of Tl-201 using Ehrlich ascites tumor cells. They found that uptake of Tl-201 by the tumor cells was inhibited using ouabain, which is known to inhibit the ATPase sodium potassium pump.

The same group also demonstrated that furosemide also inhibited thallium uptake by tumor cells. Furosemide was demonstrated to inhibit a cotransport system involving potassium and sodium, as well as the chloride ion [10]. An additive effect of both furosemide and ouabain on the inhibition of thallium uptake was also demonstrated, leading to a conclusion that at least two transport systems were involved in the uptake of thallium by tumor cells. The cotransport system for thallium was demonstrated to increases as the cells aged from the 6th day to the 12th day while, in contrast, the ATPase system fell as the cells became older. The dominant mode of cellular uptake of Tl-201 using this system was found to be in the furosemide-sensitive group, indicating that cotransport plays a dominant role in the cellular transport of Tl-201 [10].

After the inhibition of the sodium-potassium ATPase system, as well as the cotransport system, a minimal rest flow for ionic transport continued. This flow was attributed to a calcium-dependent ion channel.

Ando et al. [11] studied the biodistribution of Tl-201 in tumor-bearing animals and found thallium to be accumulated mainly by viable tumor tissue with lesser concentration abilities noted in connective tissue which contained inflammatory cells and was barely detectable in necrotic tumor tissue. In this study, Tl-201 was found mainly to exist in the free form in the fluid of the tumor, while a small fraction of thallium was located in the nuclear, myocardial, and microsenal fraction of these tissues. In addition, Tl-201 was found to be bound to a protein in these subcellular fractions. It was also noted that the biodistribution of gallium-67 was different from that of Tl-201, suggesting that the accumulation mechanisms for Tl-201 and gallium-67 in tumor tissues were independent.

Lebowitz et al. [7] implied that Tl-201 would merit evaluation for myocardial visualization as well as tumor imaging because of its physiologic and biologic properties, which were similar to potassium. This group suggested that because of the similarity of thallium to alkaline metals such as cesium, which has previously been shown concentrate in tumors, the use of radiothallium should also be evaluated for this application.

III. USE OF THALLIUM-201 IMAGING IN BREAST CANCER

Many imaging modalities are currently being employed on either a research or a clinical basis to evaluate breast cancer. These include mammography, ultrasonography, magnetic resonance imaging, and computed tomography, as well as several nuclear medicine/radiopharmaceutical techniques. While the optimum method for evaluating breast malignancy is subject to controversy, the main approach to date has been mammography and ultrasonography.

Because mammography is a highly sensitive, safe, and relatively inexpensive test, it has achieved the distinction of being the main screening modality to evaluate the breast for potential malignancy [12–18]. Diagnostic mammography has known limitations with respect to both sensitivity and specificity [18–36]. Ultrasonography in combination with mammography is used by most mammographers to direct patient management and select patients for biopsy. It is still clear, however, that many difficulties exist in the evaluation of the breast when using these conventional modalities [37].

Thallium-201 has been demonstrated to be effective in detection of many types of malignancies [5,38–62]. Hisada et al. found Tl-201 activity in two patients shown to have primary carcinoma of the breast [41]. Sehweil et al. demonstrated Tl-201 accumulation in 20 patients with primary carcinoma of the breast [51].

Waxman et al. evaluated Tl-201 in 81 women with palpable breast masses [61]. The smallest breast mass in the series was approximately 12 mm in diameter. In patients with palpable carcinoma, the sensitivity for detection of primary breast cancer was 96%. The specificity in this study was 92%. The smallest detectable cancer was an adenocarcinoma measuring $1.3 \times 1.1 \times 0.9$ cm.

Of importance was the finding that while abnormalities 12 mm and greater demonstrated a high sensitivity for thallium uptake, benign palpable masses fibrocystic disease, fat necrosis, or fibroadenoma showed a low sensitivity. This implied that benign lesions could potentially be separated from malignant lesions using Tl-201 imaging.

Lee et al. studied 40 patients including 38 women and two men in whom breast lesions were detected by physical examinations, mammography, or both [62]. A total of 39 breast lesions were evaluated. The purpose of the study was to prospectively investigate the diagnostic specificity of thallium imaging for breast cancer and to determine its value as a compliment to mammography. The study group was divided into two subgroups. The first group consisted of patients found to have breast abnormalities scheduled for biopsy or surgery. The second group were patients who were suspected to have recurrence of cancer after mastectomies or lumpectomies. The first group consisted of thallium scans performed in 32 breasts in 32 patients with pathologic diagnosis. The overall sensitivity in this group was 80% and the specificity was 96%.

The second group consisted of seven patients who were treated for breast carcinoma with surgery and radiation therapy and then underwent thallium scans because of palpable nodules at the treatment sites. Five of the seven patients in this group had true-positive posttreatment Tl-201 scans with biopsies indicating a positive recurrence of cancer. The true-positive patients in this group all had palpable masses. One patient had a false-negative scan and was found to have a microscopic focus of tumor recurrence with no palpable masses detected. Microcalcifications in this patient were noted on mammography. Since the number of patients in this group was small, there was no attempt to calculate sensitivity or specificity separately.

A combination of data from both groups (n = 39) demonstrated a sensitivity of 80% and a specificity of 96% for thallium scintigraphy in the diagnosis of breast cancer. The variance in sensitivity between the studies of Waxman and Lee were most likely due to the differences in lesion size since Waxman studied only patients with palpable masses, while Lee had a mixture of patients with palpable as well as nonpalpable masses. Of interest was the high specificity of Tl-201 for both groups.

IV.   METHODS OF BREAST IMAGING USING THALLIUM-201

Several methods of breast imaging have been suggested using Tl-201. A dose of 3 mCi of Tl-201 chloride is administered intravenously. Imaging may begin within minutes following injection, as Tl-201 is rapidly extracted by breast cancer following intravenous injection. Because of radiation considerations, the maximum dose of thallium used is 3 to 4 mCi.

Patient positioning has been variable. Waxman et al. described a supine technique with arms raised in order to evaluate both breast and axilla [61]. Multiple oblique projections including anterior and posterior obliques were obtained. The lateral views were not productive with the patients in the supine position because of the variable breast position relative to the chest wall.

Lee et al. described the use of a prone lateral position in patients able to cooperate [62]. A lateral view of the breast was taken in the prone position with the breast protruding though a hole cut through the imaging table. The surface of the collimator was positioned in the vertical position parallel to and very close to the pendulous breast. The prone view enabled the breast to be imaged without compression or distortion by gravity.

The time of imaging was variable depending on the protocol used. Waxman et al. suggested a 10-min per view technique in order to complete the sequence of anterior supine and multiple oblique projections within one hour [61]. Lee et al. employed a protocol using a preset count of 400,000 for the first view and the same exposure time used for all subsequent views using a preset time format [62]. All protocols suggested that imaging be completed within one hour following injection.

V.   THALLIUM-201 BREAST IMAGING COMPARED WITH TC-99M SESTAMIBI

Because of favorable imaging characteristics of Tc-99m using the Anger camera, Tc-99m sestamibi was suggested for tumor imaging since it appeared to have similar biodistribution characteristics to Tl-201. A favorable radiation burden for Tc-99m sestamibi, when compared to thallium-201, allowed 30 mCi of sestamibi to be used in comparison to 3 mCi for Tl-201. The added photon flux is considered an advantage for imaging.

Studies comparing Tl-201 with Tc-99m sestamibi were reported favoring the use of sestamibi over Tl-201 because of higher sensitivity. The higher sensitivity was felt mainly to be secondary to a higher photon yield. However, a higher target-to-background ratio for sestamibi when compared with thallium was also suggested as a possible explanation for the increased sensitivity [63].

Figure 1 is a Tl-201 study in a patient with a normal breast examination on both mammography as well as physical palpation. A and B are anterior supine projections with the arms raised to expose the axillary regions. A represents a 10-min acquisition beginning 2 min postinjection, while B represents a 10-min acquisition beginning 12 min postinjection. C is an LAO projection of the left breast; D is an RAO projection of the left breast.

Figure 2 is a normal Tl-201 study of the breast in a patient with a negative physical examination of the breast as well as normal mammography. The study is

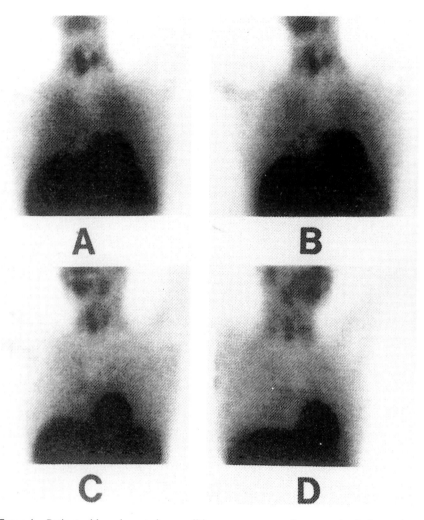

FIGURE 1   Patient with no breast abnormalities on mammography or on physical examination. Sequential 10-min Tl-201 images done in the anterior position with the arms raised (A,B). Image A was acquired between 2 and 12 min postinjection; B was acquired 12 to 22 min postinjection. Image C is an LAO projection of the left breast; D is an RAO projection. Note the gradual washout of activity from the lungs and thyroid. The left lobe of the thyroid is small in comparison to the right.

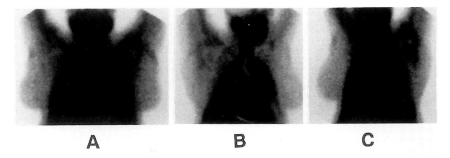

FIGURE 2   Normal Tl-201 study in a subject with no abnormalities noted on the mammogram or physical examination. Anterior (A), RAO (B), and LAO (C) projections are done with settings to optimize soft tissue visualization of the breast. Note the inability to evaluate the chest because of increased intensity. Breast studies should be evaluated on computer when possible with variable contrast settings to optimize the intensity within the region of interest.

performed in the supine position with the arms elevated. The anterior, RAO, and LAO views (A,B,C) were done at intensities which favor imaging of the breast soft tissue and tend to make the chest too dark to evaluate. It is suggested that image interpretation be done using a computer screen with the ability of the observer to modify the contrast settings in order to evaluate the specific tissue of interest with appropriate intensity settings.

Figure 3 is a patient with a 16-mm adenocarcinoma of the right breast with no pathology demonstrated in the right axilla at the time of surgery. Ten-minute anterior projections (A,B) and RAO 10-min projection of the right breast placed firmly against the collimator (C) are demonstrated. A marker view (D) is performed with a thallium marker placed over the palpable lesion of the right breast. The right axilla is normal.

Figure 4 is a comparison of a Tl-201 study (A,B) with Tc-99m-MIBI (C,D). Note the marked increase in tumor to background ratio with MIBI in both the breast (C) and left axilla (D). The patient was found to have an 18-mm adenocarcinoma of the left breast with metastases to the left axilla.

Figure 5 is a patient with a 15-mm adenocarcinoma of the right breast studied with both Tl-201 (A,B) and MIBI (C,D). The target-to-background ratio appears much higher with MIBI than with thallium.

Figure 6 is a patient with a $1.0 \times 0.7 \times 0.7$ adenocarcinoma of the right breast. The tumor is equally well demonstrated with thallium (A,B) and sestamibi (C,D). While most tumors are more readily detected using sestamibi when com-

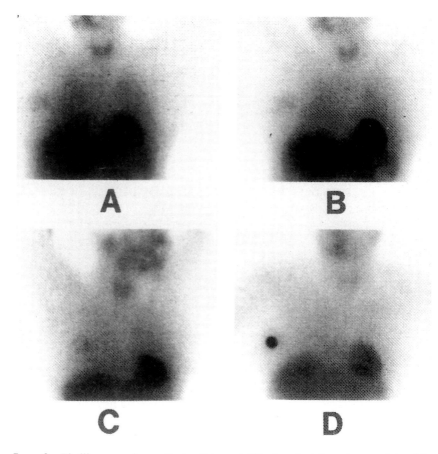

FIGURE 3   Thallium scan in a patient within an infiltrating ductal carcinoma of the right breast. The axilla at surgery was free of tumor. Ten-minute sequential anterior projections with the arms up (A,B) demonstrate the tumor in the right breast. An RAO 10-min projection with the right breast firmly against the collimator (C) demonstrates the tumor and normal axilla. A Tl-201 marker is placed over the palpable lesion of the right breast (D).

pared with thallium, several cases demonstrated thallium to be equal or slightly superior.

Figure 7 is a patient with a 25-mm adenocarcinoma of the right breast with two positive axillary nodes demonstrated at surgery. Both thallium (A,B,C) and MIBI (D,E,F) detected the primary, the axillary lymph nodes were not detected. Note the higher target-to-background ratio with Tl-201 when compared to MIBI.

Figure 8 is a patient with benign breast disease. Multiple biopsies demon-

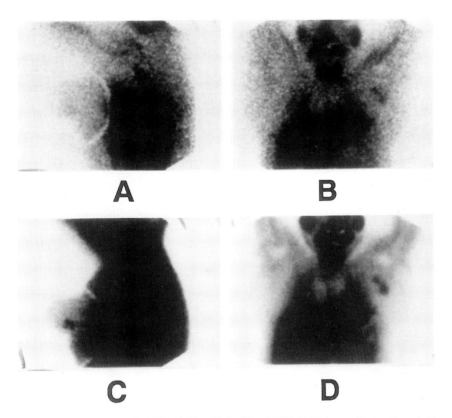

FIGURE 4   Comparison of Tl-201 (A,B) with Tc-99m-MIBI (C,D) in a patient with an infiltrating ductal carcinoma of the left breast. Note the increased target-to-background ratio in the MIBI study in both the breast and axilla when compared to thallium. Prone views (A,C) and anterior supine arm-up views (B,D) demonstrate the importance of the supine arm-up view in evaluating the axilla.

strated extensive fibrocystic changes. Note the homogenous appearance of both breasts on the 10-min sequential Tl-201 studies (A,B).

Figure 9 is a Tl-201, MIBI comparison in a patient with extensive fibrocystic changes bilaterally. Biopsy also demonstrated multiple small fibroadenomas to be present. The benign disease is detected much more readily using MIBI (C,D) than with thallium (A,B).

The poor sensitivity for benign disease with Tl-201 when compared to MIBI may improve specificity for Tl-201. However, sensitivity is compromised.

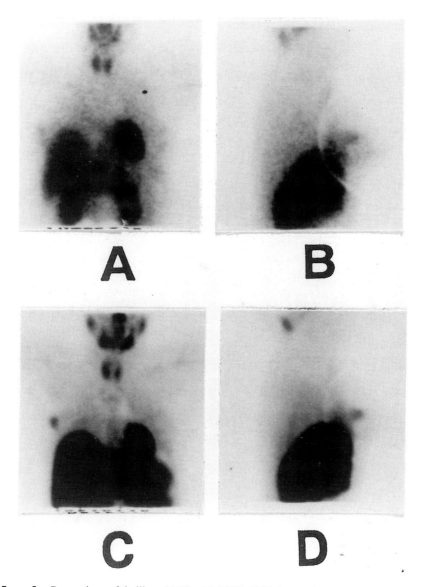

FIGURE 5   Comparison of thallium (A,B) with MIBI (C,D) in a patient with an infiltrating ductal carcinoma of the right breast with a maximum dimension of 15 mm. Target-to-background ratio is higher on the MIBI studies than with Tl-201.

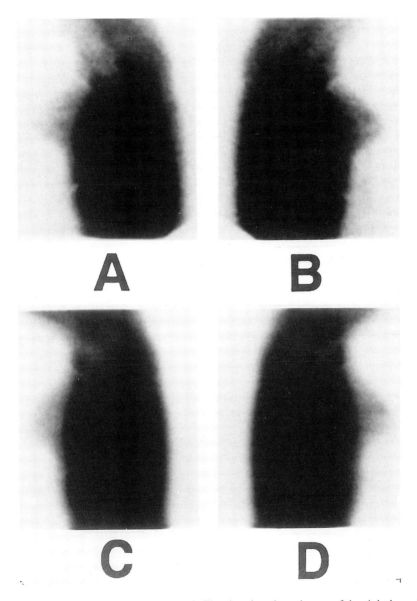

FIGURE 6   Patient with a 1.0 × 0.7 × 0.7 infiltrating ductal carcinoma of the right breast. Prone images demonstrate approximately equal tumor-to-background ratios for both Tl-201 and MIBI. A,B: thallium; C,D: sestamibi.

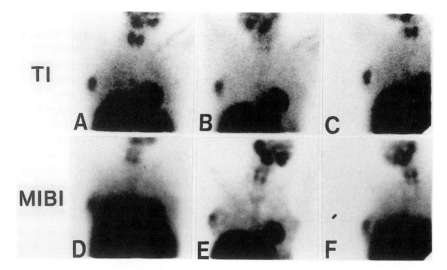

FIGURE 7   Patient with a 25-mm adenocarcinoma of the right breast. The Tl-201 (A,B,C) appears to have a slightly higher target-to-background ratio than the MIBI (D,E,F) study. The patient also was noted to have two lymph nodes in the right axilla with microscopic tumor deposits. Both Tl-201 and MIBI failed to detect the positive lymph nodes.

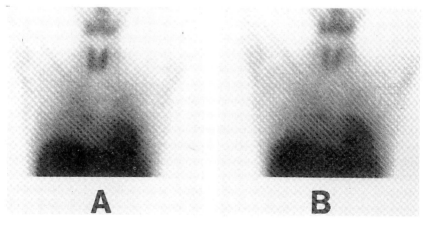

FIGURE 8   Patient with extensive palpable fibrocystic disease in both breasts. Ten-minute sequential thallium images in the supine position (A,B) failed to identify the fibrocystic abnormalities, which were demonstrated to be extensive on biopsy.

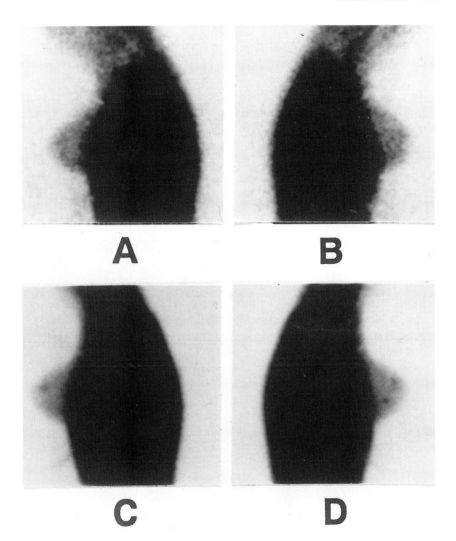

FIGURE 9   Patient with biopsy-proven extensive fibrocystic disease of both breasts with several fibroadenoma present. Prone Tl-201 (A,B) is compared with prone MIBI (C,D). Note the focal abnormalities bilaterally on the MIBI and minimally nonhomogeneous breast on Tl-201.

VI. CLINICAL RELEVANCE OF THALLIUM-201 IMAGING IN THE EVALUATION OF SUSPECTED BREAST MALIGNANCY

A clinically relevant role for Tl-201 breast imaging is difficult to define. The sensitivity for Tc-99m MIBI is superior overall to that of Tl-201 and would appear to be the radiopharmaceutical of choice at this time [64–69]. The better specificity figures for Tl-201 as compared to Tc-99m sestamibi are most likely due to the reduced photon yield with Tl-201. This would reduce sensitivity for detection of all breast lesions including malignancy as well as proliferative breast changes.

Theoretically, it would be possible to increase the imaging time for Tl-201 to 20 to 30 min per view. This may generate the total counts necessary to achieve comparable resolution to Tc-99m-MIBI if the tumor to background ratios were equal. This approach has yet to be proven and would be considered as inefficient for incorporation into the daily routine of a busy facility.

The advantages of Tl-201 over Tc-99m-MIBI are extremely limited and mainly related to the cost per dose of radiopharmaceutical. The primary disadvantage for Tl-201 is a lower photon yield due to the lower administered dose because of dosimetry considerations. Limitation of dose also limits the ability to perform adequate SPECT examinations, as inadequate photons are available for high-resolution imaging.

In summary, Tl-201 has served as an early model to demonstrate feasibility of imaging breast pathology using nuclear medicine techniques. The desirability of Tl-201 for breast imaging is less than that for other radiopharmaceuticals including Tc-99m MIBI or F-18 fluorodeoxyglucose. In areas of the world where Tc-99m Sestamibi or FDG are unavailable, then Tl-201 may serve as a less desirable alternative.

REFERENCES

1. Atkins HL, Budinger TF, Lebowitz E, et al. Thallium-201 for medical use. Part 3. Human distribution and physical imaging properties. J Nucl Med 18:133–140, 1977.
2. Tonami N, Hisda K. Clinical experience of tumor imaging with thallium-201 chloride. Clin Nucl Med 2:75–81, 1977.
3. Kaplan WD, Takvorian T, Morris JH, et al. Thallium-201 brain tumor imaging: a comparative study with pathological correlation. J Nucl Med 28:47–52, 1987.
4. Muranake A. Accumulation of radioisotopes with tumor affinity. II. Comparison of the tumor accumulation of Ga-67 citrate and thallium-201 chloride in vitro. Acta Med Okayama 35:85–101, 1981.
5. Waxman AD, Ramanna L, Said J. Thallium scintigraphy in lymphoma: relationship to gallium-67. J Nucl Med 30(5):915, 1989.

6. Gehring PJ, Hammand PB. The interrelationship between thallium and potassium in animals. J Pharmacol Exp Ther 155:187–201, 1967.

7. Lebowitz E, Greene MW, Greene R, et al. Thallium-201 for medical use I. J Nucl Med 16:151–155, 1975.

8. Bradley-Moore PR, Lebowitz E, Greene MW, Atkins HL, Ansari AN. Thallium-201 for medical use. II. Biologic behavior. J Nucl Med 16:156–160, 1975.

9. Britten JS, Blank M. Thallium activation of the (Na+,K+) activated ATPase of rabbit kidney. Biochim Biophys Acta 15:160–166, 1968.

10. Sessler MJ, Geck P, Maul FD, et al. New aspects of cellular Tl-201 uptake: Tl + Na+ –2CI. Cotransport is the central mechanism of ion uptake. J Nucl Med 25:24–27, 1986.

11. Ando A, Ando I, Katayama M, et al. Biodistribution of Tl-201 in tumor bearing animals and inflammatory lesion induced animals. Eur J Nucl Med 12:567–572, 1987.

12. Rogers JV, Powell RW. Mammographic indications for biopsy of clinically normal breasts: correlation with pathologic findings in 72 cases. AJR 115:794–800, 1972.

13. Homer MJ. Nonpalpable breast abnormalities: a realistic view of the accuracy of mammography in detecting malignancies. Radiology 153:831–832, 1984.

14. Sickles EA. Mammographic features of 300 consecutive nonpalpable breast cancers. AJR 146:661–663, 1986.

15. Pollei SR, Mettler FA, Bartow SA, et al. Occult breast cancer: prevalence and radiographic detectability. Radiology 163:459–462, 1987.

16. Stompcr PC, Davis SP, Weidner N, Meyer JE. Clinically occult, noncalcified breast cancer: serial radiologic-pathologic correlation in 27 cases. Radiology 169:621–626, 1988.

17. Basset LW, Liu TH, Guiliano AE, et al. The prevalence of carcinoma in palpable versus impalpable, mammographically detected lesions. AJR 157:21–24, 1991.

18. Kopans DB. The positive predictive value of mammography. AJR 158:521–526, 1992.

19. Mann BD, Guiliano AE, Bassett LW, et al. Delayed diagnosis of breast cancer as a result of normal mammograms. Arch Surg 118:23–25, 1983.

20. Holland R, Jan HC, Hendricks L, et al. Mammographically occult breast cancer: a pathologic and radiologic study. Cancer 52:1810–1819, 1983.

21. Feig SA, Shaber GA, Patchefskly A. Analysis of clinically occult and mammographically occult breast tumors. AJR 128:403–408, 1977.

22. Kalisher L. Factors influencing false negative rates in xeromammography. Radiology 133:297–301, 1979.

23. Burns PE, Grace MG, Lees AW, et al. False-negative mammography delays diagnosis of breast cancer. N Engl J Med 199:201–201, 1978.

24. Burns PE, Grace MG, Lees AW, et al. False-negative mammograms causing delay in breast cancer diagnosis. J Can Assoc Radiol 30:74–77, 1979.

25. Sickles EA. Mammographic features of early breast cancer. AJR 143:461–464, 1984.

26. Moskowitz M. The predictive value of certain mammographic signs in screening for breast cancer. Cancer 51:1007–1011, 1983.

27. Sadowsky N, Kopans DB. Breast cancer. Radiol Clin North Am 21:51–65, 1983.

28. Sickles EA. Mammographic features of early breast cancer. AJR 143:461–464, 1984.

29. Niloff PH, Sheiner NM. False-negative mammograms in patients with breast cancer. Can J Surg 24:50–52, 1981.

30. Spivey GH, Perry BW, Clark VA, et al. Predicting the risk of cancer at the time of breast biopsy: variation in the benign to malignant ratio. Am Surg 48:326–332, 1982.

31. Mills RR, Davis R, Stacey AJ. The detection and significance of calcifications in the breast: radiologic and pathological study. Br J Radiol 49:12–26, 1976.

32. Sickles EA. Breast calcifications: mammographic evaluation. Radiology 160:289–293, 1986.

33. Homer MJ. Nonpalpable mammographic abnormalities: timing the follow-up studies. AJR 136:923–926, 1981.

34. Meyer JE, Sonnenfeld MR, Greenes RA, et al. Preoperative localization of clinically occult breast lesions; experience at a referral hospital. Radiology 169:627–628, 1988.

35. Hermann G, Janus C, Schwartz IS, et al. Nonpalpable lesions: accuracy of prebiopsy mammographic diagnosis. Radiology 165:323–326, 1987.

36. Hall FM, Storella JM, Selverstone DZ, et al. Nonpalpable breast lesions: recommendations for biopsy based on suspicion of carcinoma at mammography. Radiology 167:353–368, 1988.

37. Kopans DB. "Early" breast cancer detection using techniques other than mammography. AJR 143:465–468, 1984.

38. Salvatore M, Carratii L, Porta E. Thallium-201 as a positive indicator for lung neoplasms: preliminary experiments. Radiology 121:487–488, 1976.

39. Tonami N, Hisda K. Clinical experience of tumor imaging with thallium-201 chloride. Clin Nucl Med 2:75–81, 1977.

40. Aneri B, Basset JY, Lonchampt MF, et al. Diagnosis of cerebral lesions by thallium-201. Radiology 128:417–422, 1978.

41. Hisada K, Tonami H, Miyame T, et al. Clinical evaluation of tumor imaging with thallium-201 chloride. Radiology 129:497–500, 1978.

42. Tonami H, Hisada K. Thallium-201 scintigraphy in postoperative detection of thyroid cancer; a comparative study with I-131. Radiology 136:461–464, 1980.

43. Winzelberg GG, Melada GA, Hydrovitz JD. False-positive thallium-201 parathyroid scan of the mediastinum in Hodgkin's lymphoma. AJR 147:819–821, 1986.

44. Stoller DW, Waxman AD, Rosen G, et al. Comparison of thallium-201, gallium-67, technetium-99m MDP and magnetic resonance imaging of muscoloskeletal sarcoma. Clin Nucl Med 12(suppl):P15, 1986. Abstract.

45. Kaplan WD, Takvorian T, Morris JH, et al. Thallium-201 brain tumor imaging: a comparative study with pathological correlation. J Nucl Med 28:47–52, 1987.

46. Waxman AD, Goldsmith MS, Greif PM, et al. Differentiation of tumor versus sarcoidosis using thallium-201 in patients with hilar mediastinal adenopathy. J Nucl Med 28:561, 1987. Abstract.

47. Ramanna L, Waxman AD, Binney G, et al. Increasing specificity of brain scintigraphy using thallium-201. J Nucl Med 28:658, 1987. Abstract.

48. Mountz JM, Stafford-Schuck, McLeever P, et al. The tumor/cardiac ratio: a new method to estimate residual high grade astrocytoma using thallium-201. J Nucl Med 28:706, 1987. Abstract.

49. Hofnagel CA, Delprat CC, Marcus HR, et al. Role of thallium-201 total body scintigraphy in follow-up of thyroid carcinoma. J Nucl Med 27:1854–1857, 1988.

50. Lee VW, Rosen MP, Baum A, Cohen SE, Colley T, Liebman HA. AIDS-related Kaposi sarcoma: findings on thallium-201 scintigraphy. AJR 151:1233–1235, 1988.

51. Sehweil AM, McKillop JH, Milroy R, et al. Thallium-201 scintigraphy in the staging of lung cancer, breast cancer and lymphoma. Nucl Med Commun 11:263–269, 1990.

52. Waxman AD, Ramanna L, Brachman MB, et al. Thallium scintigraphy in primary carcinoma of the breast: evaluation of primary and axillary metastasis. J Nucl Med 30:844, 1989.

53. Waxman AD, Ramanna L, Said J. Thallium scintigraphy in lymphoma: relationship to gallium-67. J Nucl Med 30:915, 1989. Abstract

54. Black KL, Hawkins R, Kim KT, et al. Use of thallium-201 SPECT to quantitate malignancy grade of gliomas. J Neurosurg 71:342–346, 1989.

55. Tonami N, Shuke N, Kunihiko Y, et al. Thallium-201 single photon emission computed tomography in the evaluation of suspected lung cancer. J Nucl Med 30:997–1004, 1989.

56. Ramanna L, Waxman AD, Binney G, et al. Thallium-201 scintigraphy in bone sarcoma: comparison with gallium-67 and technetium-MDP in evaluation of chemotherapy response. J Nucl Med 31:567–572, 1990.

57. Kim KT, Black KL, Marciano D, et al. Thallium-201 SPECT imaging of brain tumors: methods and results. J Nucl Med 31:965–969, 1990.

58. Kaplan WD, Wouthee ML, Annese MS, et al. Evaluating low and intermediate grade non-Hodgkin's lymphoma (NHL) with gallium-67 (Ga) and thallium-201 (Tl) imaging. J Nucl Med 31:793, 1990. Abstract.

59. Waxman AD, Ramanna L, Memsic A, et al. Thallium scintigraphy in the differentiation of malignant from benign mass abnormalities of the breast. J Nucl Med 31:747, 1990.

60. Ramanna L, Waxman AD, Braunstein G. Thallium-201 scintigraphy in differentiated thyroid cancer: comparison with radioiodine scintigraphy and serum thyroglobulin determination. J Nucl Med 32:441–446, 1991.

61. Waxman AD, Ramanna L, Memsic LD, et al. Thallium scintigraphy in the evaluation of mass abnormalities of the breast. J Nucl Med 34:18–23, 1993.

62. Lee VW, Sax EJ, McAneny DB, et al. A complementary role for thallium-201 scintigraphy with mammography in the diagnosis of breast cancer. J Nucl Med 34:2095–2100, 1993.

63. Waxman AD, Ashok G, Kooba A, et al. The use of Tc-99m methoxyisobutyl isonitrile (MIBI) in evaluation of patients with primary carcinoma of the breast: comparison with Tl-201 (Tl). J Nucl Med 34:139, 1993. Abstract.

64. Khalkali I, Mena I, Jouanne E, et al. Prone scintimammography in patients with suspicion of carcinoma of the breast. J Am Coll Surg 178:491–497, 1994.

65. Khalkali I, Mena I, Diggles I. Review of imaging techniques for the diagnosis of breast cancer: a new role of prone scintimammography using technetium-99m sestamibi. Eur J Nucl Med 21:357–362, 1994.

66. Taillefer R, Robidoux A, Lambert R, et al. Technetium-99m sestamibi prone scintimammography to detect primary breast cancer and axillary lymph node involvement. J Nucl Med 36:1758–1765, 1995.

67. Khalkali I, Cutrone JA, Mena I, et al. Technetium-99m sestamibi scintimammography of breast lesions: clinical and pathological follow-up. J Nucl Med 36:1784–1789, 1995.

68. Palmedo H, Schomburg A, Grunwald F, et al. Technetium-99m MIBI scintimammography for suspicious breast lesions. J Nucl Med 37:626–630, 1996.

69. Waxman AD. The role of Tc-99m methoxyisobutylisonitrile in imaging breast cancer. Semin Nucl Med 27:40–54, 1997.

9

Breast Imaging with
^{99m}Tc-Methylenediphosphonate

Secondo Lastoria, Sergio Piccolo, and Pietro Muto
National Cancer Institute, Naples, Italy

I. INTRODUCTION

A. Historical Background

Mammography is the mainstay for the early detection of breast abnormalities. Mammography is characterized by an elevated sensitivity but a relative low specificity in diagnosing breast cancer (1–3). Thus, a large number of patients, prevalently affected by benign diseases, undergo surgical biopsy to achieve diagnosis (4,5). A wide spectrum of imaging modalities is currently under investigation to overhelm the mammographic limitations and to reduce the number of performed biopsies. This armamentarium encompasses morphological imaging techniques: ultrasound, magnetic resonance imaging (6,7), and functional imaging techniques which are radionuclide-based. Several studies have demonstrated the ability of ^{99m}Tc-sestamibi, ^{201}Tl-chloride, ^{99m}Tc-tetrofosmin, ^{111}In-pentetreotide, labeled monoclonal antibodies, ^{18}F-FDG, and labeled steroid hormones in detecting primary breast cancer, involved axillary lymph nodes, and distant metastases (8–16). Different trials are ongoing, primarily with cathionic, lipophilic ^{99m}Tc-labeled agents.

In our laboratory, we approached breast imaging with ^{99m}Tc-sestamibi and ^{99m}Tc-methylenediphosphonate (MDP) (17,18). A significant part of our research is based on the use of ^{99m}Tc-MDP. Remarkable results were obtained introducing few methodological innovations such as time of acquisition (5–10 min after the tracer injection) and imaging the patient in prone position. In a series of 200 women, with high pretest likelihood to have breast cancer and discrete tumor nodules, the diagnostic accuracy was 90% (18). In details, the overall rate of breast cancer detection was 92%, being near to 100% for lesions ≥15 mm in diameter

301

and slightly >60% for smaller ones; the specificity was in the same order of magnitude. In the images acquired 2 hours after ^{99m}Tc-MDP injection, the sensitivity (40%) was significantly lowered (18). Tracer washout from the cancer along with increased activity in the chest cage were probably the main explanations for such difference.

B. Rationale for Clinical Use

^{99m}Tc-MDP was introduced in the early 1970s by Subramanian and McAfee. It is routinely used as bone seeking agent, because of the high tropism for remodeling bone (19). ^{99m}Tc-MDP is also concentrated in soft-tissue benign disorders (uremia, hypercalcemia, pulmonary calcinosis, chrondocalcinosis, etc.) as well as calcified tumors (20). A number of concurring processes are involved in the mechanism/s of ^{99m}Tc-MDP uptake in primary breast cancer, including increased blood flow supply, neoangiogenesis, enlarged extracellular space, cell wall damages, changes in pH and calcium content, etc. (20). Previous studies, by histochemical methods, demonstrated that increased levels of acid and alkaline phosphatase were found in benign and malignant breast tissues, without evidence of microscopic calcifications, avidly concentrating ^{99m}Tc-phosphate compounds. Chiaudauri et al. proposed a mechanism for binding of linear phosphate and diphosphonate by receptor sites on enzyme molecules (21). Similarly, the correlation between calcium content within tissues and entity of ^{99m}Tc-diphosphonate uptake has been demonstrated by Silberstein (22). The significant differences in the ^{99m}Tc-MDP uptake between benign and malignant breast lesions strongly suggest that both intratissular calcium content and the enzymatic receptor theory play pivotal roles. Furthermore, Aprile et al. found, in humans, a significantly higher effusion-to-plasma ratio of ^{99m}Tc-pyrophospate in malignant than benign effusions (23).

II. CHARACTERISTICS OF RADIOPHARMACEUTICALS

A. Chemistry/Radiolabeling

The preparation of ^{99m}Tc-MDP is well standardized in nuclear medicine radiopharmacy. Briefly, the addition of ^{99m}Tc-pertechnetate in isotonic saline to the freeze-dried mixture of MDP (as sodic salt), stannous fluoride, and sodium p-aminobenzoate causes the reduction of pertechnetate and the formation of a soluble ^{99m}Tc/MDP complex. The pH of the preparation lies in the range 5.5–7.5. When intravenously injected the complex concentrates in the skeleton, particularly in areas of osteogenic activity, as well as in soft tissues as previously reported (21,22). In our study, we used MDP vials (Amersham/Sorin Radiopharmaceuticals, Italy), obtaining five doses per vial.

B. Dosimetry

The absorbed radiation dose per 370 MBq of injected ^{99m}Tc-MDP, as reported in the manufacturer's brochure, is estimated as follows:

Skeleton	3.7–22.2 mGy
Bone marrow	3.7 mGy
Kidneys	0–11.1 mGy
Bladder wall	22–29.6 mGy
Ovaries	0–18.5 mGy
Effective dose equivalent (EDE)	0–0.08 mSv/MBq (0–0.3 rem/mCi).

C. Quality Control

The content of free ^{99m}Tc-pertechnetate in the labeled injectable MDP may be determined by thin-layer chromatography on hydroxylapatite slides, prepared as recommended by manufacturer. One drop of reconstituted ^{99m}Tc-MDP is placed 1 cm from the lower edge of the slide and developed in 0.9% (w/v) sodium chloride solution. The ^{99m}Tc-complex will remain at the origin while the top (4 cm) will contain the free ^{99m}Tc-pertechnetate. The colloidal content of the injectable material may be assessed by descending chromatography on Whatman paper (No. 541) in 0.9 (w/v) sodium chloride solution. Any colloidal material will remain at the origin, and free ^{99m}Tc-pertechnetate and ^{99m}Tc-MDP will move with the solvent front.

D. Experiences in Cell Lines

The evaluation of the ^{99m}Tc-MDP uptake in human breast cancer cell lines is under investigation in our laboratory. ^{99m}Tc-MDP uptake was evaluated at the following time points: 1, 5, 10, 40, 60, and 120 min either at 4 and 37°C. ^{99m}Tc-pertechnetate was used as control. For these experiments human breast cancer cell line MCF-7 was used. The cells were detached from the flasks and initially resuspended in 0.5 mL of RPMI 1640 medium (500,000 cells/tube), centrifuged, and washed twice with phosphate-buffered saline (PBS). The pellets containing MCF-7 cells were then resuspended in 0.5 mL of PBS and incubated with 10 µCi in 10 µL of ^{99m}Tc-pertechnetate and ^{99m}Tc-MDP at 4 and 37°C. After incubation the tubes were centrifuged, and both pellet and supernatant were counted in a γ counter. Duplicates were obtained for each experimental time point. ^{99m}Tc-MDP was concentrated in negligible amounts within human breast cancer cell lines MCF-7. Our preliminary data mirror the results of a previous study, recently published (24). However, the ^{99m}Tc-MDP cell-related activity was initially (1–10 min) higher (five- to seven-fold) than the ^{99m}Tc-pertechnetate activity, suggesting that a very early, not stable binding to the cell membranes occurs. In fact, in none of our experiments, as well as in other studies, is ^{99m}Tc-MDP internalized within the cells as occurs for sestamibi (24).

III. TECHNICAL ASPECTS

A. Image Acquisition

Each woman had physical examination by the surgeon, mammography, and eventually breast ultrasounds prior to SMM. The presence of clinical palpable lesions alone or associated with abnormal mammographic patterns which required excisional biopsy or surgery for the final diagnosis, were the main inclusion criteria adopted.

1. Mammography

Mammography was performed in all women using craniocaudal and mediolateral projections. In selected cases additional views with magnification, using coned compression, were acquired. Images were reviewed by two experienced radiologists. In women with calcifications without mass the mammograms were classified as follows:

> *Typically benign:* eggshell or rim calcifications, spherical or lucent, centered, vascular, large rodlike, coarse or popcornlike, milk of calcium
> *Less specific for malignancy or probably benign* (indeterminate coarse): amorphus or indistinct
> *Suggestive of malignancy:* pleomorphic or heterogeneous (granular) and fine and/or branching (casting)

A hook wire was positioned to mark the calcification/s, as guide for the surgeon. Resected specimens were imaged after surgery to verify the complete excision of calcifications.

2. SMM

Clinical evaluation was repeated before SMM by a nuclear medicine physician to anatomically localize the palpable masses. The interval between MMx and SMM was <1 week, while the interval between diagnostic workup and pathological evaluation was 2 weeks. SMM was performed using a single-head γ camera (Philips Tomo, Netherlands) equipped with LEHR parallel-hole collimator, interfaced with a dedicated computer. The matrix size was 128×128 pixels; the photopeak was centered at 140 keV with a symmetric 10% window to minimize the scattered radiation from the table. The lateral views of right and left breast (150–200 kcounts) were acquired 5–10 min after the IV injection of 550–740 MBq of ^{99m}Tc-MDP.

The patient was in prone position on the table of the γ camera. A self-made device allowed maintenance the breast pending and near the collimator during the acquisition. A 0.5-cm-thick guide of lead was placed between the two breasts to avoid activity from the controlateral gland impairing the quality of the imaged breast. Early (5 min) and delayed (20 min) anterior views of the chest (800 kcounts), in upright position, were acquired to better define lesions located in the inner quadrants and to eventually depict metastatic axillary nodes.

B. Data Analysis

Mammographic patterns were generally classified as *diagnostic* for cancer, *suspicious* for cancer, and *indeterminate,* as previously reported (18).

SMM findings were classified by two nuclear medicine physicians (S.L., S.P.) as positive or negative. A positive study was classified when focal or diffuse increased ^{99m}Tc-MDP uptake was seen. Disagreement was solved by consensus or with the added opinion of a third reviewer (P.M.). The results of mammography and SMM were then classified using the pathological findings as *gold standard.*

IV. CLINICAL APPLICATIONS

A. Personal Experience

In the last 4 years at the Department of Nuclear Medicine of the National Cancer Institute of Naples, more than 2000 women were investigated by SMM with ^{99m}Tc-MDP. In the initial step of the study we have investigated large breast lesions to evaluate the sensitivity and specificity of the test. The wide majority (>90%) of malignancies >10 mm was clearly detectable (18). Similarly, the accuracy of the test was >90%, with only a few benign diseases which falsely accumulated the tracer (18). However, the detection of large carcinomas only may be considered a trivial problem. Thus, we tried to address specific issues in the diagnosis of breast lesions, assessing the role of SMM with ^{99m}Tc-MDP in women: (1) with nondiagnostic mammograms, in whom biopsy was mandatory to define the nature of the lesion; (2) with mammographic evidence of calcifications without palpable masses; (3) in comparison with fine needle biopsy results; and (4) in comparison with other radiopharmaceuticals.

Preliminary experiences targeted on these issues have been published (25,26).

I. Patterns of SMM

In SMM, the ^{99m}Tc-MDP uptake has been classified in four different patterns: negative, focal, multifocal, and diffuse.

The presence of smooth, diffuse and homogeneous ^{99m}Tc-MDP uptake through the breast was classified as negative (Fig. 1a). This activity represents the background of the gland. The background activity increases during the menses and after treatment (surgery and radiotherapy). In this setting it is suggested to perform the SMM not during the cycle, and 12–16 months after radiotherapy, in order to avoid misinterpretations. A *focal* uptake was classified an area of, well-defined, increased tracer accumulation (Fig. 1b). In the majority of cases it was associated with cancer; in a small percentage, to benign diseases. The pattern characterized by two or more foci of well-defined, increased uptake was classified as *multifocal* (Fig. 1c); it was always associated with breast cancer. The pattern of *diffuse* uptake was characterized by an increased ^{99m}Tc-MDP accumulation, usually involving the wide majority of a breast; it was commonly associated with inflammatory cancer or diffuse DCIS (Fig. 1d). The evidence of skin infiltration is a distinctive, adjunctive sign of inflammatory cancer.

The intensity of ^{99m}Tc-MDP uptake and the clear contrast in the images allow an easy identification and classification of these patterns. The lack of intermediate situations helps in categorizing the SMM results. Thus, we did not use quantitative and/or qualitative scores to measure the degree of uptake.

2. SMM Overall Results

The different tumor hystotypes and grading did not influence ^{99m}Tc-MDP accumulation and results. Conversely, the tumor size influenced the rate of detection. In fact, in a series including 330 women with histologically proven carcinomas, abnormal, increased ^{99m}Tc-MDP uptake was found in 305 lesions (92%). Twenty out of 25 missed cancers were ≤10 mm and 5 ≤ 15 mm.

The relationship between the tumor largest diameter and rate of SMM detection is shown in Figure 2. However, lesions with largest diameter <10 mm were correctly recognized by SMM, as in the case shown in Figure 3. Besides the tumor size, the depth and the location of tumor nodules within inner quadrants, close to the chest wall, may impair the tumor identification. The activity, in fact, in these tumors may be masked by the surrounding tissue or covered by the background of the chest (ribs or blood pool). The anterior view of the chest is the only approach, available at the moment, to facilitate the identification of tumor deposits located in the inner quadrants. In fact, the present γ cameras do not enable the performance of craniocaudal projections of the mammary glands, and dedicated breast γ imagers are not yet commercially available.

The lack of ^{99m}Tc-MDP internalization in cultured human malignant cell lines suggested that the uptake in breast cancer is completely nonspecific and primarily related to the lesion's hypervascularization. Increased blood flow has a significant relevance in the tracer arrival to the lesions, but other factors play a role. In fact, the ^{99m}Tc-MDP uptake is still present 15 min after the injection, within

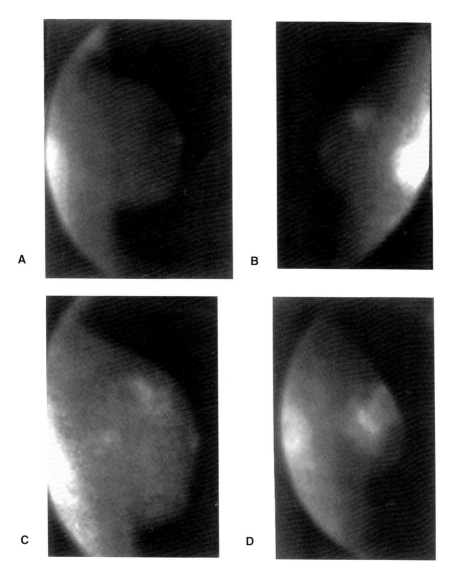

FIGURE I   Different patterns of ⁹⁹ᵐTc-MDP SMM. (A) Normal tracer distribution in a
healthy breast gland: the background activity is generally smooth, as in this case. Increased
background is seen during the menses or after recent surgery and/or radiotherapy. (B) An
example of focal, intense ⁹⁹ᵐTc-MDP uptake, due to a small infiltrating ductal carcinoma
of the left breast. (C) Multiple, distinct foci of ⁹⁹ᵐTc-MDP uptake characterize the pattern
frequently associated to plurifocal breast carcinoma as in this case. (D) A diffuse pattern of
tracer uptake involving almost the entire breast. The uptake is inhomogeneous. This pattern
is usually associated with inflammatory cancer or ductal carcinoma with a prevalent in situ
component.

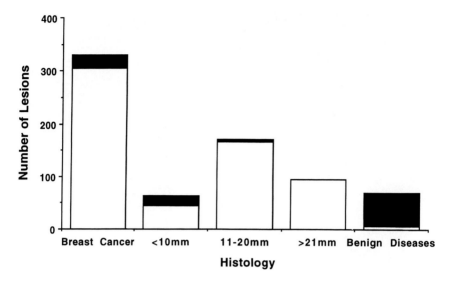

FIGURE 2   Rate of lesions detected by SMM vs. tumor size. □, Lesions detected by SMM; ■, total number of lesions.

the breast cancer; it is negligible in organs, such as liver, with high blood flow supply. The longer residency time of ^{99m}Tc-MDP within cancer deposits may be due to the trapping consequent to the enlargement of the extracellular space as well as to changes in local metabolism, pH, and calcium content. These latter mechanisms define the tracer accumulation within cancer associated with calcifications more precisely than the hypervascularization solely.

Benign breast disorders usually did not show ^{99m}Tc-MDP uptake, as shown in Figure 4. In 700 histologically proven, benign breast diseases less than 10% were classified as false-positive with a specificity >90%. False-positive ^{99m}Tc-MDP uptake was prevalently found in fibroadenomas associated with hyaline and/or mixoid degeneration; sclerotic fibroadenomas, acute inflammation, and epithelial hyperplasias associated with moderate or severe atypia. Probably, histologic features of these benign diseases facilitate the tracer uptake. In fact, fibrocystic changes, parenchymal distortion, radial scar, and other benign disorders were negative.

SMM with ^{99m}Tc-MDP correctly visualized, histologically proven metastatic axillary lymph node involvement was observed in <40% of cases, with a limited reliability in this setting. Visualized lymph nodes were clinically palpable. The poor rate of SMM in detecting metastatic axillary nodes is probably due to

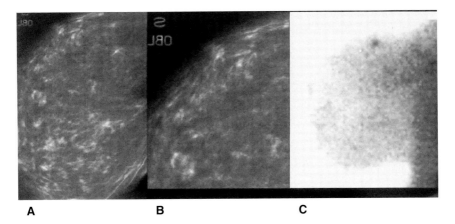

A **B** **C**

Figure 3 ^{99m}Tc-MDP SMM in small lesions. (A) Lateral mammogram, which shows a small, irregular opacity in the upper outer quadrant of the left breast, suspicious for breast carcinoma. (B) Magnified view, where the small opacity is better delineated. (C) SMM shows, in the left lateral view, increased ^{99m}Tc-MDP uptake in the small lesion, which had 6 mm largest diameter.

different causes (i.e., blood flow supply, size, depth, number of malignant cells, etc.). However, the rate of lymph nodes detected by SMM ^{99m}Tc-MDP might be improved by changing the order of images acquisition. In fact, the anterior view of the chest, which includes both axillae, is usually recorded 20–30 min after tracer injection, when the background may somehow mask the activity within lymph nodes. Nevertheless, the rate of lymph node detection appears lower than that measured by ^{99m}Tc-sestamibi and tetrofosmin in other series and in our own experience.

2. Comparison of SMM and Mammographic Findings

Biopsy was required for the diagnosis in approximately half of our patients' population, who had not had diagnostic mammograms. The most frequent causes for this finding were radio *dense* breast, parenchymal distortion, calcifications without mass, etc. In Table 1 the results of SMM, in a series of 120 women with nondiagnostic mammography, are classified according to the histological findings. The greatest incidence of nondiagnostic mammography occurred in women ranging in age from 20 to 50 years.

SMM correctly recognized 101/120 lesions with an overall accuracy of

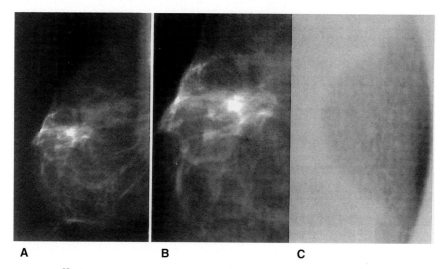

A   **B**   **C**

Figure 4 ^{99m}Tc-MDP SMM in benign breast disease. (A) By mammography an area of increased density with skin involvement, highly suspicious for locally advanced cancer, is recognized in the left breast. (B) Spot magnification confirms this pattern. (C) The lack of ^{99m}Tc-MDP uptake in this area suggest the benign nature of the lesion, as confirmed by histology (chronic mastitis) after surgery.

84%. In particular, 37/50 breast cancer concentrated ^{99m}Tc-MDP, as shown in Figure 5, while 64/70 benign lesions were truly negative (Fig. 4). The magnitude of such results clearly suggests the clinical relevance of SMM in these patients.

3.   SMM in Women with Mammographic Evidence of Calcifications Without Mass

Breast carcinoma frequently forms calcifications, which are a rare feature in other human malignancies. The exact mechanisms regulating the formation of calcium deposits in breast cancer are not fully elucidated. In some tumors the calcium is located within necrotic areas; in others, it may be produced and released by viable neoplastic cells (27).

Leborgne in 1951 first described that calcifications may be the only mammographic manifestation of a breast carcinoma (28). The percentage of nonpalpable breast carcinomas associated with calcifications is extremely high, ranging from 30% to 50% (29,30). Thus, the identification of clustered and/or isolated calcifications, without associated mass, has been largely used to diagnose clinically occult breast cancer. In fact, a wide majority of nonpalpable ductal carcinoma in situ (DCIS) and 70% of infiltrating cancer <5 mm were seen as microcalcifications alone (31,32). The challenge to radiologists is not only to recognize

Table 1 Scintimammographic Results in Women with
Nondiagnostic Mammography

Histology size (mm)	No. cases	SMM results	
		Positive	Negative
Carcinoma	**50**	**37**	**13**
<10	15	7	8
11–20	26	21	5
>21	9	9	0
Benign lesions	**70**	**6**	**64**
Adenoma	21	0	21
Fybrocistic dysplasia	22	0	22
Fybrocistic dysplasia with severe atypia	4	3	1
Masthytis	5	0	5
Intracystic papilloma	4	0	4
Mixoid fibroadenoma	3	2	1
Sclerotic fibroadenoma	3	1	2
Radial scar	2	0	2
Fat necrosis	2	0	2
Papillomatosis	4	0	4

the presence of these tiny particles but also to assess the likelihood of malignancy to avoid unnecessary biopsies (33).

Benign and malignant calcifications may produce similar mammographic patterns, and there are not specific criteria to diagnose breast cancer when isolated clusters of microcalcifications occur (34). The specificity ranged between 20% and 30% (35). The success or failure of the mammographic calcification analysis scheme primarily depends on image quality and radiologist's expertise (33). Nevertheless, indeterminate calcifications, apart from dense, mastopathic breasts, are the greatest unsolved diagnostic problem for mammography. The recommendation by a radiologist to perform a biopsy of calcifications indicates an unequivocal concern that the lesion may be malignant (35). The complete excision of a mammographic abnormality permits the pathologist to evaluate the entire lesion and to determine the benign or malignant nature (36,37). On the other hand, less than complete excision of a nonpalpable lesion or incisional biopsy may often present a management dilemma for both the clinician and the radiologist, especially when histologic analysis proves the specimen to be benign (37).

Correlation between mammographic and pathologic findings indicates an average cancer occurrence in about 33% of cases (32–43). Fine needle aspiration (FNA) biopsy or core biopsy of calcifications may be inconclusive. In fact, the

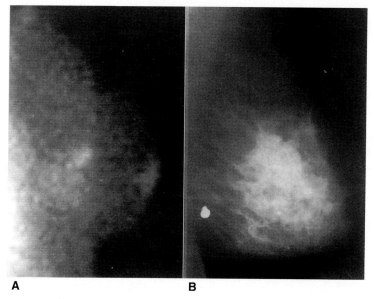

A   **B**

FIGURE 5 ^{99m}Tc-MDP SMM in woman with an indeterminate mammogram. (A) The ^{99m}Tc-MDP uptake in the posterior part of the right breast, in the area of palpable mass, is highly diagnostic for breast carcinoma. (B) The mammogram cannot demonstrate, in this dense breast, the morphological aspects of the palpable lesion.

calcium deposits, which are the mammographic target, may not be within the malignant tissue. Thus, the aspiration of cells in areas of microcalcifications could miss the adjacent tumor, leaving it undiscovered and therefore untreated.

There is the possibility that excised benign tissue is not representative of the entire lesion and that undiagnosed malignancy has been left within the breast. Thus, open biopsy is mandatory for definitive diagnosis. On the other hand, this approach has proven to be costly, cosmetically disfiguring to the breast, and psycologically traumatic to patients.

SMM with ^{99m}Tc-MDP had a significant impact in detecting and differentiating malignant from benign breast calcifications without palpable masses in a series of 186 women (mean age of 52 ± 10 years; 38% were in premenopausal and 62% in postmenopausal status) with isolated and/or clustered calcifications. Cytology or histology diagnosed carcinoma in 65 women and benign breast diseases in 121. The spectrum of malignant and benign histotypes is summarized in Table 2.

Malignant calcifications, in this series, were frequently associated to DCIS (55%; 36/65 cases); less frequently, to LCIS (7.7%; 5/65). Tumor largest diameter, when measured by gross anatomy, ranged between 4 and 55 mm. Benign cal-

Table 2   SMM Results in Patients with Evidence of Calcifications Without Mass According to Histological Diagnosis

Histology	No. cases	SMM			
		TP	TN	FP	FN
Malignant lesions	**65**	**60**	**0**	**0**	**5**
DCIS	36	34	0	0	2
Comedo type	20	19	0	0	1
Noncomedo type	16	15	0	0	1
Invasive ductal Ca	14	13	0	0	1
Mixed Ca	8	7	0	0	1
LCIS	5	5	0	0	1
Invasive lobular Ca	2	2	0	0	0
Benign lesions	**121**	**0**	**109**	**12**	**0**
Typical ductal hyperplasia	50	0	47	3	0
Fibrocystic dysplasia	46	0	46	0	0
Atypical epithelial hyperplasia	9	0	4	5	0
Fibrosis	5	0	5	0	0
Fibroadenoma	4	0	2	2	0
Papillomatosis	4	0	4	0	0
Chronic Inflammation	3	0	1	2	0

cifications were frequently associated with both typical ductal hyperplasia (41%) and fibrocystic dysplasia (38%).

In 34 women mammography was classified "typically benign," being present in egg shell, or rim, or spherical and/or lucent-center calcifications. Pathological or clinical follow-up findings were concordant to mammographic pattern in all these cases, selected as *control group* to evaluate the specificity of SMM.

In 40 cases mammography was classified "probably benign," being present in linear or amorphous or indistinct calcifications. In this subgroup, pathology diagnosed 15 malignant and 25 benign lesions.

In 112 patients mammography was classified "having high probability for cancer," being present pleomorphic or heterogeneous and/or fine or branching calcifications. The histologic diagnosis was of breast carcinomas in 50 women (27 DCIS, 21 invasive ductal, and two invasive lobular carcinomas) and benign lesions in 62.

SMM was positive in 60 of 65 histologically proven breast cancer, the missing five lesions being classified as false-negative. The histotypes of missed malignancies were DCIS (two cases), LCIS (one), infiltrating ductal (one), and mixed carcinoma (one); the largest diameter was <12 mm. The overall sensitivity was

92%. The majority (109/121) of patients with calcifications associated with benign breast lesions had negative SMM. The histotypes of benign disorders which showed ^{99m}Tc-MDP uptake were atypical ductal hyperplasia (five), typical ductal hyperplasia (three), fibrocystic dysplasia (two), and inflammation (two). The overall specificity was 90%. Predictive positive and negative values of SMM were respectively 83% and 95%.

The comparison of pathological, mammographic, and scintigraphic results is summarized in Table 3. The pattern of ^{99m}Tc-MDP uptake was focal in 58, plurifocal in 10, and diffuse in four cases. Focal ^{99m}Tc-MDP uptake was seen in patients with either isolated or grouped calcifications associated with breast cancer in 46 and to benign breast disorders in 12 women. In Figure 6 is shown an example of focal ^{99m}Tc-MDP uptake occurring in an invasive carcinoma, mammographically detected as clustered calcifications suspicious for cancer.

Multifocal and diffuse patterns of ^{99m}Tc-MDP uptake occurred only in patients with histologically proven breast cancer, primarily ductal carcinoma with a prevalent in situ component, as shown in Figure 1d. The extent of tracer uptake was usually larger than the extension of calcifications, mirroring more precisely the size of the lesion as defined by gross anatomy. SMM with ^{99m}Tc-MDP allowed also differentiation of malignant from benign calcifications within the same breast, suggesting that cancer produces substantial modifications within the glandular tissue.

The results of mammography and SMM were concordant in the 34 patients of the control group. Conversely, in the women with mammographic patterns classified as probably benign or having high probability for breast cancer, the scintigraphic results were significantly discordant (Table 3).

The benign-to-malignant lesions ratio of 2:1 did not bias the sensitivity (92%) and the specificity (90%) of SMM in this cohort of patients and corroborates the evidence that this test is extremely accurate in differentiating the nature of lesions associated with calcifications without palpable mass. Thus, SMM seems

TABLE 3   Summary of Mammographic, Scintigraphic, and Pathological Results in Women with Calcifications Without Mass

Mammography	Typically benign (34 cases)	Low probability for BC (40 cases)		High probability for BC (112 cases)	
	↓	↓		↓	
Histology	34 BD	25 BD	15 BC	62 BD	50 BC
	↓	↓	↓	↓	↓
SMM	34 TN	21 TN	14 TP	54 TN	46 TP
		4 FP	1 FN	8 FP	4 FN

BC = breast cancer; BD = benign disease; TN = true negative; TP = true positive; FP = false positive; FN = false negative.

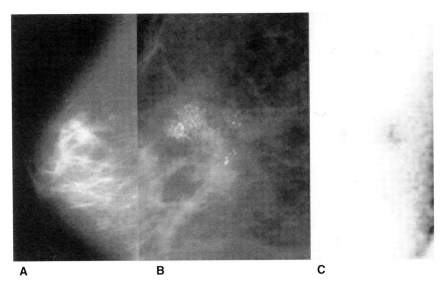

A   **B**   **C**

Figure 6 ^{99m}Tc-MDP SMM in woman with mammographic evidence of calcification without mass. (A) The mammogram identifies calcification in the left breast. (B) The magnified spot, after compression, enables to define the calcification type (cluster) which was considered suspicious for cancer. (C) The ^{99m}Tc-MDP uptake in the breast region characterized by calcification corroborated the suspicion of malignancy.

a reliable, complementary test to mammography in women with patterns not diagnostic for benign diseases. The correct diagnosis of calcifications is, in our opinion, one most promising niche where SMM with ^{99m}Tc-MDP will have a major impact in the patients' management, reducing the number of unnecessary biopsies and changing the surgical strategy. For instance, the evidence of multicentric tumor deposits in different quadrants is a contraindication for breast-conserving surgical therapy. Multifocal tumors in one quadrant require extension of the operation to a quadrantectomy rather than a simple tumorectomy. Since US and MRI with specific contrast agents use different substrates from mammography, these are investigated as alternative and/or adjunctive tests to mammography, to differentiate malignant versus benign/normal breast tissues. Unfortunately, both modalities have significant limits in the characterization of calcifications.

Among the other radiopharmaceuticals used for the SMM, namely sestamibi and tetrofosmin, few data are available in addressing this specific issue. A previous report from Maffioli et al. faced this topic using sestamibi in a small series of patients with calcifications either associated or not with masses (45). The reported specificity was high, but the sensitivity was <50%. Probably, the mechanisms of sestamibi uptake, mainly intracellular, are a drawback when small tumors or discrete clusters of malignant cells are associated or adjacent to calcifications.

4. Comparison of SMM and FNA Biopsy Results

In a subset of 139 patients with microcalcifications without mass and/or indeterminate mammograms, SMM findings have been compared with FNA biopsy results. The rationale for such approach was based on the evidence that FNA may be disfiguring; it is not well accepted by the women and accounts 3–7% false-negative results (46). Furthermore, a constant limitation is represented by insufficient material, which in different series ranged from 8% to 26% (36,38,44,47,48). In addition, the lack of well-defined cytological criteria to differentiate benign, premalignant, and malignant lesions and the overlapping features among different diseases are significant diagnostic drawbacks.

In our study protocol, the women underwent FNA a few days after the SMM. The FNA was US-guided in nonpalpable masses sonographically evident; otherwise, it was performed under sterotaxic mammographic guidance. The results showed that SMM was truly negative in 43 of 44 women with FNA negative for cancer, truly positive in all 34 FNA positive for cancer (49). The most important part of the study was in the 60 cases where FNA was inconclusive. In fact, according to the histology 25 were malignant and 35 benign lesions, as summarized in Table 4. In these 60 cases, SMM gave 21 TP, 27 TN, 4 FN (tumor size <10 mm), and 8 FP. The sensitivity of SMM was again positively correlated to the tumor size, as shown in Table 5. That these results may significantly affect the patients' management is evident by the comparison of the statistical figures of both SMM and FNA, shown in Table 6.

5. Comparison with Other Radiopharmaceuticals

In a preliminary report, we have investigated the sensitivity and specificity of both tracers in a group of 65 women (50). Forty-seven of 50 carcinomas were correctly recognized by the two agents, with a 94% sensitivity. Conversely, in the evalua-

TABLE 4   Histological Diagnosis in 60 Women with Suspicious FNAB

Tumor type (No.)	Benign disease (No.)
Invasive ductal Ca (12)	Fibroadenoma (13)
Invasive lobular Ca (6)	Fibrocystic dysplasia (13)
Inflammatory Ca (2)	Adenosis (5)
Intraductal Ca (2)	Chronic mastitis (1)
Mixed carcinoma (1)	Atypical epith. hyperpl. (1)
Mucinous carcinoma (1)	Granuloma (1)
Papillary carcinoma (1)	Ductal ectasia (1)

TABLE 5   Relationship Between Tumor Size and
SMM Findings

Size (mm)	No. lesions	SMM positive
<10	2	1 (50%)
10–20	25	23 (92%)
20–50	23	23 (100%)
>50	2	2 (100%)
Not measured	8	7 (87%)

tion of 15 women with benign disorders, ^{99m}Tc-MDP had a higher specificity than sestamibi (93% vs. 53%). The rate of metastatic axillary lymph nodes correctly detected was higher by sestamibi (17/24 pts.; 73%) than by MDP (5/24; 21%). We have extended this protocol to 90 patients. The results are shown in Table 7.

The statistical figures for both breast cancer agents are substantially unmodified. The limited number of enrolled women does not allow final conclusions, and larger series should be investigated. However, the trend indicates that a relatively lower number of benign, highly cellular lesions concentrated ^{99m}Tc-MDP than ^{99m}Tc-sestamibi. Such difference is justified from the different behavior of the tracers, mainly intracellular for sestamibi and prevalently extracellular for MDP. Comparative studies are needed to compare MDP with tetrofosmin. Comparative studies between SMM and PET (using as tracers FDG and ^{11}C-Met) are ongoing. Such studies will more likely face biological parameters than clinical diagnostic aspects of breast cancer for the relative limited diffusion of PET units and for the still elevated cost of these studies.

In our institution we have analyzed, in a small series of patients, the feasibility of detecting primary breast carcinoma with fluorine-18 (^{18}F) (51). The rationale to use this positron emitter, bone-seeking nuclide is the same used for ^{99m}Tc-MDP. The results show a similar behavior in the distribution of ^{99m}Tc-MDP and

TABLE 6   Comparison of Cytological and
SMM Findings

	Cytology		SMM	
Sensitivity	34/60	(57%)	56/60	(93%)
Specificity	44/79	(56%)	70/79	(89%)
Accuracy	78/139	(56%)	126/139	(91%)
PPV	44/70	(63%)	70/74	(94%)
NPV	34/69	(49%)	56/65	(91%)

TABLE 7   Comparative Results of SMM with ^{99m}Tc-MDP and Sestamibi

SMM	Malignant	Benign	SENS	SPEC
MDP			95%	88%
Positive	62	3		
Negative	3	22		
Sestamibi			94%	64%
Positive	61	4		
Negative	9	16		

^{18}F within cancer. The maximal ^{18}F uptake within cancer was seen between 2 and 5 min after the injection. This immediate uptake is strictly related to the small size of this ion. The tumor-to-background ratios were as high as sixfold. The washout of ^{18}F from lesions was faster than that of ^{99m}Tc-MDP. Metastatic axillary lymph nodes were detected earlier and in larger number by PET with ^{18}F than by conventional SMM. The evidence that metastatic lymph nodes were visualized earlier than primary tumors suggested modifying the sequence of image acquisition during SMM with ^{99m}Tc-MDP by anticipating the anterior view of the chest before the two lateral views in prone position.

B. Review of Medical Literature

The current approach in imaging breast cancer by ^{99m}Tc-MDP follows the pioneering studies of the early 1970s (52–55). These studies were interrupted because of the low impact in the diagnosis of breast cancer. The significant technological improvement in the nuclear medicine equipment and the changes in the protocol of acquisition have substantially modified the rate of breast cancer detection by this radiopharmaceutical. The current literature is prevalently composed by the experiences of our group (18,25,26). However, in the past 2 years other groups have been testing this procedure.

C. Conclusions

The SMM with ^{99m}Tc-MDP, as demonstrated by the results of our experience in numerically significant groups of women, may be clinically useful in some certain indications:

> Characterization of palpable nodules with a not diagnostic mammographic pattern
> Characterization of calcifications without palpable masses

Characterization of nonnodular abnormalities with indeterminate mammograms.

SMM as a role in characterizing palpable nodules, >10 mm in size, with not diagnostic mammographic patterns, having a diagnostic accuracy >90% (18,25, 26). Therefore, a positive SMM is highly indicative for cancer and surgical treatment; conversely, a negative SMM will suggest a follow-up, whose interval may be established case by case. In both circumstances FNA may be avoided, with significant advantages for both clinicians and patients. Few false-positive cases may occur in lesions which were surgically removed (fibroadenomas and fibrocystic changes with atypia). For lesions <10 mm, the rate of detection is approximately 60%, making this modality not reliable to diagnose or to rule out the presence of cancer. Thus, only a limited number of patients, with very small lesions, might really benefit from a scintigraphic study. In these women FNA or open biopsy is strongly recommended.

SMM has to follow mammography in characterizing all nondiagnostic cases, especially nonpalpable lesions and nonnodular images.

In women with mammographic evidence of calcifications (but not diagnostic) the use of SMM immediately after mammography might better define their nature and reduce the number of FNA.

FNA should be required only when SMM is negative; surgery should be considered when SMM is positive. In Table 8 is summarized the diagnostic scheme currently applied, using SMM with ^{99m}Tc-MDP, in our institution.

SMM with ^{99}Tc-MDP is under investigation in these other conditions and it may be only suggested, at the moment for:

Early identification of recurrent breast cancer (in women previously operated and/or irradiated, and in women with implants)
Monitoring of response to neoadjuvant chemotherapy in patients with advanced breast cancer.

Preliminary results in the early detection of recurrent breast cancer have shown very promising insights. The timing and the frequency in performing the test are the problems to solve in these patients. SMM should be avoided in the first 3–6 months after extensive surgery and up to 1 year after radiotherapy. The increased background activity within the remaining mammary tissue might mask the recurrence. The early detection of recurrent disease in women with breast implants has been studied in a few cases. The encouraging results mirror the experience reported with other tracers, but again the trend has to be confirmed in larger series.

In monitoring neoadjuvant chemotherapy, the use of sestamibi or tetrofosmin seems preferable because both these lipophilic agents are substrates of the P-glycoprotein 170 (Pgp-170), which regulates one of the mechanisms of the multidrug resistance (MDR) phenomenon (56,57). Recent studies have demonstrated

Table 8   Diagnostic Algorithm Suggested for the Proper Use of SMM

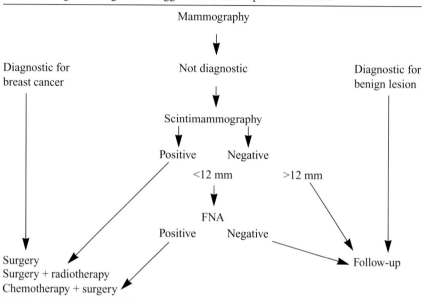

that the in vivo efflux rate of sestamibi from breast cancers is positively correlated with the levels of Pgp-170 expressed on the neoplastic cells (58,59). Thus, performing studies with sestamibi and measuring the differences in the uptake before and after neoadjuvant chemotherapy, tumor regression or onset of the MDR may be diagnosed. This is not a trivial problem, allowing in time modification of the therapeutic regimen, sparing from ineffective treatment patients with elevated Pgp-170 expression on the tumor cells. Nevertheless, preliminary results with ^{99m}Tc-MDP showed promising insights.

The routine clinical use of SMM should represent a goal for nuclear medicine physicians. To capitalize on the present, increasing interest of clinicians, surgeons, and radiologists for SMM and to minimize the risks of a reduced use in the near future, the following rules should be followed:

Proper application of the test in specific, well-circumscribed diagnostic niches, where the other imaging modalities are generally less accurate
Correct execution of the test
Necessary training for technologists in performing the test and for physicians in reading the images.

The use of SMM only in the above-mentioned niches avoids misleading results and delays in the diagnosis.

The proper execution of the test is mandatory to avoid the risks of poor-quality exams, which increase the chances of error in the interpretation of the images. In this setting, we should keep in mind the lesson learned from mammography, where poor quality still represents one of the major diagnostic drawbacks. In fact, moving from investigational purposes to clinical practice, the increasing number of tests to perform daily may affect the quality. Finally, a correct report of the SMM may not be done without performing an accurate physical examination, collecting the patient's data, comparing the scintigraphic images of both breasts, between them, and with the mammograms.

V. SUMMARY

The SMM is a simple, noninvasive, and accurate test to depict breast cancer and to characterize some peculiar biologic parameters. The different tracers currently used allow definition of the cellularity and perfusion (sestamibi, tetrofosmin, thallium chloride), the calcium metabolism (MDP),the receptor (octreotide, hormones), and the antigenic profile (monoclonal antibodies) (8–14,18,25,26). Besides investigational aspects, the clinical impact of SMM has been proven, at least for sestamibi and MDP, in large series of women as an adjunctive test to mammography to ameliorate the accuracy in the diagnosis of carcinoma.

Experience with ^{99m}Tc-MDP in more than 2000 women at the National Cancer Institute of Naples faced different aspects of breast imaging. The results allow suggesting this approach to characterize breast abnormalities in the following cases: palpable nodules (>10 mm) with a nondiagnostic mammographic pattern; calcifications without palpable masses, and lesions with indeterminate mammogram in nonnodular abnormalities. The cost of SMM with ^{99m}Tc-MDP ($150 U.S.) is significantly lower than those proposed or charged for other tracers ($600–800 U.S. for sestamibi, octreotide, and PET with FDG). Since the high diagnostic accuracy obtained by SMM with ^{99m}Tc-MDP, the limited cost is a further, not secondary, advantage over the other radiopharmaceuticals for clinical utilization.

REFERENCES

1. Sickels EA. Breast masses: mammographic evaluation. Radiology 1989; 173:297–303.
2. Donegan WL. Evaluation of palpable breast masses. N Engl J Med 1992;327:937–942.
3. Adler DD. Mammographic evaluation of masses. In: Syllabus: A Categorical Course

in Breast Imaging. Kopans DB, Mendelson EB, eds. RSNA Publ, Oak Brook, IL, 1995:107–116.

4. Sickles EA. Management of probably benign lesions. In: Syllabus: A Categorical Course in Breast Imaging. Kopans DB, Mendelson, EB, eds. RSNA Publ, Oak Brook, IL, 1995:133–138.

5. Teixidor HS, Wojsatek DA, Reiches AM, Santos-Buch CA, Minick CR. Fine-needle aspiration of breast biopsy specimens: correlation of histologic and cytologic findings. Radiology 1992;184:55–58.

6. Gordon PB. US for problem solving in breast imaging: tricks of the trade. In: Syllabus: A Categorical Course in Breast Imaging. Kopans DB, Mendelson EB, eds. RSNA Publ, Oak Brook, IL, 1995:121–131.

7. Kaiser WA, Zeitler E. MR imaging of the breast: fast imaging sequences with and without Gd-DTPA. Radiology 1989;170:681–686.

8. Khalkhali I, Cutrone JA, Mena I, et al. Scintimammography: the complementary role of Tc-99m sestamibi prone breast imaging for the diagnosis of breast carcinoma. Radiology 1995;196:421–426.

9. Taillefer R, Robidoux A, Lambert R, Turpin S, Laperriére J. Technetium-99m-sestamibi prone scintimammography to detect primary breast cancer and axillary lymph node involvement. J Nucl Med 1995;36:1758–1765.

10. Waxman AD, Ramanna L, Memsic LD, et al. Thallium scintigraphy in the evaluation of mass abnormalities of the breast. J Nucl Med 1993;34:18–23.

11. Lee VW, Sax EJ, McAneny DB. A complementary role for thallium-201 scintigraphy with mammography in the diagnosis of breast cancer. J Nucl Med 1993;34:2095–2100.

12. Mansi L, Rambaldi PF, Procaccini E, et al. Scintimammography with ^{99m}Tc tetrofosmin in the diagnosis of breast cancer and lymph node metastases. Eur J Nucl Med 1996;23:932–939.

13. Van Eijck C, Krenning E, Bootsma A, Oet H, van Pel R. Somatostatin receptor scintigraphy in primary breast cancer. Lancet 1994;343:640–643.

14. Sivolapenkow GB, Douli V, Bekhtasides D, et al. Breast cancer imaging with radiolabelled peptide from complementarity-determining region of antitumor antibody. Lancet 1995;346:1662–1666.

15. Adler LP, Crowe JP, Al-Kaisi NK, Sunshine JL. Evaluation of breast masses and axillary lymph nodes with 18-F2-deoxy-2-fluoro-d-glucose PET. Radiology 1993;187:743–750.

16. Scheidauer K, Muller S, Smolarz K, et al. Tumorszintigraphie mit J-123 markiertem Ostradiol beim mammakarzinon-rezeptorszintigraphie. Nucl Med 1991;30:84–99.

17. Lastoria S, Varrella P, Mainolfi C, et al. Technetium-99m-sestamibi scintigraphy in the diagnosis of primary breast cancer. J Nucl Med 1994;35s:79.

18. Piccolo S, Lastoria S, Mainolfi C, Muto P, Bazzicalupo L, Salvatore M. Technetium-99m-methylene diphosphonate scintimammography to image primary breast cancer. J Nucl Med 1995;36:718–724.

19. Subramanian G, McAfee JG, Blair RJ, Kallfelz FA, Thomas FD. Technetium-99m methylene diphosphonate a superior agent for skeletal imaging: comparison with other technetium complexes. J Nucl Med 1975;16:744–755.

20. Worsley DF, Lentle BC. Uptake of technetium-99m-MDP in primary amyloidosis with a review of the mechanisms of soft-tissue localization of bone-seeking radiopharmaceuticals. J Nucl Med 1993;34:1612–1615.

21. Chauduri TK, Gulesserian HP, Christie TH, Tonami N. Extraosseous noncalcified soft-tissue uptake of ^{99m}Tc-polyphosphate. J Nucl Med 1974;15:1054–1056.

22. Silberstein EB, Francis MD, Tofe AJ, Siough CL. Distribution of ^{99m}Tc-Sn-diphosphonate and free ^{99m}Tc-pertechnetate in selected soft and hard tissues. J Nucl Med 1975;16:58–61.

23. Aprile C, Bernardo G, Carena M, et al. Accumulation of ^{99m}Tc-Sn-pyrophosphate in pleural effusions. Eur J Nucl Med 1978;3:219–222.

24. Maffioli L, Seregni E, Chiti A, et al. Radiopharmaceuticals for breast cancer imaging. Tumori 1997;83:512–514.

25. Piccolo S, Lastoria S, Muto P, et al. Scintimammography (SMM) with ^{99m}Tc-MDP: an overview of the experience at the National Cancer Institute of Napoli. Tumori 1997;83:515–519.

26. Piccolo S, Lastoria S, Muto P, et al. Scintimammography with ^{99m}Tc-MDP in the detection of primary breast cancer. Q J Nucl Med 1997; 41:225–230.

27. Homer MJ, Safaii H, Smith TJ, Marchant DJ. The relationship of mammographic microcalcification to histologic malignancy: radiologic-pathologic correlation. AJR 1989;153:1187–1189.

28. Leborgne R. Diagnosis of tumors of the breast by simple roentgenography: calcifications in carcinoma. AJR 1951;65:1–11.

29. Feig SA Galkin BM, Muir HD. Evaluation of breast microcalcifications by means of optically magnified tissue specimen radiographs. Recent Results Cancer Res 1987; 105:111–124.

30. D'Orsi CJ, Reale FR, Davis MA, Brown VJ. Breast specimen microcalcifications: radiographic validation and pathologic-radiologic correlation. Radiology 1991; 180:397–400.

31. Feig SA, Shaber GS, Patchefsky A. Analysis of clinically occult and mammographically occult breast tumors. AJR 1977;128:403–408.

32. Moskowitz M. The predictive value of certain mammographic signs in screening for breast cancer. Cancer 1983;51:1007–1011.

33. Feig SA. Mammographic evaluation of calcifications. In: Syllabus: A Categorical Course in Breast Imaging. Kopans DB, Mendelson EB, eds. RSNA Publ, Oak Brook, IL, 1995: 93–105.

34. de Lafontan B, Daures JP, Salicru B, et al. Isolated clustered microcalcifications: diagnostic value of mammography-series of 400. cases with surgical verification. Radiology 1994;190:479–483.

35. Sickles EA. Breast calcifications: mammographic evaluation. Radiology 1986;160: 289–293.

36. Fajardo LL, Davis JR, Wiens JL, Trego DC. Mammography-guided stereotactic fine-needle aspiration cytology of nonpalpable breast lesions: prospective comparison with surgical biopsy results. AJR 1990;155:977–981.

37. Homer MJ. Nonpalpable breast microcalcifications: frequency, management, and results of incisional biopsy. Radiology 1992;185:411–413.

38. Ciatto S, Rosselli del Turco M, Bravetti P. Nonpalpable breast lesions: stereotaxic fine-needle aspiration cytology. Radiology 1989;173:57–59.

39. Lev-Toaff AS, Feig SA, Saitas VL, Finkel GC, Schwartz GF. Stability of malignant breast microcalcifications. Radiology 1994;192:153–156.

40. D'Orsi CJ, Reale FR, Davis MA, Brown VJ. Breast specimen microcalcifications: radiologic validation and pathologic-radiologic correlation. Radiology 1991;180: 397–401.

41. Holland R, Hendriks JHCL. Microcalcifications associated with ductal carcinoma in situ: mammographic-pathologic correlation Semin Diagn Pathol 1994;1:181–192.

42. Evans A, Pinder S, Wilson R, et al. Ductal carcinoma in situ of the breast: correlation between mammographic and pathologic findings. AJR 1994;162:1307–1311.

43. Sickles EA. Further experience with microfocal spot magnification mammography in assessment of clustered breast microcalcifications. Radiology 1980;137:9–14.

44. Wainreb JE. MR imaging of the breast. Radiology 1995;196:593–610.

45. Maffioli L, Agresti R, Chiti A, et al. Prone scintimammography in patients with non-palpable breast lesions. Anticancer Res 1996;16:1296–1274.

46. Moskowitz M. Minimal breast cancer, redux. Radiol Clin North Am 1983;21:93–113.

47. Meyer JE, Kopans DB, Stomper PC, Lindfors KK. Occult breast abnormalities: per-cutaneous preoperative needle localization. Radiology 1984;150:335–337.

48. Rosenberg AL, Schwartz GF, Feig SA, Patchefsky AS. Clinically occult breast lesions: localizations and significance. Radiology 1987;162:167–170.

49. Piccolo S, D'Aiuto G, Lastoria S, et al. Can Tc-99m MDP scintimammography diag-nose breast lesions in women with suspicious mammographic and cytological results? J Clin Oncol 1997;16:131A. Abstract.

50. Lastoria S, Piccolo S, Varrella P, et al. Comparative results of technetium-99m MIBI and technetium-99m methylenediphosphonate scintimammography in patients with breast abnormalities. J Nucl Med 1995;36(s):51P. Abstract.

51. Lastoria S, Varrella P, Mainolfi C, et al. Fluorine-18 PET imaging of primary breast cancer: preliminary results. J Nucl Med 1997;38(s):243P. Abstract.

52. Berg GR, Kalisher L, Osmond JD, et al. Technetium-99m-diphosphonate concentra-tion in primary breast cancer. Radiology 1973;109:393–394.

53. Ross McDougall I, Pistenma DA. Concentration of ^{99m}Tc-diphosphonate in breast tis-sues. Radiology 1974;112:655–657.

54. Burnett KR, Lyons KP, Theron-Brown B. Uptake of osteotropic radionuclides in the breast. Semin Nucl Med 1984;14:48–49.

55. Hobbs S, Neumann RD, Merino MJ, et al. Localization of Tc-99m-MDP in cystosar-coma phyllodes. Clin Nucl Med 1992;17:58–60.

56. Piwnica-Worms D, Chiu ML, Budding M, et al. Functional imaging of multi-drug resistant P-glycoprotein with an organotechnetium complex. Cancer Res 1993; 53:977–984.

57. Ballinger JR, Banneman J, Boxen I, et al. ^{99m}Tc-tetrofosmin as a substrate for P-gly-coprotein: in vivo studies in multidrug-resistant breast tumor cells. J Nucl Med 1996;37:1578–1581.

58. Del Vecchio S, Ciarmiello A, Potena MI, et al. In vivo detection of multidrug-resistant (MDR1) phenotype by ^{99m}Tc-sestamibi scan in untreated breast cancer patients. Eur J Nucl Med 1997;24:150–159.

59. Del Vecchio S, Ciarmiello A, Pace L, et al. Fractional retention of technetium-99m-sestamibi as an index of P-glycoprotein expression in untreated breast cancer patients. J Nucl Med 1997;38:1348–1351.

10

Uptake Mechanisms of ^{99m}Tc-Labeled Perfusion Imaging Agents in Detection of Breast Cancers

JEAN MAUBLANT
Centre Jean Perrin, Clermont-Ferrand, France

I. INTRODUCTION

Initially designed in order to mimic ^{201}Tl, the ^{99m}Tc-labeled myocardial perfusion imaging agents have exhibited unexpected properties that eventually led to their use in tumor imaging, in particular in breast cancer. The in vitro approach has allowed to elucidate the mechanism of cellular accumulation of ^{99m}Tc-sestamibi and has eventually led to a better understanding of the pathophysiological process underlying the scintigraphic aspect. It has also suggested clinical applications which were not initially expected and which provide great promise for the use of these agents in tumor functional imaging.

II. ACCUMULATION OF ^{99m}TC-SESTAMIBI IN MYOCARDIAL CELLS

^{99m}Tc-sestamibi (Cardiolite Du Pont) has been the first ^{99m}Tc-labeled agent available for the evaluation of myocardial perfusion. The clinical and experimental observations of its tumorous accumulation were conducted almost simultaneously with the in vitro studies which allowed elucidation of its mechanism of cellular uptake. Because of its indications in myocardial perfusion imaging, this tracer was initially studied in vitro on models of cardiac cells.

^{99m}Tc-sestamibi is a stable compound formed of a Tc(I) core encased in a lipophilic structure into which the cationic charge is delocalized. The explanation of the intimate mechanism of cellular accumulation of this small, lipophilic, and cationic radiopharmaceutical came from experiments conducted by Piwnica-Worms et al. in 1990 [1] in cultured embryonic chick ventricular myocytes. Their transmembrane electrical potentials were altered by modifying the extracellular potassium concentration or using the potassium ionophore valinomycin or protonophores such as 2-4-dinitrophenol and a cyanide derivative. The membranes were also hyperpolarized through the use of the K^+/H^+ ionophore nigericin and the ATP synthetase inhibitor rotenone. Globally, there was a clear relationship between the changes in the cellular accumulation of ^{99m}Tc-sestamibi and the expected degree of the electrical transmembrane potential alterations (Fig. 1), even if these potentials were only estimated from the known effects of these agents in similar conditions. The possibility of a nonspecific binding to cell components could be excluded since the cellular accumulation was very low in dead cells. Another proof that this mechanism of uptake differs from ^{201}Tl is that exposure to ouabain did not result into a decreased accumulation, but rather in an increased uptake, a likely expression of the secondary hyperpolarization of the mitochondrial membrane in this condition. It was therefore suggested that ^{99m}Tc-sestamibi accumulation was due to a transmembrane diffusion allowed by the lipophilicity of the molecule, and driven by the electrical potential allowed by the cationic charge.

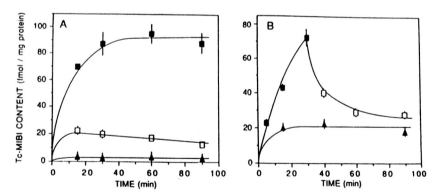

FIGURE 1 Effect of modifications of the transmembrane electrical potential of cultured chick heart cells on the kinetics of accumulation of ^{99m}Tc-sestamibi. Panel A: net uptake in control conditions (dark squares) and with a high concentration (130 mmol.L^{-1}) of K^+ in the medium without (open squares) or with (dark triangles) valinomycin. Panel B: buffer with a high concentration of K^+ from the beginning of the accumulation phase (triangles) or only after 30 min of incubation (squares). From Ref. 1.

It is known that the negative transmembrane electrical potential is lower at the mitochondrial inner matrix than at the sarcolemmal level (between −100 and −150 mV vs. between −50 and −100 mV, respectively). Consequently it can be expected that, intracellularly, 99mTc-sestamibi is preferentially sequestered into the mitochondria, the intracellular sites of energy production. This has been verified by Crane et al. [2] in the heart of guinea pigs. Ten minutes after the in vivo injection of 99mTc-sestamibi, the mitochondrial fraction of myocardial homogenates contained 80% to 90% of the overall cellular activity. Eventually, the direct proof of the intramitochondrial accumulation of 99mTc-sestamibi was provided by Backus et al. [3]. The analysis of freeze-dried cryosections of cultured embryonic chick heart cells by quantitative electron-probe X-ray revealed an overconcentration of up to 1000 times in the mitochondria relatively to the extracellular medium. An interesting demonstration that a transmembrane electrical potential is sufficient to drive by itself the accumulation of 99mTc-sestamibi has been obtained with artificial unilamellar vesicles [4]. After having been electrically charged by being placed in a solution underconcentrated in potassium and containing 99mTc-sestamibi, these artificial bags with a lipidic membrane accumulated 99mTc-sestamibi in direct relation with the electrical potential calculated by the Nernst equation (Fig. 2).

These observations apparently support the statement that the mechanism of cellular accumulation of 99mTc-sestamibi is through passive diffusion [5] since no ATP is directly consumed during this process. However, in living organisms, the transmembrane chemical and electrical gradients represent stores of energy. They are the end results of the metabolic activity and are generated mostly through the consumption of ATP. Consequently, since a part of this energy is dissipated in order to accumulate 99mTc-sestamibi, its mechanism of accumulation corresponds more appropriately, in our opinion, to the so-called secondary active transport [6].

III. ACCUMULATION OF 99mTC-SESTAMIBI IN TUMOR CELLS

Following the inadvertent discovery of the tissular accumulation of 99mTc-sestamibi in a lung cancer [7], in vitro experiments have confirmed its ability to truly overconcentrate in tumor cells. The first experimental report originated from Delmon-Moingeon et al. [8] in 1990. In a series of nine human carcinoma cell lines and two normal cell types (hamster lung fibroblasts and human lymphocytes), these authors observed a maximal cellular concentration of 99mTc-sestamibi ranging between 5% to 28% of the external medium activity in the tumor cells lines, and of <2% in the normal cells. The maximum level was reached after 1 hour, and the time to half-maximum was 10 min, a kinetics similar to what is observed in cultured myocardial cells. Depolarization of the plasma transmembrane potential

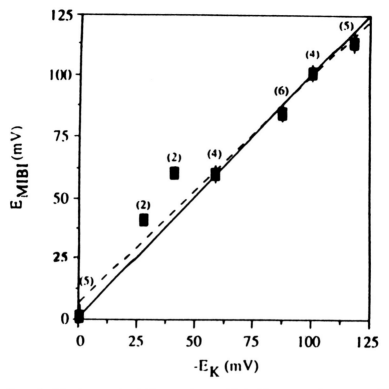

FIGURE 2   Membrane potential in accordance with the Nernst equation from the ^{99m}Tc-sestamibi distribution (–EMIBI) into large unilamellar vesicles plotted against the potassium diffusion potential (EK). From Ref. 4.

induced by a high concentration of K^+ in the incubation medium reduced the ^{99m}Tc-sestamibi uptake by 60%. Incubation with valinomycin, an ionophore that dissipates the mitochondrial membrane electrical potential, eliminated 80% to 85% of ^{99m}Tc-sestamibi uptake; incubation with nigericin, which increases this potential, also increased ^{99m}Tc-sestamibi uptake. At this point, there was a strong suggestion that, as in the myocardial cells, ^{99m}Tc-sestamibi tumor concentration could also be linked to the presence of mitochondria. In fact this agent shows a biological behavior similar to that of other lipophilic cations already used experimentally for the measurement of transmembrane plasma and mitochondrial potentials in living cells [9]. In particular, tritiated tetraphenylphosphonium and fluorescent rhodamine-123 had been utilized for that purpose in MCF-7 cells (derived from human breast carcinoma) and in epithelial cells [10]. By depolarizing and hyperpolarizing the mitochondrial or plasma membranes through chemical interventions such as the modification of the extracellular potassium concentration or the action of ionophores, their overaccumulation into the MCF-7 cells had been demonstrated to be the direct consequence of the transmembrane electrical potentials. A comparison between ^{99m}Tc-sestamibi and these agents was the starting point of the original study by Piwnica-Worms et al. [1].

Finally, in tumor cells as in myocardial cells, ^{99m}Tc-sestamibi accumulates by transmembrane diffusion in response to an electrical potential. Because tumor cells have a higher mitochondrial density and probably also a higher transmembrane electrical potential than the surrounding epithelial cells, ^{99m}Tc-sestamibi accumulates more intensely into the tumor cells, and hence more intensely in the malignant tumors than in their surrounding epithelial tissue. But this nonspecific mechanism opens the possibility of an increased accumulation in nontumorous cells with a high metabolic activity or a high density of mitochondria, a situation encountered in atypical hyperplasia.

IV. OTHER ^{99m}TC-LABELED LIPOPHILIC CATIONS

^{99m}Tc-teboroxime (Cardiotec, Bracco) is a highly lipophilic neutral agent with a low retention time in the heart [11]. Its cellular accumulation has been compared with that of ^{99m}Tc-sestamibi and ^{201}Tl in four series of tumor cell lines, including MCF7, and four series of nontumorous cell lines, including myocytes from newborn rats [12]. Since the tracer accumulation was measured in steady-state conditions, i.e., with a constant extracellular concentration and 1 hour of incubation, the differences in retention times could not affect the results. It was demonstrated that, in these conditions, ^{99m}Tc-teboroxime accumulation does not differ significantly among the various cell lines, a behavior which is not surprising since this agent also strongly binds to the membranes of dead cells. So ^{99m}Tc-teboroxime is the only one of the available ^{99m}Tc-labeled perfusion imaging agents to behave only as a function of blood flow delivery. But no overconcentration can be expected in vivo in malignant tumors besides the one related to a possible increased blood flow. This probably explains why no clinical study has been launched with this agent.

^{99m}Tc-tetrofosmin (Myoview, Amersham), a lipophilic phosphine cation, is a more recently introduced perfusion imaging compound [13]. Even if limited to two, the in vitro studies strongly suggest that its mechanism of cellular accumulation in myocardial cells is essentially similar to ^{99m}Tc-sestamibi. In adult rat ventricular homogenates prepared after an in vivo injection and submitted to differential centrifugation, the uptake of the cellular fraction was decreased by the simultaneous action of the glycolysis inhibitor iodoacetic acid and of the mitochondrial uncoupler 2,4-dinitrophenol [14]. Modification of the mitochondrial electrical potential by ionophores influenced accordingly the concentration of

^{99m}Tc-tetrofosmin in the mitochondrial fraction. In a different approach, mitochondria were first isolated and subsequently incubated with ^{99m}Tc-tetrofosmin [15]. The mitochondrial accumulation was found to be nonsaturable over a wide range of concentrations, but to be quickly affected by a depolarizing maneuver such as the addition of 2,4-dinitrophenol or of calcium ions. This study remains the sole example of the direct measurement of the intramitochondrial accumulation of a ^{99m}Tc-labeled perfusion imaging agent, but it does not preclude of the possibility of the presence of an extramitochondrial intracellular fraction of the tracer.

In tumor cells, one study has addressed a comparison among ^{99m}Tc-tetrofosmin, ^{99m}Tc-sestamibi, and ^{201}Tl [16] in two tumor cell lines (HBL-2 and SW-13). The net uptake of ^{99m}Tc-tetrofosmin was constantly lower than that of ^{99m}Tc-sestamibi. The effects of metabolic inhibition were more pronounced on ^{99m}Tc-sestamibi than on ^{99m}Tc-tetrofosmin, with a stronger increase in the presence of nigericin ($P < .05$) and a larger decrease in the presence of a cyanide derivative (73% vs. 33% release, respectively). The authors suggest that a larger fraction of the tracer accumulates inside the mitochondria with ^{99m}Tc-sestamibi than with ^{99m}Tc-tetrofosmin. A novel observation concerning the ^{99m}Tc-labeled perfusion agents was that ouabain induced a 22% to 31% inhibition of ^{99m}Tc-tetrofosmin uptake in both cell lines, and a 21% to 26% inhibition of ^{99m}Tc-sestamibi uptake in the SW13 cell line. It is suggested that the uptake of these agents, and more specifically of ^{99m}Tc-tetrofosmin, could be partly mediated by the Na$^+$/K$^+$ pump.

^{99m}Tc-Q12 (Technescan Q12, Mallinckrodt) is a mixed ligand complex of the "Q" series initially developed by Deutsch et al. [17] and involving nonreducible Tc(III) cations. In animals, its myocardial uptake is related to myocardial blood flow and there is no evidence of redistribution [18]. In isolated rat hearts, ^{99m}Tc-Q12 and ^{99m}Tc-sestamibi show close maximum and net extraction (E_{max} and E_{net}) values (respectively 29.5 ± 3.1 and 25.6 ± 0.7 for E_{max}, and 14.2 ± 3.3 and 19.7 ± 1.2 for E_{net}), which are, however, lower than for ^{201}Tl (70.1 ± 3.6 for E_{max} and 31.1 ± 2.1 for E_{net}) [19]. ^{99m}Tc-Q12 has been utilized successfully for myocardial blood flow imaging in humans [20]. Like ^{99m}Tc-sestamibi and ^{99m}Tc-tetrofosmin, the mechanisms of cellular accumulation of ^{99m}Tc-Q12 seem to be mostly related to its cationic and lipophilic properties. Comparative uptake measurements in suspensions of myocytes and mitochondria have shown that mitochondria accumulation on a per-gram basis is five to 10 times higher than in intact cells and is lowered by the addition of the uncoupler FCCP 5 mM [21]. For tumor imaging, clinical results are still lacking. However, experimentally, the kinetics of uptake of ^{99m}Tc-Q12 has been compared with ^{99m}Tc-sestamibi and ^{99m}Tc-tetrofosmin in cultures of adenocarcinoma breast cell lines MCF-7 and ZR-75 [22]. In all series, ^{99m}Tc-sestamibi uptake was significantly higher than ^{99m}Tc-tetrofosmin, which was itself higher than ^{99m}Tc-Q12 uptake (highest values in % dose/mg protein were 15.9 ± 0.5, 6.8 ± 0.6 and 3.2 ± 0.1, respectively). These differences do not seem to be related to differences in the E_{max} and E_{net}. In another study with six tumor cell lines, ^{99m}Tc-sestamibi also showed the highest uptake. For instance, in MCF7 cells, percent uptake was 1.72 ± 0.09 for ^{99m}Tc-sestamibi, 1.32 ± 0.10 for ^{99m}Tc-tetrofosmin, and 1.14 ± 0.11 for ^{99m}Tc-furifosmin [23]. In conclusion, there are some indications that these agents behave slightly differently, which is not surprising since they do not show exactly the same physical chemical properties.

V. FROM IN VITRO RESULTS TO IN VIVO IMAGING

Predicting the in vivo behavior of a tumor-avid radiopharmaceutical from in vitro results is a difficult task since numerous factors intervene between the site of injection and the cellular or mitochondrial accumulation. The membrane transport is only one step in this complex process. If this step corresponds to a totally passive diffusion or nonspecific binding, as for ^{99m}Tc-teboroxime for example, it can be predicted with a high degree of confidence that this agent will be of little use to detect a malignant tumor. Knowing that an active, metabolism-related mechanism or a specific binding is involved is a favorable property, but it does not allow by itself to predict that a tracer will be an efficient in vivo tumor imaging agent.

A key point in scintigraphic imaging is to attain a high enough target-to-background ratio. With agents having a fast blood clearance, this can be achieved only if they show a high extraction fraction from the capillary bed. This parameter involves the value of the transmembrane electrical or chemical gradient, but also the possibility for the molecule to be transported rapidly across the capillary, plasma, and mitochondrial barriers, since the blood concentration remains high for only a few minutes after injection. The role of enhancing molecules that could facilitate the tissue extraction by modifying the transmembrane electrical potential profile is under investigation in vitro for ^{99m}Tc-sestamibi [24], but their in vivo applications remain a remote perspective.

VI. MULTIDRUG RESISTANCE AND ^{99M}TC-LABELED AGENTS

A. Expression and Mechanism of the Multidrug Resistance

A well-known observation in cancer chemotherapy is that patients treated with a drug often become eventually resistant not only to that drug but also to a series of other, structurally related but different drugs. This crossresistance, called multidrug resistance, or MDR, has been linked to the overexpression of a transmembrane P-glycoprotein of 170-kD (P-gp 170) through the activation of a mammalian *MDR1* gene. It has been demonstrated that P-gp 170 is in fact present in several normal tissues—for instance, kidney tubules, bile canaliculi, and adrenal glands [25]. It acts by actively expelling small molecules which are not "recognized" as being normal intracellular components. The substrates of this ATP-dependent process are molecules which do not necessarily share any structural or functional property but which are always small, cationic, and hydrophobic [26]. This is for instance the case of cytotoxic drugs like adriamycin, vincristine, and daunorubicin. It has also been demonstrated that the effect of P-gp 170 can be reversed in vitro by the action of molecules like the calcium entry blocking agent verapamil [27], tamoxifen, or cyclosporins which act through various mechanisms of action. The use of such agents could be of first importance to restore chemosensitivity in patients in whom chemoresistance has developed. But the in vivo evaluation of both the expression of P-gp 170 and the functional efficacy of a reversing agent remain in the research domain. In effect, the expression of P-gp 170 is usually detected by immunohistochemistry on tissue samples [28]. The assessment of the functional value of the basal, chemotherapeutically induced, or reversed P-gp 170 activity by a noninvasive method has led to the tentative development of labeled analogs of anthracyclines, but none is currently available in clinical practice.

An interesting property of P-gp 170 is that fluorescent dyes such as rhodamine-123 are also recognized as substrates. The observed rapid release of this fluorescent molecule from resistant cells [29] suggested that, on the one side, the accepted use of fluorescent dyes for the in vitro determination of the transmembrane electrical potential was very likely of limited value in resistant cells [30] but that, on the other side, this property could help to identify in vitro, on cells from tissue samples, the P-gp-mediated resistance to chemotherapy [31,32].

B. Multidrug Resistance and ^{99m}Tc-Labeled Lipophilic Cations

Being also a small lipophilic cationic molecule, ^{99m}Tc-sestamibi has the expected attributes to be also recognized as a substrate by P-gp 170. This hypothesis was tested by Piwnica-Worms et al. in a series of cultured cells expressing low, intermediate and high levels of P-gp 170 [33]. At steady state, the content in ^{99m}Tc-sestamibi was >25 times higher in cells with low levels than in cells with high levels of P-gp 170 (Fig. 3). At contrast, incubation in presence of the reversing agent verapamil or cyclosporin A multiplied by 200 the tracer accumulation in the cells with a high level of P-gp 170 expression. It was therefore suggested by these authors that ^{99m}Tc-sestamibi could be utilized in vivo to rapidly characterize P-gp expression in tumors and to target reversal agents. A direct proof that ^{99m}Tc-sestamibi is a substrate for P-gp 170 has been provided by Rao et al. when they

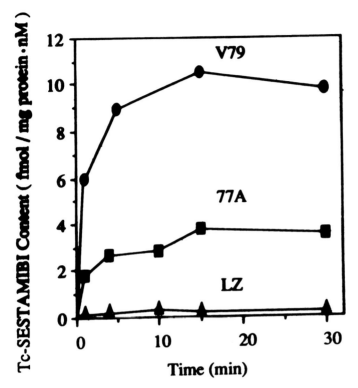

FIGURE 3   Kinetics of accumulation of ^{99m}Tc-sestamibi in drug-sensitive V79 lung fibro-blasts and in the 77A and LZ derivative cell lines expressing intermediate and high levels of P-gp 170, respectively. From Ref. 33.

infected P-gp-free insect cells with a recombinant virus containing the human *MDR1* gene so that high levels of P-gp 170 were produced [34]. The ^{99m}Tc-ses-tamibi net uptake was reduced by 97% in the infected cells, an effect that was par-tially reversible in the presence of verapamil.

These observations have been confirmed by others. In a rat breast adenocar-cinoma cell line and its doxorubicin-resistant variant, a 16-fold difference of ^{99m}Tc-sestamibi concentration was reported, a value which decreased by a twofold when the resistant line was treated by a nonimmunosuppressive cyclosporin A analog, PSC833 [35]. In rats bearing these tumors, the most noticeable difference was a faster washout in the resistant than in the nonresistant tumors (time to half-maximum of 37 ± 5 min vs. 105 ± 6 min, respectively; P < .001). In a series of nine human breast tumor cell lines among which one line was expressing a high level of P-gp 170, Cordobes et al. noticed a more than 100-fold difference in ^{99m}Tc-sestamibi concentration, and a tracer concentration increase by a factor of 12 in the presence of verapamil in the resistant line [36].

Since ^{99m}Tc-sestamibi shares with ^{99m}Tc-tetrofosmin and ^{99m}Tc-furifosmin its cationic and hydrophobic properties, it could be expected that they also share the same properties with regard to P-gp 170. In fact, with the same experimental model that the one used with ^{99m}Tc-sestamibi [35], Ballinger et al. observed a 26-fold difference in tracer concentration between the nonresistant and resistant cell lines [37]. It became 2.5-fold when the PSC833 reverser was present, mostly because an 11-fold increase uptake in the resistant line. Recent results also suggest that ^{99m}Tc-furifosmin is indeed also a substrate of P-gp 170 [38]. Ongoing research projects are aimed at defining new Tc-99m-labeled compounds with an optimized behavior as P-gp 170 transport substrates for functional imaging in vivo [39].

In summary, the results of the in vitro experiments suggest that, as was expected from the physical chemical properties of the cationic ^{99m}Tc-labeled perfusion imaging agents, these compounds can provide access to the functional evaluation of the MDR expression. However, the crossresistance to chemotherapy is not limited to the sole expression of P-gp 170. Overexpression of the multidrug-resistance-associated protein (*MRP*) gene, encoding for a 190-kD protein [40] and of the anionic glutathione-S-transferase (*GST*) gene [41], linked to melphalan resistance, have also been described. In a study comparing parental, adriamycin-resistant, and melphalan-resistant MCF7 cell lines, ^{99m}Tc-sestamibi accumulation was found to be decreased in the adriamycin-resistant line but significantly increased in the line overexpressing the *GST* gene (3.1% $\pm$ 0.6% in the parental line, 1.86% $\pm$ 0.5% in the adriamycin-resistant, and 5.93% $\pm$ 1.7% in the melphalan-resistant) [42]. Reversal of melphalan resistance through the action of buthiomine sulfoximine, an agent that depletes the cellular glutathione content, did not modify the cellular concentration of ^{99m}Tc-sestamibi. This study has important implications since it would indicate that the presence of ^{99m}Tc-sestamibi accumulation in a tumor does not imply that this tumor is sensitive to chemotherapy. On the other side, there is evidence from the previous study and also from more recent results [43,44] that ^{99m}Tc-sestamibi is also a substrate of MRP.

In conclusion, the MDR phenotype appears as a complex multifactorial phenomenon. Only clinical studies correlating the uptake or the rate of release of these ^{99m}Tc-labeled agents with the response to chemotherapy or, even more interestingly, to the prognosis, will possibly be able to demonstrate the predictive value of scintimammography. Nevertheless, being able to detect the level of resistance of a tumor by scintigraphy could open an innovative way of testing quickly the effect of the so-called reversing or modulation agents on a patient-per-patient basis.

REFERENCES

1. Piwnica-Worms D, Kronauge JF, Chiu ML. Uptake and retention of hexakis (2-methoxyisobutyl isonitrile) technetium(I) in cultured chick myocardial cells. Mitochondrial and plasma membrane potential dependence. Circulation 82:1826–1838, 1990.
2. Crane P, Laliberté R, Heminway S, Thoolen M, Orlandi C. Effect of mitochondrial viability and metabolism on technetium-99m-sestamibi myocardial retention. Eur J Nucl Med 20:20–25, 1993.
3. Backus M, Piwnica-Worms D, Hockett D, et al. Microprobe analysis of Tc-MIBI in heart cells: calculation of mitochondrial membrane potential. Am J Physiol 265:C178–C187, 1993.
4. Chernoff DM, Strichartz GR, Piwnica-Worms D. Membrane potential determination in large unilamellar vesicles with hexakis(2-methoxyisobutylisonitrile) technetium(I). Biochim Biophys Acta 1147:262–266, 1993.
5. Mousa SA, Williams SJ, Sands H. Characterization of in vivo chemistry of cations in the heart. J Nucl Med 28:1351–1357, 1987.
6. Maublant J. Tc-99m-sestamibi cellular uptake: passive or secondary active transport? (Letter to the Editor.) J Nucl Med 38:1170, 1997.
7. Campeau RJ, Kronemer KA, Sutherland CM. Concordant uptake of Tc-99m-sestamibi and Tl-201 in unsuspected breast tumor. Clin Nucl Med 17:936–937, 1992.
8. Delmon-Moingeon LI, Piwnica-Worms D, Van den Abbeele AD, Holman BL, Davison A, Jones AG. Uptake of the cation hexakis (2-methoxyisobutyl-isonitrile)-technetium-99m by human carcinoma cell lines in vitro. Cancer Res 50:2198–2202, 1990.
9. Lichtshtein D, Kaback HR, Blume AJ. Use of a lipophilic cation for determination of membrane potential in neuroblastoma-glioma hybrid cell suspensions. Proc Natl Acad Sci USA 76:650–654, 1979.
10. Davis S, Weiss MJ, Wong JR, Lampidis TJ, Chen LB. Mitochondrial and plasma membrane potentials cause unusual accumulation and retention of rhodamine-123 by human breast adenocarcinoma-derived MCF-7 cells. J Biol Chem 260:13844–13850, 1985.
11. Narra RK, Nunn AD, Kuczynski BL, Feld T, Wedeking P, Eckelman WC. A neutral technetium-99m complex for myocardial imaging. J Nucl Med 30:1830–1837, 1989.
12. Maublant J, Zhang Z, Rapp M, Ollier M, Michelot J, Veyre A. In vitro uptake of technetium-99m teboroxime in carcinoma cell lines and normal cells: comparison with technetium-99m-sestamibi and thallium-201. J Nucl Med 34:1949–1952, 1993.
13. Kelly JD, Forster AM, Higley B, et al. Technetium-99m-tetrofosmin as a new radiopharmaceutical for myocardial perfusion imaging J Nucl Med 34:222–227, 1993.
14. Platts EA, North TL, Pickett RD, Kelly JD. Mechanism of uptake of technetium-tetrofosmin. I. Uptake into isolated adult rat ventricular myocytes and subcellular localization. J Nucl Cardiol 2:317–326, 1995.
15. Younès A, Songadele JA, Maublant J, Platts E, Pickett R, Veyre A. Mechanism of uptake of technetium-tetrofosmin. II. Uptake into isolated adult rat heart mitochondria. J Nucl Cardiol 2:327–333, 1995.
16. Arbab AS, Koizumi K, Toyama K, Araki T. Uptake of technetium-99m-tetrofosmin, technetium-99m-MIBI and thallium-201 in tumor cell lines. J Nucl Med 37:1551–1556, 1996.

17. Deutsch E, Libson K, Jurisson S, Lindoy L. Technetium chemistry and technetium radiopharmaceuticals. Prog Inorg Chem 30:75–139, 1983.

18. Gerson MC, Millard RW, Roszell NJ, et al. Kinetic properties of ^{99m}Tc-Q12 in canine myocardium. Circulation 89:1291–1300, 1994.

19. McGoron AJ, Biniakiewicz DS, Roszell NJ, Gerson MC, Washburn LC, Millard RW. Extraction and retention of ^{99m}Tc-Q12, ^{99m}Tc-sestamibi and ^{201}Tl imaging agents in isolated rat heart during acidemia. Circulation 92:I–181, 1995. Abstract.

20. Rossetti C, Vanoli G, Paganelli G, et al. Human biodistribution, dosimetry and clinical use of technetium(III)-99m-Q12. J Nucl Med 35:1571–1580, 1994.

21. Roszell NJ, McGoron AJ, Biniakiewicz DS, Gerson MC, Ahmed S, Millard RW. ^{99m}Tc Q12 handling by isolated rat cardiac myocytes and mitochondria. Circulation 92:I–181, 1995. Abstract.

22. de Jong M, Bernard BF, Breeman WAP, et al. Comparison of uptake of ^{99m}Tc-MIBI, ^{99m}Tc-tetrofosmin and ^{99m}Tc-Q12 into human breast cancer cell lines. Eur J Nucl Med 23:1361–1366, 1966.

23. Wolf H, Frieling B, Brenner W, Henze E. Uptake of Tc-99m-sestamibi, Tc-99m-tetrofosmin and Tc-99m-furifosmin in sensitive and multidrug-resistant carcinoma cells. J Nucl Med 38:241P.1997. Abstract.

24. Piwnica-Worms D, Kronauge JF, Chiu ML. Enhancement by tetraphenylborate of technetium-99m-MIBI uptake kinetics and accumulation in cultured chick myocardial cells. J Nucl Med 32:1992–1999, 1991.

25. van der Valk P, van Kalken CK, Ketelaars H, et al. Distribution of multi-drug resistance-associated P-glycoprotein in normal and neoplastic human tissues. Ann Oncol 1:56–64, 1990.

26. Pearce HL, Safa AR, Bach NJ, Winter MA, Cirtain MC, Beck WT. Essential features of the P-glycoprotein pharmacophore as defined by a series of reserpine analogs that modulate multidrug resistance. Proc Natl Acad Sci USA 86:5128–5132, 1989.

27. Tsuruo T, Iida H, Tsukagoshi S, Sakurai Y. Increased accumulation of vincristine and adriamycin in drug-resistant P388 tumor cells following incubation with calcium antagonists and calmodulin inhibitors. Cancer Res 42:4730–4733, 1982.

28. Verrelle P, Meissonnier F, Fonck Y, et al. Clinical relevance of immunohistochemical detection of multidrug resistance P-glycoprotein in breast carcinoma. J Natl Cancer Inst 83:111–116, 1991.

29. Neyfakh AA. Use of fluorescent dyes as molecular probes for the study of multidrug resistance. Exp Cell Res 174:168–176, 1988.

30. Kessel D, Beck WT, Kukuruga D, Schutz V. Characterization of multidrug resistance by fluorescent dyes. Cancer Res 51:4665–4670, 1991.

31. Mazzanti R, Gatmaitan Z, Croop JM, Shu H, Arias IM. Quantitative image analysis of Rhodamine 123 transport by adriamycin-sensitive and resistant NIH 3T3 and human hepatocellular carcinoma (Alexander) cells. J Cell Pharmacol 1:50–56, 1990.

32. Gros P, Talbot F, Tang-Wai D, Bibi E, Kaback R. Lipophilic cations: a group of model substrates for the multidrug-resistance transporter. Biochemistry 31:1992–1998, 1992.

33. Piwnica-Worms D, Chiu ML, Budding M, Kronauge JF, Kramer RA, Croop JM. Functional imaging of multidrug-resistant P-glycoprotein with an organotechnetium complex. Cancer Res 53:977–984, 1993.

34. Rao VV, Chiu ML, Kronauge JF, Piwnica-Worms D. Expression of recombinant human multidrug resistance P-glycoprotein in insect cells confers decreased accumulation of technetium-99m-sestamibi. J Nucl Med 35:510–515, 1994.
35. Ballinger JR, Hua HA, Berry BW, Firby P, Boxen I. Tc-99m-sestamibi as an agent for imaging P-glycoprotein-mediated multi-drug resistance: in vitro and in vivo studies in a rat breast tumour cell line and its doxorubicin-resistant variant. Nucl Med Commun 16:253–257, 1995.
36. Cordobes MD, Starzec A, Delmon-Moingeon L, et al. Technetium-99m-sestamibi uptake by human benign and malignant breast tumor cells: correlation with mdr gene expression. J Nucl Med 37:286–289, 1996.
37. Ballinger JR, Bannerman J, Boxen I, Firby P, Hartman NG, Moore MJ. Technetium-99m-tetrofosmin as a substrate for P-glycoprotein: in vitro studies in multidrug-resistant breast tumor cells. J Nucl Med 37:1578–1582, 1996.
38. Crankshaw CL, Marmion M, Burleigh BD, Deutsch E, Piwnica-Worms D. Non-reducible mixed ligand Tc(III) cations (Q complexes) are recognized as transport substrates by the human multidrug resistance (MDR) P-glycoprotein. J Nucl Med 36:130P, 1995. Abstract.
39. Luker GD, Crankshaw CL, Piwnica-Worms D. Tc-99m-Q58 and Tc-99m-Q63 show transport selectivity for *MDR1* over *MDR3* P-glycoprotein. J Nucl Med 38:87P, 1997. Abstract.
40. Cole SPC, Bhardwaj G, Gerlach JH, et al. Overexpression of a transporter gene in a multidrug-resistant human cancer cell line. Science 258:1650–1654, 1992.
41. Tew KD. Glutathione-associated enzymes in anticancer drug resistance. Cancer Res 54:4313–4320, 1994.
42. Kabasakal L, Ozker K, Hayward M, et al. Technetium-99m sestamibi uptake in human breast carcinoma cell lines displaying glutathione-associated drug-resistance. Eur J Nucl Med 23:568–570, 1996.
43. Hendrikse NH, Franssen EJF, van der Graaf WTA, Meijer C, de Vries EGE. Reduced ^{99m}Tc-sestamibi accumulation in P-gp positive and MRP positive cell lines. Proc Am Assoc Cancer Res 36:358, 1995. Abstract.
44. Duran Cordobes M, Moretti JL, de Beco V, et al. Sestamibi Tc-99m (MIBI) uptake in human cell lines exhibiting multidrug resistance related to MDR or MRP genes. J Nucl Med 38:253P, 1997. Abstract.

11
Breast Imaging with
99mTc-Tetrofosmin

Enrico del Vecchio, Luigi Mansi, Pier Francesco Rambaldi, Vincenzo Cuccurullo, Biagio Pecori, Mario Quarantelli, Decio Capobianco, and Marco Bresciani

Second University of Naples, Naples, Italy

I. HISTORICAL BACKGROUND

99mTc-tetrofosmin (TF) is a lipophilic diphosphine routinely used for myocardial scintigraphy and currently proposed for extracardiac utilization mainly in the field of oncology. The use of lipophilic compounds in oncology started with a series of studies demonstrating uptake, both in myocites and in neoplastic cells, of radiocompounds such as ^{123}I-rhodamine [1,2] but is mainly related to similarities with [201]thallium-chloride (Tl-201). In fact, 99mtechnetium-labeled lipophilic compounds proposed for scintimammography have all been developed as radiotracers for myocardial scintigraphy. They are characterized, as Tl-201, by an intracellular uptake proportional to coronary blood flow.

Interesting results obtained with Tl-201 in the diagnosis of malignant tumors strongly supported the clinical use in this field of the isonitrile 99mTc-sestamibi (MIBI), both because of better physical characteristics of 99mTc with respect to Tl-201 and because of in vitro studies, demonstrating higher uptake in neoplastic cells [3]. Many studies demonstrated both pathophysiological premises and clinical usefulness of MIBI in Oncology [4–10]. On the other hand, another family of radiocompounds, boronic acid adducts of technetium dioximes (BATO) and in particular teboroxime, met with no clinical interest both because the unfavorable kinetics made it unsuitable for nuclear cardiology, and because in vitro studies demonstrated worse results with respect to MIBI [3].

TF is the product of a radiochemical research regarding the third main family of technetium-labeled tracers for myocardial scintigraphy, i.e., diphosphines, including also Q12 (furifosmin). Its use in oncology has been proposed after the demonstration of the clinical usefulness in this field of Tl-201 and MIBI. The rationale for a role in patients with breast cancer is mainly based on its similarities with MIBI, as demonstrated by the clinical use in nuclear cardiology and by in vitro experiments suggesting similar uptake mechanisms.

II. CHARACTERISTICS OF THE RADIOPHARMACEUTICAL

A. Chemistry

Tetrofosmin (1,2-bis[bis(2-ethoxyethyl)phosphino]ethane) is a newly developed compound of the diphosphine group forming a lipophilic cation complex with technetium (as $[^{99m}Tc(tetrofosmin)_2 O_2]^+$). The molecule has a linear trans-oxo core with the four phosphorous atoms of the two bidentate diphosphine ligands forming a perfectly planar array (Fig. 1) [11].

B. Radiolabeling

TF is supplied as vials containing sterile lyophilized powder for reconstitution with sodium pertechnetate (^{99m}Tc). Each vial contains 0.23 mg tetrofosmin, 0.03 mg stannous chloride dihydrate, 0.32 mg disodium sulphosalicylate, 1.0 mg sodium D-gluconate, and 1.8 mg sodium hydrogen carbonate, sealed under nitrogen. Prior to reconstitution, TF vials must be stored at 2 to 8°C and protected from light. Each vial has to be reconstituted with 4 to 8 ml of a ^{99m}Tc solution at a radioactive concentration not exceeding 1.1 GBq/ml (30 mCi/ml), prepared by diluting the eluate from a ^{99m}Tc generator with a 0.9% sodium chloride injectable

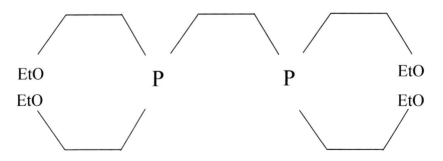

FIGURE 1   Molecular structure of tetrofosmin. EtO: ethoxy-ethyl.

solution. The vial should then be gently shaken to ensure complete dissolution of the lyophilized power and allowed to stand at room temperature (15 to 25°C) for 15 min. Radiochemical purity should be determined prior to use. The reconstituted solution can be stored at room temperature and used within 8 hours.

C.   Quality Control

Applying a 10 to 20-µl sample of the reconstituted solution at one end of a Gelman ITLG/SG strip (2 × 20 cm), placed vertically in a tank with 35:65 v/v acetone/dichloromethane, free pertechnetate runs to the top of the strip, Tc-99m tetrofosmin migrates to the center, while reduced hydrolyzed ^{99m}Tc and hydrophilic complex impurities remain at the bottom end. The strip should then be cut at 3 and 12 cm from the bottom end. Radiochemical purity is calculated as percentage of the activity of the central part of the strip divided by the total activity of all three pieces. A radiochemical purity >90% is required for clinical use.

D.   Dosimetry

The principal sites of absorbed radiation dose are the excretory organs, in particular gallbladder, upper and lower large intestines, small intestine, and urinary bladder. Doses to the higher-dosed organs are approximately 30% lower after exercise because of the lower rate of excretion. Literature data concerning tetrofosmin dosimetry showed that it is more favorable when compared with that reported for ^{201}Tl, and, in many respect, also with sestamibi. In fact, in comparison with ^{201}Tl, even in the worst case for ^{99m}Tc-tetrofosmin (i.e., at rest) the dosimetry is more favorable, allowing the administration of up to 20 times the thallium activity for a similar effective dose [12].

With respect to MIBI, a lower dose to ovaries, testes, small intestine, upper large intestine, lower large intestine, liver, lungs, kidneys, spleen, and thyroid derives from a more rapid excretion of TF [12].

Concerning breasts, it is not known whether ^{99m}Tc is secreted in human milk; therefore, if administration is considered necessary, formula feeding should be substituted to breast feeding for at least 12 hours. Table 1 summarizes radiation doses to various organs from TF iv administration [12].

E.   Side Effects and Toxicology

No serious adverse reactions to TF have been reported. A slight feeling of warmth in the whole body immediately after the initial injection, vomiting (12 to 24 hours postinjection), a transient metallic taste, disturbance of smell, and a mild burning sensation in the mouth after injection have been observed rarely. Transient rises in white blood cell counts have been reported in a small number of patients. More

TABLE I   Absorbed Radiation Dose
(μGy/MBq)

Gallbladder	48.6
Upper large intestine	30.4
Urinary bladder	19.3
Kidney	12.5
Salivary glands	11.6
Ovaries	9.6
Uterus	8.4
Thyroid	5.8
Red marrow	4.0
Testes	3.1
Liver	4.2
Breasts	1.8
Total body	3.7

recently, with the widespread use in clinical routine, a few cases of flushing and urticarial or erythematous rash have been noticed. At present no toxic effects are known in humans.

III.   RATIONALE FOR CLINICAL USE

Tetrofosmin uptake mechanisms are not completely understood. An intracellular distribution has been demonstrated and concentration is present only in viable tissue and depends both on flow and on the metabolic status of cells [13,14]. Many similarities with MIBI have been observed, but a possible role of mechanisms that are not dependent on mitochondria has been hypothesized. In vitro studies are mainly derived from cell culture systems, on both myocites and neoplastic cells, but experimental data have also been obtained in subcellular structures such as isolated adult rat mitochondria [14]. It is hypothesized that TF crosses the cell membrane in a nonspecific manner which is dependent on its lipophilicity and driven by membrane potentials. Even if blood flow is a limiting factor [13,15], tissue retention can only occur if these potentials are preserved, i.e., in viable and metabolically active cells [16].

Data from the literature regarding the possible role of Na-K ATPase, i.e., of the main, albeit not exclusive, mechanism involved in [201]thallium chloride uptake, is not univocal [16–20]. In a study performed in adult rat ventricular myocites no significant effect on the uptake has been shown by Na+ and K+ channel inhibitors [20]. In partial contrast with this data, Arbab, in the Epstein-Barr virus-negative lymphoma B-cell line HBL2 and in the small-cell carcinoma of the adrenal cortex cell line SW-13 [16], demonstrated that cellular TF uptake depends both on cell membrane (Na+/K+ pump) and mitochondrial potentials. This paper is relevant because it demonstrates the existence of differences in uptake mechanisms between TF and MIBI. In this study it was also observed that only a small fraction of TF accumulates inside the mitochondria while most of the MIBI has an intramitochondrial location.

A primary role of mitochondria in TF uptake mechanism is, however, supported by many studies. Most of the significant information comes from studies performed on isolated adult rat mitochondria, suggesting that the cellular uptake of TF is driven by the sarcolemmal and mitochondrial transmembrane potentials [14]. Metabolically active cells are required for an optimal uptake that cannot be explained on the basis of simple diffusion. Uptake is temperature-dependent, is decreased by metabolic inhibitors, and reaches values exceeding those achievable with simple diffusion [16,20,21].

It has been demonstrated in different neoplastic cell culture systems that TF shares with MIBI the property of being a substrate for P-glycoprotein (P-gp), a membrane transporter responsible for the multidrug resistance [22–26]. A similar behavior has also been hypothesized with respect to the multidrug resistance-associated protein (MRP), an alternative transporter discovered by Cole [27]. Ballinger [22,23] studied TF and MIBI uptake in wild-type and doxorubicin-resistant variants of the rat MatB and human MCF-7 breast tumor cell lines. Wolf evaluated TF uptake in comparison with MIBI, Tl-201 and ^{99m}Tc-furifosmin in human drug-sensitive breast and gastric carcinoma cells and in multidrug-resistant cells of breast, gastric, and pancreatic carcinoma [21,24,26,28].

Nakamura carried out experiments on human anaplastic thyroid carcinoma (KB3-1) and on two human recombinant cell lines: MDR1-transferred KB-G2, and MRP-transferred C-A500 [25]. Nakamura also performed in vivo studies on cell lines implanted in athymic mice, concluding that both TF and MIBI report the functional expression mediated by P-gp as well as by MRP, although MIBI seems to be a more sensitive tool.

Studies in tumor-bearing mice have also been performed by Schomäcker [29] and Amano [30]. Schomäcker [29] evaluated biokinetics of MIBI, TF, ^{99m}Tc-Q-12, and Tl-201 in DBA/2N mice transplanted with a CaD2-mamma carcinoma, individuating higher T/Bkg ratios for MIBI. Amano [30] compared ^{18}F-fluorodeoxyglucose (FDG), ^{18}F-methyltyrosine (FMT), TF, MIBI, and Tl-201 behavior in the MCF-7 breast carcinoma-bearing mice. In these experiments, while uptake values were significantly higher for FMT, there were no significant differences among TF, MIBI, and ^{201}Tl uptake in the tumors.

A comparison between TF and MIBI in cell culture systems has been also published by De Jong, who compared MIBI, TF, and ^{99m}Tc-Q-12 in human breast adenocarcinoma MCF-7 and ZR-75 cell lines [31] and by Seregni, who evaluated the uptake of MIBI, TF, ^{99m}Tc-medronate (MDP), FDG, and free ^{99m}Tc in MCF-7 mammary carcinoma cell lines both in basal conditions and during cell growth [32]. In the first paper [31] MIBI showed the highest cellular uptake, followed by TF and Q-12. The uptake of MIBI and TF was inhibited at low temperatures, and the outflow processes of the radiolabelled compounds were similar. Seregni [32] demonstrated that there is a high uptake of MIBI and TF in tumor cells (50% of activity being released after <30 min) while uptake of MDP is lower and comparable to that of pertechnetate. The relationship between the uptake of the different radiotracers and the cell proliferation ratio is variable.

While no differences in MIBI and TF cellular uptake with respect to growth rates have been observed. FDG concentration is higher in fast growing cells [31,32]. Data related to glucose metabolism are agreement with those obtained by us comparing uptake of (^{3}H)-2-deoxyglucose (^{3}H-2d-Gle) in chick embryo fibroblasts cultures both infected by Rous sarcoma virus (CEF-RSV) and uninfected (CEF) [19]. In this system, in which (^{3}H)-thymidine uptake was also used as marker of cell multiplication, similar results with respect to ^{3}H-2d-Glc have been obtained with Tl-201, Ga-67 citrate, and Co-57 Bleomicin. The effect of transformation per se and of the growing rate on Tl-201 and ^{3}H-2d-Glc uptake has been confirmed in rat thyroid carcinoma cells compared with normal thyroid cells [18,19].

On the basis of experimental data, we can hypothesize that TF uptake mechanisms, not completely understood at present, are similar to those of MIBI, mainly depending on blood flow and on the metabolic status of cells. Comparative studies demonstrated that accumulation of TF is lower than that of MIBI, probably reflecting differences in the responsiveness of the two tracers to membrane potentials [16,31,33]. Differences are related to the lower influence of mitochondrial activity on TF uptake and to the partial dependence of TF uptake on the Na+/K+ pump. This last mechanism is also involved, together with others, in Tl uptake. However, it has to be pointed out that a clinical role for TF scintimammography cannot be based exclusively on experimental studies performed in vitro or on animals, because the T/Bkg ratio is also dependent on parameters that are evaluable only in humans.

An important role is played by the pharmacokinetics; by the possible formation of different radiochemical forms after labeling or caused by in vivo metabolism; by pathophysiological parameters such as blood flow, blood volume, and permeability; and by technical aspects related to attenuation, scatter, etc. With respect to MIBI, TF presents the advantage of a room temperature reconstitution. Its stability and radiochemical purity are demonstrated until 8 hours after reconstitution also in unrefrigerated conditions [34,35].

In vivo similarities between TF and MIBI have been clearly demonstrated. TF has a clinical role as a routine tracer in the analysis of patients with coronary artery disease with results overlapping those obtained with MIBI [36,37]. A similar whole-body distribution and slight pharmacokinetic differences have been observed. For TF no significant cardiac washout and a more favorable clearance from the lungs and liver have been observed, allowing an earlier myocardial scan than with MIBI [12,38,39]. Faster hepatic clearance could determine an advantage in the evaluation of tumors located in the inferior hemisphere of right breast, determining a lower background, but data supporting this hypothesis have not been published. The more favorable pharmacokinetics of TF with respect to MIBI is also expressed in a lower dosimetry, mainly due to more rapid body clearance [12].

T/Bkg ratio at the level of breast lesions could also be determined by differences in blood clearance or in tumor wash out affecting uptake mechanisms. Similar results have also been obtained with TF and MIBI in the oncological field despite some pharmacokinetic differences [40–62]. In particular, a different pattern has been observed in parathyroid adenomas, with an higher late parathyroid adenoma/thyroid ratio for MIBI, due to a more favorable differential washout. This behavior does not seem dependent on free perthecnetate [63]. Nevertheless, we prefer to perform MIBI or TF parathyroid scintigraphy [45,64] after perchlorate administration, especially if a quality control at the injection time is not available.

The possible presence of free ^{99m}Tc after radiolabeling or in vivo administration of TF has to be carefully considered. In fact, pertechnetate has been proposed as a tracer for scintimammography, mainly because of differences in permeability between benign and malignant tumors [65]. Data derived from parathyroid scintigraphy and from the use of TF in differential diagnosis of brain tumors [48] are in disagreement with a significant contribution of free ^{99m}Tc to breast tumor imaging. In fact, neither thyroid nor choroid plexus uptake is affected by perchlorate. Nevertheless a blood-brain barrier rupture is a necessary premise to a pathological TF cerebral uptake, but a concentration is not possible in absence of cells. This behavior, i.e., cellular uptake, represents a major advantage of TF scintimammography in the evaluation of local relapse after surgery and/or radiotherapy over other procedures, which are more dependent on extracellular uptake mechanisms, such as those utilizing MDP or contrast media at MRI or ultrasounds. Using these approaches, a differential diagnosis of recurrence is difficult in the first year following treatment, on account of an specific uptake due to increased permeability. Using TF scintimammography, an accurate differential diagnosis can be achieved at the first follow-up control, i.e., at 3 to 6 months after surgery and/or radiotherapy.

The presence of cells is fundamental for uptake to occur, and this creates the premise for a differential diagnosis of primary tumors based on cellularity. No significant uptake is possible in benign cystic and/or in predominantly acellular lesions. Moreover, concentration is present in the viable part of the tumor but not in the necrotic one. This behavior, which does not determine a higher rate of false-negative results since necrosis occurs mainly in large tumors, has to be taken into account when an accurate quantitative evaluation is requested, and could also stimulate the use of TF as a tracer for a radioguided biopsy of the viable part of the tumor when a complex structure is present [66,67]. While uptake is impossible in acellular lesions, concentration can occur in cellular lesions in the absence of malignancy.

The clinical use of TF in the detection of parathyroid adenomas is based on the uptake in benign cellular lesions. Moreover, TF uptake has been reported in other benign tumors such as functioning and nonfunctioning thyroid adenomas [42], pneumonia, and active tuberculosis [68].

In our experience in breast cancer, using planar dedicated projections, no significant TF focal uptake has been observed in cellular benign tumors, such as four fibroadenomas, one granuloma, one papilloma, and three proliferative fibrocystic dysplasia, even if larger than the strongly concentrating malignant ones. No uptake has been observed in three patients with fibrocystic dysplasia or in a woman with a steatonecrosis.

A slight diffuse uptake not corresponding to the mammographic image has been observed in a case with proliferative fibrocystic dysplasia and in a fibroadenoma (Fig. 2). Because the scintimammographic pattern was clearly different from that observed in malignant tumors, we defined these studies as true-negative. In partial disagreement with our experience, other authors presented false-positive results mainly in fibroadenoma. In particular, Lind [69] reported in a group of 48 patients a 74% specificity due to the presence of uptake in one of the 12 cases with fibrocystic disease and in all of five fibroadenomas. It has to be pointed out that in two of the six false-positive primary lesions (one fibrocystic disease, one fibroadenoma), TF uptake was only demonstrated at SPET. In the remaining four fibroadenomas there was also a "more or less clear uptake" in the planar views, that was considered definitely positive only in one case and "probably" positive in three. In a more recent paper from the same group [70], in which 84 patients were studied, false-positive results were obtained in only nine out of the 18 fibroadenomas evaluated.

At first we can hypothesize that a discrepancy with our data can derive from differences dependent on country [71] or histology [72], as already suggested for MIBI. A different accuracy, with main reference to specificity, however, is more probably related to the evaluation procedure and to how the odds of malignancy are defined. As example, at present, no reliable advantages seem to be related to SPET, mainly because of the possibility of a worst specificity. The definition of qualitative, quantitative, or semiquantitative criteria to define a study "positive" are also a very important issue in defining the accuracy. Interesting suggestions can be derived from the experience of Hoh and co-workers using FDG [73], suggesting that values have to be adjusted so that different sensitivity and specificity along the ROC curve can be selected depending on the clinical application. For these reasons a methodological goal of TF scintimammography could be the def-

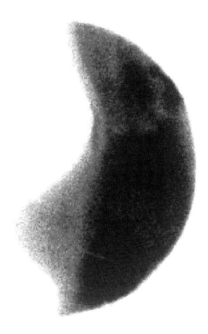

FIGURE 2 Left prone projection in a 24-year-old patient with a 7-cm fibroadenoma. A diffuse uptake of the radiotracer, with a weak focal activity not corresponding to the mammographic image, can be seen stressing the windowing condition. The study was considered negative.

inition of a tumor/background threshold supporting diagnosis of malignancy also in presence of a slight uptake in benign lesions.

A quantitative analysis has to be carefully defined considering many parameters with main reference to the acquisition procedure, to size and location of the tumor and of the corresponding region of interest (ROI), scatter contribution, attenuation, and presence of necrosis [74,75]. Attenuation and scatter correction, information derived from phantoms, new cameras, beds or mattress, more objective analysis methodologies, or new procedures concerning both planar acquisition and SPET can increase the accuracy of the exam [76–80]. With respect to SPET, a significant improvement, with main reference to the evaluation of lymph node involvement, could be obtained optimizing the acquisition procedure. In particular, interesting perspectives can be derived from the evaluation of the best patient positioning and from the definition of the best are of rotation orbit in agreement with clinical experience, not only in myocardial scintigraphy but also in the evaluation of other organs [81].

We evaluated the influence of tumor location in detection capability using a

66-mm cylinder filed with a solution of ^{99m}Tc providing the same counting rate as the "in vivo" breast [74]. A 17-mm cylinder containing activities ranging from 0 to 10 times higher than Bkg was located in medial, intermediate, and lateral position. Using this system we demonstrated that lateral lesions are identifiable starting from activity rates >200% of Bkg, while medial and intermediate ones can be detected only when lesion concentration is >300%. In our experience, anterior and lateral breast lesions are better detectable than those located in medial hemispheres or close to the thoracic wall.

Correction of quantitative values on the basis of size and presence of necrosis (Fig. 3) may also be important for the definition of a threshold between benign and malignant lesions. Information on tumor dimension for a possible correction of T/Bkg values could be achieved not only from scintimammography but also from measurements performed at Rx mammography and/or ultrasounds. To have a better definition of an uptake threshold between benign and malignant tumors in the presence of necrosis, values have to be calculated not only on the whole lesion but also on the most active part.

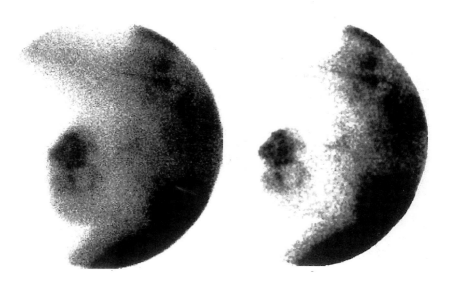

FIGURE 3   Left lateral projection acquired in a patient with a 10.0 × 7.0 cm ductal infiltrating carcinoma of the outer upper quadrant. Inhomogeneous uptake at the level of the tumor, in the presence of necrosis, is shown. Ipsilateral axillary uptake at the level of metastatic lymph nodes is also evident. T/Bkg ratio ranged from 2.5 to 1.6 for the part of the tumor with the higher activity and for the necrotic part, respectively. Average T/Bkg ratio was 1.8. From Ref. 88.

The role of lesion size in tumor detection with TF is clearly demonstrated by the lower sensitivity observed in T1 patients with respect to T2 and T3. The evaluation of the role of the histology in determining TF uptake, as suggested for MIBI [72], is more difficult at present, due to the absence of studies analyzing this relationship. In our experience a false-negative result in patients with tumor >1 cm has been observed only in a woman with a 3-cm mucinous papillary carcinoma, the only one with this histology in our series. A low cellularity, a very slow growing rate, and the absence of a desmoplastic reaction were observed in this case. A false negative corresponding to a mucinous carcinoma has been reported also by Adalet [82]. In our experience, a clear uptake was present not only in case of infiltrating ductal carcinomas, which are the large majority in our series, but also in a medullary carcinoma, a mixed carcinoma, in two lobular infiltrating carcinomas, and in an ovarian metastasis.

In tumor detection a major parameter to be taken into account is background activity, which is determined mainly by liver, heart, skeletal muscle, bowel and, to a lower extent, thyroid and lung TF concentration, which varies over time (e.g., decreases in the liver and increases in the bowel) or can be modified by physical activity and/or drugs (e.g., at skeletal and myocardial muscular level). Because of a higher background, conditioning the achievable T/Bkg ratio, lymph node evaluation is more difficult in comparison with primary tumors. Pathological uptake at level of distant metastases has been demonstrated both in patients with breast cancer and with other tumors [42,74]. However, a whole-body analysis may be difficult to read because of the presence of many areas with specific activity.

IV. TECHNICAL ASPECTS

A. Dose Administration

We did not observe a significant influence of different phases of the menstrual cycle in TF scintimammography accuracy, also if an effect on T/Bkg value cannot be excluded. Because of the possibility of nonspecific uptake, we suggest performing scintimammography preferably at least 3 months after surgery or radiotherapy. Nevertheless, nonspecific uptake has low probability to be present in absence of active scar 1 month after surgery. For the same reason TF scintimammography should be performed before or at least 7 days after fine needle aspiration.

No preparation, fasting or drug wash out is requested. We inject a bolus of 15 to 20 mCi (555 to 740 MBq) into the antecubital vein of the arm contralateral to the affected breast. When bilateral lesions are suspected or in follow-up after surgery, injection in a dorsal pedis vein is preferred to better evaluate axillary lymph nodes because of the possibility of nonspecific uptake due to a subcutaneous injection.

B.   Acquisition Time

No diagnostic information is added by dynamic acquisition, which may play a role in defining prognostic parameters. Acquisition is started 5 to 10 min after IV injection. In our experience scans performed 2 hours after injection did not improve diagnostic accuracy. However, the acquisition of early and late scans could define the presence of tumor washout, probably related to chemoresistance, as already observed for MIBI [83]. In this case an acquisition such as that proposed by Del Vecchio with a 15-min dynamic study followed by static planar images at 0.5, 1, 2, and 4 hours could be preferred to obtain a better quantitative analysis. A two-points study (10 and 120 min) could be probably sufficient to separate tumors with a different behavior. In fact, because of the decrease of the T/Bkg ratio with time, it seems better not to start TF scintimammography later than 30 min after injection [74].

C.   Data Acquisition

All our patients have been studied using planar projections. SPET studies have been acquired only in selected patients as in the case of a previously mastectomized woman presenting at CT enlarged lymph nodes at the level of the internal mammary chain [74]. Whole-body scans have been used when clinically indicated, as in a case of a solitary bone metastasis of the foot [74] and in a patient with a diffusely metastatic ovarian cancer presenting a breast metastasis and a pleural effusion. Whole-body scans have also been performed in a small series of patients with arthrosis undergoing myocardial scintigraphy with TF and bone scan to evaluate differential uptake at level of benign "hot" spot at MDP scan.

Our preference for planar images has been also supported by practical reasons. We wanted, in fact, to compare prone projection with our original approach utilized since 1993 using Tl-201 and/or MIBI [84], which included two anterior and four lateral projections with additional images acquired 2 hours after injection when a washout study was performed, thus leaving no extra time for a SPET study. Planar images are obtained using a 256×256 matrix with a large-field camera equipped with a high-resolution collimator. A 15% window centered at the 140 keV photopeak is set. Five-minute scans and/or at least 1.5 million counts are taken. No zoom is utilized. Our experimental protocol has been based on two supine anterior and four lateral views, with further delayed scans performed 2 hours after the IV injection when a washout analysis was requested.

In the lateral view as originally proposed by our group [74,84], the patient is placed in lateral recumbence, with homolateral arm raised, and the camera located under the table; a thin lead shield is placed between the two mammary glands, slightly compressing the relevant one onto the table (Fig. 4). Using this approach, we achieve a better T/Bkg ratio, both because of the reduction of back-

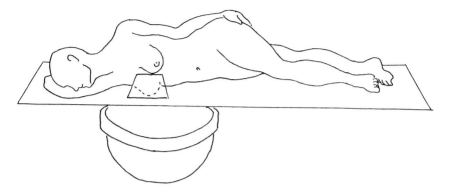

FIGURE 4   Patient position for lateral view.

ground due to the lowering of counts from the contralateral breast and because of increased tumor counts due to the "mammographic" effect (i.e., the smaller distance of the tumor from the detector). The prone lateral projection is used with the patient lying prone and the homolateral arm raised. This approach is better performed using a dedicated table or a mattress with holes for the mammary glands.

As regards supine anterior projections, we prefer to use two separate anterior views of right and left hemithorax, the patient lying supine with the arms raised above the head, including in the field of view breast, axilla, supraclavear region, and sternum, minimizing counts deriving from heart, liver, and bowel. Useful information, mainly in the evaluation of medial lesions, can be obtained using oblique views. An interesting approach is that proposed by Zerva et al. [85] with the patient rotated 30° to the left and then to the right to provide breast images without chest wall interference as much as possible. An evaluation in orthostatism can be helpful, mainly in the analysis of lymph node involvement. Special approaches such as that suggested by Maurer for craniocaudal breast imaging [86] can be occasionally utilized.

The same parameters utilized for MIBI SPET acquisition can be used for TF. We perform SPET with the patient supine; 64 30-sec projections are acquired using a 64 × 64 matrix over a 180° circular orbit from −90° to +90°. A 20% window centered on the 140 keV photopeak is chosen. Reconstruction is performed using a Butterworth filter (0.7 cutoff and 10.0 order number) without attenuation correction (Fig. 5).

In our experience, mainly for lymph node evaluation, in presence of a satisfactory counting rate, we prefer to acquire more views in a shorter time. For routine clinical purposes sufficient information can be obtained utilizing only a supine anterior view including both axillas and two lateral (right and left) projections

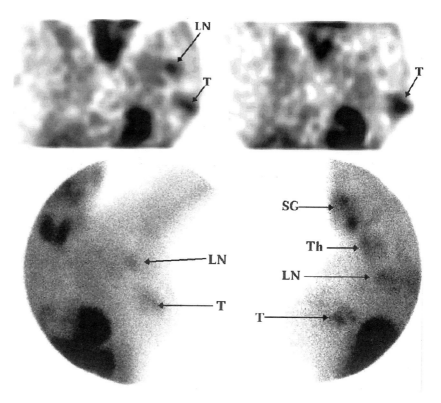

FIGURE 5   Left anterior and left prone projection (lower row) in 64-year-old patient with a ductal infiltrating carcinoma in the outer upper quadrant with concomitant lymph node involvement, confirmed by the analysis of the coronal SPECT reformat (upper row). LN: lymph nodes; SG: salivary gland; T: tumor; Th: thyroid.

acquired with the patient prone or in lateral recumbence. Further views are strongly suggested when dubious images are present.

The analysis of axilla has to be done in studies acquired with arm raised (Fig. 6A). A comparison with contralateral axilla and the evaluation of the possibility of aspecific uptake due to extravasation at the injection site are mandatory.

A correct diagnosis of axillary lymph nodes involvement is helped by the interactive image analysis on monitor (Fig. 6B) by the number of analyzed images and by the experience of the observer. Significant help in defining accuracy is related to the evidence of uptake by the primary tumor. Further help can be also derived by clinical evaluation of breast and axilla, yet taking into account the possible presence of false-negative and positive results at palpation. Important information is obtained from comparison with mammography, ultrasounds, and other diagnostic procedures.

D. Data Analysis

When available, analogical images can be helpful. In the analysis of digital images, different parameters have to be utilized for breast and lymph node evaluation. The gray and/or color scale window has to be optimized for tumor detection maximizing the tumor/normal breast contrast, not taking into any account the external areas presenting high count rate such as heart, thoracic wall, liver, and bowel. The use of an analysis with more than one scale, such as a linear and a nonlinear one, could be helpful. In this way it is possible to improve both sensitivity and specificity.

The best qualitative evaluation is achieved when scintimammography is first analyzed blindly and then revised on the basis of the comparison with clinical and instrumental data. For quantitative analysis it is very important the choice of the region of interest (ROI). A quantitative analysis concerning the primary tumor has been performed by our group, utilizing an irregular ROI for the background defined over all the breast to minimize statistical noise; the tumor region after a 50% increase in size is automatically excluded from the Bkg (Fig. 7) [74].

In the presence of necrosis, as in the case presented in Figure 3, differences in tumor values are clearly present between the whole lesion and its viable part. As previously described, quantitative analysis gave us the possibility, comparing early and late scans, to demonstrate the presence of a tumor washout, as already demonstrated for MIBI [83], and to compare different values achievable using different projections.

V. CLINICAL APPLICATION

At present we have evaluated with TF scintimammography about 200 patients since 1994, when we observed an intense TF uptake by the primary tumor and involved axillary lymph nodes in a patient undergoing myocardial scintigraphy [87]. At the beginning of our experience we also analyzed, as normal controls, women undergoing myocardial scintigraphy without breast disease [74,87–90]. Scintimammography with TF has been possible in all patients also when Rx mammography was not diagnostic, i.e., in presence of dense breast, after mastectomy and radiotherapy, in presence of breast implant. No side effects or discomfort were observed in any patient.

In this chapter we present the results from a series of 53 patients (mean age 51, range 18–74) with 62 breast lesions (0.4 to 10 cm in size), including four women with clinical suspicion of recurrence. Diagnosis was always confirmed at histology

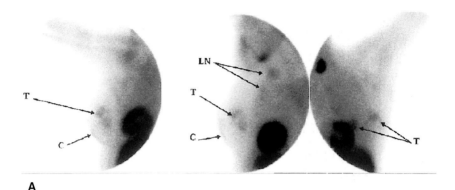

A

FIGURE 6   (A) Left lateral, prone, and anterior projection acquired in a 67-year-old patient with a multifocal ductal infiltrating carcinoma in the outer upper quadrant and inner lower quadrant of 2 and 3 cm diameter, respectively, with concomitant lymph node involvement and cutaneous involvement. In this case, mainly due to incorrect positioning of the patient's arm, cutaneous and lymph nodal involvement are more evident if appropriate windowing is chosen. C: cutaneous involvement; LN: lymph nodes; T: tumor. (B) Same as in 6A, prone projection, but using a different window. Lymph node and cutaneous involvement are more advantageously displayed using an appropriate window.

in primary tumors and in axillary metastases. Malignant lesions were 33 infiltrating ductal CA, two lobular infiltrating CA, one mucinous papillary CA, one medullary CA, one intraductal CA, one mixed CA, and one ovarian metastasis. Benign lesions included three proliferative fibrocystic dysplasias, three fibrocystic dysplasias, one steatonecrosis, four fibroadenomas, one granuloma, and one papilloma.

In our series Mx was not diagnostic in 24% of patients, including four women with suspicion of local relapse after mastectomy. In the evaluated patients a 92.0% sensitivity, a 63.6% specificity, a 78.7% accuracy, a 74.0% positive predictive value, and an 87.5% negative predictive value were obtained. Scintimammography with TF detected 44 out of 46 malignant lesions in 38 out of 40 patients with cancer. Two false-negative results were related to a 0.4-cm intraductal carcinoma, which was also negative at Mx, and to a 3-cm mucinous papillary carcinoma. The smallest detected lesion corresponded to a 0.6-cm infiltrating ductal carcinoma. No uptake was observed in the contralateral normal breast of tumor patients or in the normal controls.

In mastectomized patients, uptake was observed in two patients with recurrence (Fig. 8) but not in two women without local relapse, despite clinical suspicion. A 95.6% sensitivity, a 93.7% specificity, a 95.2% accuracy, a 97.8% positive predictive value and a 88.2% negative predictive values were calculated for TF scintimammography.

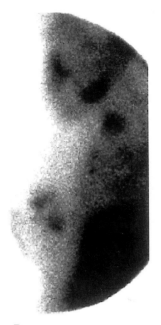

B

FIGURE 6   Continued

Axillary uptake was detected in 19 out of 20 patients with lymph node involvement. A false-negative and a false-positive result were present. The false-positive result corresponded to a patient with a cytological diagnosis of primary breast cancer showing uptake at the level of palpable axillary lymph nodes. No metastases were detected at surgery performed after neoadjuvant chemotherapy. Nevertheless, it cannot be excluded in this case that lymph node TF uptake may have been a true-positive result at the moment of scintimammography, as suggested by the 40% reduction of the mass of the primary tumor determined by therapy. A 95% value was calculated for sensitivity, specificity, accuracy, and positive and negative predictive values for the diagnosis of axillary lymph node involvement. Clinical evaluation of axillary lymph nodes yielded five false-negative and four false-positive results. An internal mammary chain metastasis was also detected in one patient and suspected in another woman.

We did not observe a different accuracy evaluating separately lateral projections acquired prone or in lateral recumbence. Differences can be observed in multifocal and/or heterogeneous tumors, but neither lateral view is consistently superior to the other. At the opposite, the poorest information is in general obtained

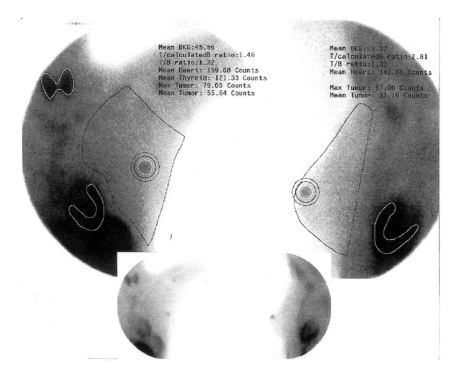

Mean BKG:45.56
T/calculatedB ratio:1.46
T/B ratio:1.22
Mean Heart: 159.08 Counts
Mean Thyroid: 121.33 Counts
Max Tumor: 79.00 Counts
Mean Tumor: 55.64 Counts

Mean BKG:23.37
T/calculatedB ratio:2.81
T/B ratio:1.33
Mean Heart: 142.88 Counts

Max Tumor: 57.00 Counts
Mean Tumor: 31.19 Counts

FIGURE 7   TF scintimammography in a patient with a 1.8 × 1.6 cm ductal infiltrating carcinoma. Intense tetrofosmin uptake is evident at the level of the outer upper quadrant. Region
of interest placement over the anterior and prone view. Irregular regions are used for background, thyroid, and heart. A circular region is placed over the lesion. Automated background selection (the area between two concentric circles with a radius twice and 1.5 times
the tumor region, calculated Bkg) is not feasible for peripheral tumors (in this case the
automated background fell out of the breast, giving an artificially high T/Bkg ratio).

using the anterior view. Nevertheless the anterior projection is important mainly
for the diagnosis of recurrence in mastectomized patients and of lymph node
involvement, providing information on the location of the primary tumor.

Concerning quantitative analysis, we demonstrated in the analysis of 27
patients that T/Bkg ratios are significantly higher in lateral and prone projections
than in anterior views. Values of 1.31 ± 0.21, 1.68 ± 0.20, and 1.59 ± 0.10 have
been obtained respectively for anterior, lateral in lateral recumbence, and prone
projection. Although differences between lateral and prone projections did not
reach statistical significance in this group of patients, higher T/Bkg ratios in lateral view have been obtained for tumors located in superior or medial hemi-

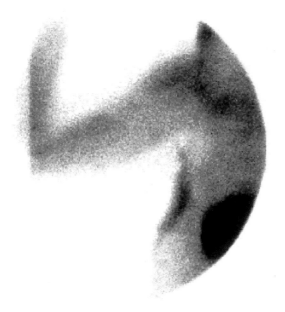

F<small>IGURE</small> **8**   Left lateral projection in a patient (lateral recumbent position) who previously underwent total mastectomy for ductal infiltrating carcinoma. A 12.0 (2.0 cm) ulcerative lesion with clinical signs of relapse is present. Intense uptake at level of the recurrence is shown. From Ref. 88.

spheres. Moreover, differences have been found in tumors located in the left breast (1.7 ± 0.35 vs. 1.5 ± 0.08) but not in the right mammary gland.

We performed delayed scans to obtain information on the presence of TF tumor washout. Preliminary data demonstrate the presence of changes of T/Bkg ratios in the presence of decreasing values of both T and Bkg (Fig. 9). Ratios obtained at 2 hours are lower than those calculated at 10 min, supporting the need for an early acquisition after injection. The presence of tumor washout and the heterogeneity of the values measured in different lesions support the hypothesis of a possible use of TF-scintimammography for the functional imaging of chemoresistance, as already demonstrated for MIBI [83].

Data derived from the comparison with MDP bone scan demonstrate that TF can be a reliable radiotracer for differential diagnosis of solitary bone metastases [74]. Moreover, the evidence in a patient of an intense TF uptake by involved lymph nodes at the level of the internal mammary chain, disappearing after radiotherapy, is in agreement with a predictive value of a therapeutic response [74]. Preliminary data seem to suggest a similar behavior for chemotherapy response.

T/Bkg Ratio

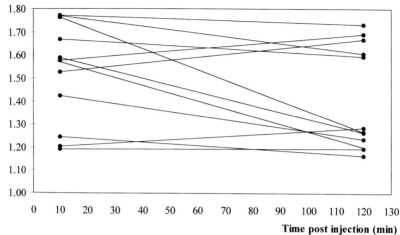

Time post injection (min)

FIGURE 9   Tumor/background ratios at 10 min and 120 min in 12 patients. Heterogeneous behavior is observed with respect to washout.

VI. REVIEW OF MEDICAL LITERATURE

Vieira and Weinholtz [91] reported their experience in TF scintimammography in 27 patients with suspected breast cancer. While a 0.8-cm malignant lesion was not detected, a 0.4-cm carcinoma was visualized. Moreover, a 53% sensitivity in detecting lymph node metastases was reported. No false-positive results were obtained in this study.

As reported above, a lower specificity has been referred by Lind [69], presenting in a group of 48 patients a 91% sensitivity because of a false-negative result in an infiltrating ductal CA. A low specificity (74%) was mainly determined by the presence of uptake in all of the five fibroadenomas. More recently [70] the same authors, evaluating a series of 84 patients with both SPET and planar images, reported a 93% sensitivity and a 80% specificity, with uptake at level of only nine out of 18 fibroadenomas evaluated. A 71% positive predictive value and a 96% negative predictive values were reported. In another paper [92], concerning nine patients evaluated with planar views, a concentration in seven malignant tumors and the absence of uptake in two benign lesions has been reported. Madariaga [93] compared TF scintimammography and mammography in 15 patients. Sensitivities of 100% and 60% and specificities of 80% and 100% were obtained for TF and mammography respectively. Schillaci [94] evaluated 55 patients reporting a

93% sensitivity and a 93% specificity. The same group [95] in a comparative study with MIBI reported overlapping results.

Interesting data can be found in the paper published by Adalet [82] on 18 patients presenting 19 mammary lesions. Uptake observed in 13 out of 14 malignant lesions with the exception of a patient affected with a mucinous carcinoma. No uptake was seen at level of two patients with fibrocystic disease and two fibroadenomas, while accumulation was present in a case of chronic mastitis. Cases of patients with breast cancer presenting TF uptake have been also published by Berghammer [49] and Adachi [96].

TF scintimammography is a promising procedure to detect primary breast cancer and axillary lymph node metastases. Different values in sensitivity and specificity in the literature are mainly due to differences in acquisition procedures or in the examined population. As an example, in a group of 30 patients with suspicious breast masses [97], TF gave true-positive results in 16/26 patients with primary breast cancer and true-negative in 3/4 patients with fibroadenoma, corresponding to a sensitivity of 61% and a specificity of 75%. But planar static images were started only 60 min after the injection of TF, not considering a possible washout, thus decreasing sensitivity.

A 100% sensitivity and 82% specificity was obtained in 50 patients studied at the Ankara Numune Hospital in Turkey [98]. Zerva [85], in 36 patients, utilizing an original oblique projection, obtained a 85% sensitivity and a 88% specificity in detection of malignant tumors. Spanu [57] published a study demonstrating SPET ability to improve sensitivity in the detection of lymph node involvement.

A comparison between TF and MIBI performed by Ivancevic [99] demonstrated similar diagnostic results, with a sensitivity depending strongly on tumor stage, falling from 100% for TF and 80% for MIBI with T2, T3 tumors to 42% and 46%, respectively, with <T2 tumors. These data have been further on confirmed [100]. Moreover, mainly because interpretation was more difficult, in this series SPET did not prove to be superior to planar imaging. The same group [101], in comparison of FDG and TF in planar scintimammography and in SPET, further confirmed dependence of tumor detection from size. FDG has an higher sensitivity using SPET.

Comparison between TF and MIBI have also been reported in the evaluation of other tumors. Concordant results have been observed in the analysis of patients with thyroid diseases [42,62], lung cancer [51], nasopharyngeal carcinomas [52], and musculoskeletal sarcomas [59].

Interesting information can be derived from the paper by Kostakoglu [52]. Even if there was no statistically significant difference between the two imaging techniques in the detection of the primary disease, MIBI was superior to TF on the detection of regional lymph node metastases, presenting a 95% sensitivity, vs. 79% for TF. At the opposite, in the evaluation of nine patients with suspicion of residual/recurrent tumor MRI presented five false-positive results, TF 2 and MIBI

3. TF, MIBI, and MRI had specificity of 78%, 67%, and 44% and accuracy of 87.5%, 81% and 69%, respectively.

A small but not significant difference in favor of MIBI has been reported in musculoskeletal sarcomas [59] and in lung cancer [51]. At the opposite, MIBI showed significantly lower T/Bkg ratios and detections rates than TF in the follow-up of patients with differentiated thyroid carcinomas treated with thyroidectomy and high dose I-131 therapy [62].

On the basis of the present experience we can conclude that TF is a reliable radiocompound for the evaluation of patients with breast cancer. While not indicated for screening, an important complementary role with respect to mammography can be played, mainly in cases where this procedure is not diagnostic. Useful information can be obtained in the detection of lymph node involvement and in the differential diagnosis of distant metastases. TF can have an important clinical role in follow-up for the evaluation of tumor relapse. Interesting perspective that have to be evaluated further on could regard the predictive value of the procedure to assess the therapeutic response.

Many similarities with MIBI are evident, but no data at the moment give a clear evidence of the superiority of one over the other. The choice may depend on which agent is used routinely for myocardial studies in the laboratory. Further studies are mandatory to define an identical or a different clinical use for these two compounds. To better define indications in diagnostic and/or prognostic field, further research has to compare the effect of parameters such as number and activity of mitochondria, pharmacokinetics, and effect of drugs.

VII. SUMMARY

^{99m}Tc-tetrofosmin (TF) is a lipophilic diphosphine compound, routinely used for myocardial scintigraphy, also proposed for the evaluation of patients with malignant neoplasms and in parathyroid adenomas. Concerning uptake mechanisms, the importance of flow and the metabolic status of cells have been hypothesized. The intracellular uptake depends on mitochondria and the Na+/K+ pump. Similarities with ^{99m}Tc-sestamibi regarding both uptake mechanisms and the property of being a substrate for P-glycoprotein (P-gp), a multidrug resistance transporter, have been published. Scintimammography with TF is a useful procedure mainly in patients with equivocal results at mammography. A role can be also individualized to avoid or guide surgery and/or biopsy.

Many studies reported a satisfactory sensitivity and specificity in the detection of primary tumors. Nevertheless unsatisfactory values are obtained for lesions <1 cm. The possibility of uptake in benign lesions with main reference to fibroadenomas has been reported. TF is reliable tracer also for diagnosis of local recurrence and of axillary lymph node metastases. Its capability to detect distant metastases has been also demonstrated.

ACKNOWLEDGMENTS

Experimental work has been partially supported by a CNR grant.

REFERENCES

1. Summerhayes IC, Lampidis TJ, Bernal SD, et al. Unusual retention of rhodamine-^{123}I by mitochondria in muscle and carcinoma cells. Proc Natl Acad Sci USA 79:5292–5296, 1982.
2. Nadakavukaren KK, Nadakavukaren JJ, Chen LB. Increased rhodamine-123 uptake by carcinoma cells. Cancer Res 45:6093–6097, 1985.
3. Maublant JC, Zheng Z, Rapp M, Ollier M, Michelot J, Veyre A. In vitro uptake of ^{99m}Tc teboroxime in carcinoma cell lines and normal cell lines: comparison with ^{99m}Tc-sestamibi and 201-Tl. J Nucl Med 34:1949–1952, 1993.
4. Khalkhali I, Cutrone JA, Mena IG, et al. Scintimammography: the complementary role of Tc-99m sestamibi prone breast imaging for the diagnosis of breast carcinoma. Radiology 196:421–426, 1995.
5. Hassan IM, Sahweil A, Constantinides C, et al. Uptake and kinetics of Tc-99m-hexakis-2-methoxy-isobutyl-isonitrile in benign and malignant lesions in the lungs. Clin Nucl Med 14:333–340, 1989.
6. O'Tuama LA, Packard AB, Treves SD. Spect imaging of pediatric brain tumor with hexakis (methoxyisobutylisonitrile)technetium (I). J Nucl Med 31:2040–2041, 1990.
7. Caner B, Kitapcl MN, Unlu M, et al. Technetium-99m-MIBI uptake in benign and malignant bone lesions: a comparative study with technetium-99m-MDP. J Nucl Med 33:319–324, 1992.
8. Balon HR, Fink Bennett D, Stoffer SS. Technetium-99m-sestamibi uptake by recurrent Hurthle cell carcinoma of the thyroid. J Nucl Med 33:1393–1395, 1992.
9. Baillet G, Albuquerque L, Chen Q, Poisson M, Delattre JY. Evaluation of single-photon emission tomography imaging of supratentorial brain gliomas with technetium-99m-sestamibi. Eur J Nucl Med 21:1061–1066, 1994.
10. Delmon-Moingeon LI, Piwnica-Worms D, Van den Abeele AD, Holman BL, Davidson A, Jones AG. Uptake of the cation hexakis (2-methoxyisobutyl-isonitrile)-technetium-99m by human carcinoma cell lines in vitro. Cancer Res 50:2198–2202, 1990.
11. Kelly JD, Forster AM, Higley B, et al. Technetium-99m-tetrofosmin as a new radiopharmaceutical for myocardial perfusion imaging. J Nucl Med 34:222–227, 1993.
12. Higley B, Smith FW, Smith T, et al. Technetium-99m-1,2-bis [bis (2-ethoxyethyl) phosphino] ethane: human biodistribution, dosimetry and safety of a new myocardial perfusion imaging agent. J Nucl Med 34:30–38, 1993.
13. Sinusas AJ, Shi Q, Saltzberg MT, et al. Technetium-99m-tetrofosmin to assess myocardial blood flow: experimental validation in an intact canine model of ischemia. J Nucl Med 35:664–671, 1994.
14. Younes A, Songadele JA, Maublant J, Platts E, Pickett R, Veyre A. Mechanism of

uptake of technetium-tetrofosmin. II. Uptake into isolated adult rat heart mitochondria. J Nucl Cardiol 2:327–333, 1995.

15. Koplan BA, Glover D, Ruiz M, et al. Comparison between Tl-201 and Tc-99m tetrofosmin uptake under experimental conditions of sustained low flow and profound systolic dysfunction. J Nucl Med 35(suppl):47P, 1994. Abstract.

16. Arbab AS, Koizumi K, Toyama K, Araki T. Uptake of technetium-99m-tetrofosmin, technetium-99m-MIBI and thallium-201 in tumor cell lines. J Nucl Med 37:1551–1556, 1996.

17. Sessler MJ, Geck P, Maul FD, Hor G, Munz DL. New aspects of cellular thallium uptake: Tl+,Na+,–2Cl-cotransport is the central mechanism of ion uptake. Nuklearmedizin 25:24–27, 1986.

18. Venuta S, Ferraiuolo R, Ambesi-Impiombato FS, Morrone G, Mansi L, Salvatore M. The uptake of Tl-201 in normal and transformed cell lines. J Nucl Med All Sci 4:163–166, 1979.

19. Salvatore M, Mansi L, Morrone G, Ferraiuolo R, Venuta S. In vitro techniques to study the transport of radiotracers. In: Colombetti LG, ed. Biological Transport of Radiotracers. Boca Raton, FL: CRC Press, 1982:289–309.

20. Platts EA, North TL, Pickett RD, Kelly JD. Mechanism of uptake of technetium-tetrofosmin: uptake into isolated adult rat ventricular myocites and subcellular localization. J Nucl Cardiol 2:317–326, 1995.

21. Wolf H, Kaiser K, Nacke C, et al. Uptake mechanism of Tc-99m tetrofosmin in tumour cell cultures. Eur J Nucl Med 23:1252, 1996. Abstract.

22. Ballinger JR, Bannemann J, Boxen I, et al. Accumulation of Tc-99m tetrofosmin in breast tumour cells in vitro: role of multidrug resistance p-glycoprotein. J Nucl Med, 36(suppl):202P, 1995. Abstract.

23. Ballinger JR, Banneman J, Boxen I, et al. Tc-99m-tetrofosmin as a substrate for P-glycoprotein: in vivo studies in multidrug-resistant breast tumor cells. J Nucl Med 37:1578–1581, 1996.

24. Wolf H, Frieling B, Nacke C, et al. Tc-99m tetrofosmin accumulation in sensitive and multidrug resistant tumour cells with and without verapamil. Eur J Nucl Med 23:1095, 1996. Abstract.

25. Nakamura K, Sugawara I, Satake S, Kubo A, Takamj H. Comparison of Tc-99m-MIBI and Tc-99-m-tetrofosmin uptakes in anaplastic thyroid carcinoma. Eur J Nucl Med 23:1142, 1996. Abstract.

26. Wolf H, Frieling B, Brenner W, Henze E. Uptake mechanism of Tc-99m sestamibi. Tc-99m tetrofosmin and Tc-99m furifosmin in sensitive and multidrug-resistant carcinoma cells. J Nucl Med 38(suppl)241P, 1997. Abstract.

27. Cole SPC, Bhardwaj G, Gerlach JH, et al. Overexpression of a transporter gene in a multidrug-resistant human cancer cell line. Science 258:1650–1654, 1992.

28. Wolf H, Nacke C, Kaiser K, et al. Uptake of Tc-99m tetrofosmin, Tc-99m sestamibi and Tl-201 in chemotherapy sensitive and resistant tumour cell lines. Eur J Nucl Med 23:1252P, 1996. Abstract.

29. Schomäcker K, Lohr H, Scharl A, et al. Comparison of Tc-99m MIBI, Tc-99m tetrofosmin, Tc-99m Q-12 and Tl-201: biokinetics on tumour bearing mice. J Nucl Med 38(suppl):241P, 1997. Abstract.

30. Amano S, Inoue T, Tomiyoshi K, et al. In vivo comparison of radiopharmaceuticals

for PET and SPECT in detecting breast cancer. J Nucl Med 38:233, 1997. Abstract.

31. De Jong M, Bernard BF, Breeman WAP, et al. Comparison of uptake of ^{99m}Tc-MIBI, ^{99m}Tc-tetrofosmin and ^{99m}Tc-Q12 into human breast cancer cell lines. Eur J Nucl Med 23:1361–1366, 1996.

32. Seregni E, Botti C, Molteni Nerini S, et al. Uptake of Tc-99m sestamibi, Tc-99m tetrofosmin, Tc-99m medronate and F-18 FDG in breast cancer cell line. Q J Nucl Med 40:67, 1996. Abstract.

33. Piwnica-Worms D, Chiu ML, Budding M, Kronauge JF, Kramer RA, Croop JM. Functional imaging of multidrug-resistant P-glycoprotein with an organotechnetium complex. Cancer Res 53:977–984, 1993.

34. Jones JM, Evans WD, Middleton GW, Richards AR The radiochemical purity of Tc-99m tetrofosmin: effect of generator elution and storage at room temperature. Eur J Nucl Med 22:944, 1995. Abstract.

35. Baravelli R, Ferraguti L, Marini B, Perri A, Bentivoglio R. The stability of Tc-99m tetrofosmin labelling at room temperature (22°C). Eur J Nucl Med 23:1258, Abstract.

36. Flamen P, Bossuyt A, Franken PR. Technetium-99m-tetrofosmin in dipyridamole-stress myocardial SPECT imaging: intraindividual comparison with technetium-99m-sestamibi. J Nucl Med 36:2009–2015, 1995.

37. Widding A, Hesse B, Gadsboll N. Technetium-99m sestamibi and tetrofosmin myocardial single-photon emission tomography: can we use the same reference data base? Eur J Nucl Med 24:42–45, 1997.

38. Zaret BL, Rigo P, Wackers JT, et al. Myocardial perfusion imaging with Tc-99m-tetrofosmin. Comparison to Tl-201 imaging and coronary angiography in a Phase III multicenter trial. Circulation 91:313–319, 1995.

39. Jain D, Wackers FJT, Mattera J, McMahon, Sinusas AJ, Zaret BL. Biokinetics of technetium-99m-tetrofosmin: myocardial perfusion imaging agent implications for a one-day imaging protocol. J Nucl Med 34:1254–1259, 1993.

40. Basoglu T, Sahin M, Coskun C, Koparan A, Bernay I, Erkan L. Tc-99m-tetrofosmin uptake in malignant lung tumours. Eur J Nucl Med 22:687–688, 1995.

41. Kosuda S, Yokoyama H, Katayama M, YokoKawa T, Kusano S, Yamamoto O. Tc-99m tetrofosmin and Tc-99m sestamibi imaging of multiple metastases from differentiated thyroid carcinoma. Eur J Nucl Med 22:1218–1220, 1995.

42. Klain M, Maurea S, Cuocolo A, et al. Technetium-99m tetrofosmin imaging in thyroid diseases: comparison with Tc-99m-pertechnetate, thallium-201 and Tc-99m-methoxyisobutylisonitrile scans. Eur J Nucl Med 23:1568–1574, 1996.

43. Nemec J, Nyvltova O, Preiningerova M, et al. Positive thyroid cancer scintigraphy using Tc-99m-tetrofosmin (Myoview): a preliminary report. Nucl Med Commun 16:694–697, 1995.

44. Rambaldi PF, Mansi L, Di Lieto E, et al. Tc-99m tetrofosmin SPET in primary lung tumor. J Nucl Med 37(suppl):264P, 1996. Abstract.

45. Mansi L, Rambaldi PF, Marino G, Pecori B, Del Vecchio E. Kinetics of Tc-99m sestamibi and Tc-99m tetrofosmin in a case of parathyroid Adenoma. Clin Nucl Med 21:700–703, 1996.

46. Giordano A, Meduri G, Marozzi P. Parathyroid imaging with Tc-99m-tetrofosmin. Nucl Med Commun 17:706–710, 1996.

47. Ishibashi M, Nishida H, Kumabe T, et al. Tc-99m tetrofosmin. A new diagnostic tracer for parathyroid imaging. Clin Nucl Med 20:902–905, 1995.

48. Soricelli A, Cuocolo A, Tedeschi E, et al. Evaluation of brain tumours with Tc-99m tetrofosmin and thallium-201: a preliminary report. Eur J Nucl Med 21(suppl):S6, 1994. Abstract.

49. Berghammer P. Wiltschke, Sinzinger H, Zielinski CC. Tc-99m tetrofosmin soft tissue scanning and metastatic disease Lancet 348:1169–1170, 1996.

50. Kaya HH, Cobaner R, Isik R, Seyigit A, Yilmaz S, Coskunsel M. Tetrofosmin accumulation in the malign pleural mesothelioma. Eur J Nucl Med 23:1214, 1996. Abstract.

51. Tutas A, Nardah M, Gulmez I, Silov G, Kibar M, Karahacioglu E. Evaluation of primary lung cancer with Tc-99m tetrofosmin in comparison to Tc-99m MIBI uptake. Eur J Nucl Med 23:1212, 1996. Abstract.

52. Kostakoglu L, Uysal U, Ozyar E, et al. A comparative study of Tc-99m sestamibi and Tc-99m tetrofosmin single-photon tomography in the detection of nasopharyngeal carcinoma. Eur J Nucl Med 24:621–628, 1997.

53. Giordano A. Meduri G. Differences between Tc-99m tetrofosmin and Tc-99m sestamibi in parathyroid scintigraphy. Eur J Nucl Med 24:347, 1996. Abstract.

54. Aigner RM, Feuger GF, Nicoletti R. Parathyroid scintigraphy: comparison of Tc-99m MIBI and Tc-99m tetrofosmin studies. Eur J Nucl Med 23:693–696, 1996.

55. Lind P. Parathyroid imaging with Tc-99m labelled cationic complexes: which tracer and which technique should be used? Eur J Nucl Med 24:243–245, 1997.

56. Pastore V, Mansi L, Rambaldi PF, et al. Tc-99m tetrofosmin uptake in lung carcinoma. Proceedings of the 2nd International Congress on Lung Cancer, Bologna, 1996:193–196.

57. Spanu A, Ginesu F, Dettori G, et al. Tc99m-tetrofosmin scan in lung and breast cancer detection. Eur J Nucl Med 23:1212P, 1996. Abstract.

58. Aigner RM, Sill H, Zinke W, Fueger GF. Tc-99m tetrofosmin scintigraphy in Hodgkin's disease. Nuc Med Commun 18:252–257, 1997.

59. Soderlund V, Jacobsson H, Brosjo O, Bauer HC, Johnsson C. Comparison of Tc-99m MIBI and Tc-99m tetrofosmin uptake by musculoskeletal sarcomas. J Nucl Med 38:682–686, 1997.

60. Ishibashi M, Hayabuchi N, Meno S, Ohzono H, Fujimoto K. Tc-99m tetrofosmin uptake in mediastinal tumours. Br J Radiol 69:1134–1138, 1996.

61. Lind P, Gomez I, Mikosch P, Kresnik E, Langsteger W, Gallowitsch HJ. Tc-99m tetrofosmin whole body scintigraphy in the follow-up of differentiated thyroid carcinoma. J Nucl Med 38:348–352, 1997.

62. Gallowitsch HJ, Lind P, Gomez I, Pipam W, Mikosch P, Kresnik E. Tc-99m tetrofosmin scintigraphy: an alternative scintigraphic method for following up differentiated thyroid carcinoma: preliminary results. Nuklearmedizin 35:230–235, 1996.

63. Civelek AC, Durski K, Shafique I, et al. Failure of perchlorate to inhibit Tc-99m isonitrile binding by the thyroid during myocardial perfusion studies. Clin Nucl Med 16:358–361, 1991.

64. Mansi L, Golia R, Spadafora M, Mazzarella G, De Rimini ML, Miletto P. A new

approach to parathyroid scintigraphy with Tc-99m MIBI. J Nucl Biol Med 38:259–260, 1994.

65. Cancroft ET, Goldsmith SJ. Technetium-99m-pertechnetate scintigraphy as an aid in the diagnosis of breast masses. Radiology 106:441–444, 1973.

66. Raylman RR, Ficaro EP, Wahl RI. Stereotactic coordinates from ECT sinograms for radionuclide-guided breast biopsy. J Nucl Med 37:1562–1567, 1996.

67. Wagner RH, Karesh SM, Dillehay GL, Henkin RE. Accuracy of needle localization of scintigraphic abnormalities using a radio-directed biopsy system (RDBS). J Nucl Med 38(suppl):22P, 1997. Abstract.

68. Atasever T, Unlu M, Ozturk C, Cetin N, Vural G, Gokcora N. Evaluation of malignant and benign lung lesions with Tc-99m tetrofosmin. Nucl Med Commun 17:577–582, 1996.

69. Lind P, Gallowitsch HJ, Kogler D, Kresnik E, Mikosch P, Gomez I. Tc-99m tetrofosmin scintimammography: a prospective study in primary breast lesions. Nuklearmedizin 35:225–229, 1996.

70. Lind P, Gallowitsch HJ, Gomez I, Kresnik E, Mikosch P. Tc-99m tetrofosmin scintimammography: a prospective study in patients with primary breast lesions. J Nucl Med 38(suppl):233P–234P, 1997. Abstract.

71. Cwikla JB, Buscombe JR, Kelleher SM, et al. Poor specificity of scintimammography in primary breast cancer in patients in U.K. J Nucl Med 38(suppl):21P–22P, 1997. Abstract.

72. Cwikla JB, Barlow RV, Buscombe JR, et al. Size or histology? Factors affecting uptake of Tc-99m sestamibi in breast lesions in patients with suspected primary breast cancer. J Nucl Med 38(suppl):234P, 1997. Abstract.

73. Hoh CK, Glaspy JA, Seltzer MA, et al. Application of Bayes' theorem in various methods for measuring FDG uptake in breast lesions. J Nucl Med 38(suppl):242P, 1997. Abstract.

74. Mansi L, Rambaldi PF, Cuccurullo V, et al. Diagnostic and prognostic role of ^{99m}Tc-tetrofosmin in breast cancer. Q J Nucl Med. 41:239–250, 1997.

75. Mansi L, Rambaldi PF, Cuccurullo V, Quarantelli M, Laprovitera A, Procaccini E. Semiquantitative analysis of Tc-99m scintimammography: assessment of the acquisition protocol. Eur J Nucl Med. 24:1048, 1997. Abstract.

76. Buyat I, De Sousa MC, Di Paola M, Lumbroso J, Ricard M, Aubert B. Impact of scatter correction on tumor detection in planar scintimammography: a phantom study. J Nucl Med 38(suppl):66P–67P, 1997. Abstract.

77. Pamplona R, Joaquim AI, Brunetto SQ, et al. Mammoscintigraphy: a new mattress for simultaneous acquisition of both breasts with a dual head camera. J Nucl Med 38(suppl):209P–210P, 1997. Abstract.

78. Costa M, Moura L. Automatic assessment of scintimamographic images using a novelty filter. Proc Annu Symp Comput Appl Med Care (US) 1995:537–541.

79. Doshi NK, Basic M, Cherry SR, Pang LJ. Development of a realistic multimodality breast and axillary node phantom. J Nucl Med 38(suppl):203P–204P, 1997. Abstract.

80. Ivancevic V, Marnitz S, Wandke E, Reisinger I, Munz DL. Phantom study on the validity of the tumour/background ratio in planar prone scintimammography. Eur J Nucl Med 23:1092, 1996. Abstract.

81. Peng NJ, Chiou YH, Kwok CG, et al. Comparative study of Tc-99m DMSA SPECT

with 180° and 360° data collection in detection of renal scars. J Nucl Med 38(suppl):49P–50P, 1997. Abstract.

82. Adalet I, Cantez S, Bozfakioglu Y, Muslumanoglu M, Demirkol MO. Tc-99m tetrofosmin scintigraphy in the evaluation of palpable breast masses. Nucl Med Commun 18:118–121, 1997.

83. Del Vecchio S, Ciarmiello A, Potena MI, et al. In vivo detection of multidrug-resistant (MDR1) phenotype by Tc-99m sestamibi scan in untreated breast cancer patients. Eur J Nucl Med 24:150–159, 1997.

84. Golia R, Miletto P, Spadafora M, et al. An improved technique for mammary scintigraphy in patients with breast cancer. J Nucl Biol Med 38:236–237, 1997.

85. Zerva C, Sabali C, Kiriaki D, Kitsou E, Gogas I, Alevizou V. Tc tetrofosmin imaging in breast tumours suspicious for malignancy. Eur J Nucl Med 23:1224P, 1996. Abstract.

86. Maurer AH, Caroline DF, Jadali FI, et al. Limitations of craniocaudal thallium-201 and technetium-99m sestamibi mammoscintigraphy J Nucl Med 36:1696–1700, 1995.

87. Rambaldi PF, Mansi L, Procaccini E, Di Gregorio F, Del Vecchio E. Breast cancer detection with Tc-99m tetrofosmin. Clin Nucl Med 20:703–705, 1995.

88. Mansi L, Rambaldi PF, Procaccini E, et al. Scintimmammography with Tc-99m tetrofosmin in the diagnosis of breast cancer and lymph node metastases. Eur J Nucl Med 23:932–939, 1996.

89. Mansi L, Rambaldi PF, Cuccurullo V, et al. ^{99m}Tc-tetrofosmin in breast cancer: experience of the Second University of Naples. Tumori. 83:523–525, 1997.

90. Mansi L, Rambaldi PF, Laprovitera A, Di Gregorio F, Procaccini E. Tc-99m uptake in breast tumors. J Nucl Med 36(suppl):83P, 1995. Abstract.

91. Vieira MR, Weinholtz JHB. Technetium-99m-tetrofosmin scintigraphy in the diagnosis of breast cancer. Eur J Surg Oncol 22:331–334, 1996.

92. Batista JF, Sanchez E, Stusser RJ, et al. Usefulness of Tc-99m tetrofosmin scintimammography in palpable breast tumours. Nucl Med Commun 18:338–340, 1997.

93. Madariaga P, Perez Vazquez JM, Trampal C, et al. Tc-99m tetrofosmin scintigraphy to evaluate breast lesions. Anticancer Res 17:1619–1621, 1997.

94. Schillaci O, Colella AC, Cannas P, et al. Scintimammography with Tc-99m tetrofosmin in suspected brast cancer. Anticancer Res 17:1623–1626, 1997.

95. Schillaci O, Scopinaro F, Danieli R, et al. Tc-99m tetrofosmin (TF) scintimammography (SMM): accuracy in patients with suspicion of breast cancer and comparison with Tc-99m MIBI. Eur J Nucl Med 23:1223, 1996. Abstract.

96. Adachi I, Ohtake Y, Tamoto S, et al. Two cases of breast cancer detected by Tc-99m tetrofosmin myocardial scintigraphy. Kaku Igaku 33:531–536, 1996.

97. Bohuslavizki KH, Brenner W, Bolling C, et al. Scintimammography using Tc99m-tetrofosmin in preoperative work-up of breast cancer. Eur J Nucl Med 23:1094P, 1996. Abstract.

98. Yagcioglu H, Ibis S, Naldoken S. Differentiation of malignant and benign breast mass using Tc-99m-tetrofosmin: comparison with mammography, ultrasonography and biopsy. Eur J Nucl Med 23:1094, 1996. Abstract.

99. Ivancevic V, Marnitz S, Winzer K-J, et al. Intraindividual comparison of Tc-99m sestamibi and Tc-99m tetrofosmin in prone and supine scintimammography. Eur J Nucl Med 23:1223, 1996. Abstract.

100. Ivancevic V, Marnitz S, Winzer K-J, et al. Tc-99m sestamibi and ^{99m}Tc tetrofosmin in

planar scintimammography and SPECT: intraindividual comparison. J Nucl Med 38(suppl):233P–234P, 1997. Abstract.
101. Ivancevic V, Marnitz S, Wolter A, et al. Intraindividual comparison of F-18 fluo-rodeoxiglucose and Tc-99m tetrofosmin in planar scintimammography and SPECT. J Nucl Med 38(suppl):68P–69P, 1997. Abstract.

12

Role of ^{99m}Tc Sestamibi Scintimammography for the Evaluation of Breast Lesions

IRAJ KHALKHALI AND JORGE TOLMOS
Harbor-UCLA Medical Center, Torrance, California

LINDA DIGGLES
Harbor-UCLA Medical Center, Torrance and California State University, Dominiguez Hills, California

I. INTRODUCTION

Breast cancer is the second most common malignancy among women in the United States, with a projected 180,200 cases in 1997 [1]. It ranks second only to lung cancer in cancer-related mortality. It is estimated that approximately 43,900 women will die of breast cancer in the United States in 1997 [1]. In fact, it is the leading cause of death among women aged 30 to 70 years, and its incidence is rising 3% per year [1]. The lifetime risk of a woman developing invasive breast cancer is one in eight [2].

Early diagnosis permits a high rate of cure with multimodality therapy [3]. Early breast cancer can be detected as a nonpalpable lesion with the aid of mammography, which remains the only imaging screening test of proven value for the detection of clinically occult breast cancer [4–6]. Screening mammography has been shown to significantly reduce breast cancer mortality and to allow treatment options such as breast conservation therapy [7–13].

The presence of malignancy in a mammographically detected abnormality must be confirmed by a breast biopsy, which is associated with significant physical discomfort and emotional stress [14]. The risk and cost of performing biopsies are also to be taken into consideration [15]. Mammography has a positive predictive value for detection of breast cancer of 10% to 30%, meaning that 70% to 90% of patients will have a breast biopsy for a benign disease [6,16]. Furthermore, 10% of patients with breast cancer present with normal mammograms, and the false-negative rate is even higher in younger patients because of the increased incidence of radiographically dense breast tissue in young women [17]. Mann et al. showed that a false-negative mammographic study may result in considerable delay in the decision to biopsy a patient subsequently shown to have carcinoma of the breast. This delay significantly increases the probability of axillary lymph node metastasis [18].

A noninvasive technique to select those patients who would benefit most from breast biopsy and reduce the number of negative biopsies is clearly of value. Newer imaging techniques, including nuclear medicine imaging, are therefore assuming an increasing role in detection strategies. This chapter will review the current status of Tc-99m sestamibi scintimammography for the detection and staging of breast cancer.

II. HISTORY OF RADIONUCLIDE TUMOR IMAGING

The first published report of radionuclide breast scanning was in 1946 by Low-Beer in which 25 patients with breast masses were evaluated with a radioactive pure β-emitter phosphorus (^{32}P). Of the 17 patients with proven carcinoma, 16 patients showed a 25% increase in counts in the area of the malignancy when compared with the corresponding area of the opposite breast and adjacent normal areas of the same breast [19,20]. Since the maximum range of the beta emissions of ^{32}P in body tissue is about 8 mm, this method could not detect lesions deeper than 5 mm and thus was abandoned. During the following years several radionu-clides, including ^{42}K [21], ^{86}Rb [22], ^{197}Hg chlormeridin [23], ^{67}Ga [24], and ^{206}Bi-citrate [25], were investigated for external counting over breast masses. It was not until 1966 that Whiley et al. reported increased uptake of ^{99}Tc-pertechne-tate in a case of breast carcinoma [26]. In 1974, Siegel et al. reported increased breast uptake of ^{99m}Tc-HEDSPA (1-hydroxy-ethylidene-1,1-disodium phospho-nate) during routine bone scanning of patients with known breast cancer [27]. The sensitivity for the detection of breast carcinoma was generally high, but the speci-ficity was low using these tracers, limiting their clinical use.

In 1976, Cox et al. reported an incidental finding of increased uptake of ^{201}Tl in a patient with left lung carcinoma during routine myocardial perfusion imaging [28]. This finding suggested that nuclear scanning might play a role for detection of malignancy in an asymptomatic patient. Subsequently, Hisada et al. reported a series of 173 malignant tumors of all types, including two breast can-cers, as well as 76 benign lesions with increased uptake of ^{201}Tl [29].

The first uses of ^{99m}Tc-sestamibi for tumor imaging were reported by Muller et al. [30] and Hassen et al. [31]. At many institutions, ^{99m}Tc-sestamibi has been effectively used in primary malignant as well benign tumors: parathyroid adeno-mas [32–34], carcinoma of the thyroid [35], brain gliomas [36], and bone tumors [37,38].

Recent reports of radionuclide imaging of the breast have utilized the non-specific tumor imaging agents Thallium-201 (^{201}Tl) [39] and ^{99m}Tc sestamibi (MIBI), as well as the bone scanning agents ^{99m}Tc methylene diphosphonate (MDP) [40] ^{99m}Tc polyphosphate [41], and ^{99m}Tc HMDP [42]. The mechanisms of uptake of these nuclear tracers in malignant tissue are not well understood. Attempts to formulate radiotracers more specific for breast carcinoma have included biologically active peptides such as indium-labeled (^{III}In) somatostatin analogs which are targeted to specific receptors and radiolabeled monoclonal antibodies to breast cancer cells [43,44]. This chapter focuses on 99mTc-ses-tamibi, the radiopharmaceutical most extensively used for nuclear medicine breast imaging.

III. ^{99m}-TC SESTAMIBI (MIBI) SCINTIMAMMOGRAPHY

^{99m}Tc-labeled hexakis (2-methoxyisobutyl isonitrile) technetium (I) (^{99m}Tc-ses-tamibi or MIBI) is a gamma-emitting lipophilic monovalent cationic metallophar-maceutical radiotracer that concentrates in cardiac mitochondria [45,46]. MIBI localizes in the myocardium in proportion to the amount of blood flow and is widely used for the scintigraphic assessment of myocardial perfusion in the eval-uation of patients with known or suspected coronary artery disease [47,48]. Cel-lular uptake in myocardial cells is related to retention of the MIBI cation by intra-cellular mitochondria [45,49]. Chiu et al. and Piwnica-Worms et al. indicated the driving force of MIBI accumulation in tissue culture cells to be a strong electro-static attraction between the positive charge of the lipophilic ^{99m}Tc-MIBI mole-cule and the negative charge of the mitochondria [50].

Delmon-Moingeon et al. showed that approximately 90% of ^{99m}Tc-ses-tamibi activity is found within the mitochondria [51]. Mitochondrial retention of MIBI does not appear to be organ-specific and may thus account for MIBI accu-mulation in tumors such as breast carcinoma [52,53]. MIBI has recently been val-idated as a P-glycoprotein transport substrate, which could be one of the mecha-nisms responsible for the uptake of MIBI in breast tumor cells [54].

Hallmarks of breast carcinoma, like many malignancies, include increased mitotic activity of tumor cells, the development of neovascularization (angiogen-esis) as a means of obtaining nutrients for growth and invasion, and the develop-ment of intense fibrosis (desmoplasia). While increased mitotic activity is seen in both in situ and invasive tumors, angiogenesis and desmoplasia signal tumor inva-siveness [55,56]. Cutrone et al. found that the degree of MIBI uptake in breast lesions appears to be related more to the degree of desmoplastic activity and cel-lular proliferation than neovascularity and mitochondrial density [57].

Maublant et al. have demonstrated that malignant breast tumors strongly concentrate ^{99m}Tc-sestamibi at a ratio of nearly 6:1 compared with the surrounding normal breast or fat tissue. Interestingly, in this study scintimammography did not show focal uptake in four malignant tumors in vivo, whereas in vitro studies showed the presence of ^{99m}Tc-sestamibi [58]. Two of the tumors were smaller than 8 mm, and the other two, 10 and 25 mm, were located in the lower inner quadrant of the left breast. The author concluded that tumor size is one limitation of scintimammography, but a medial location and possible superimposition of the myocardium can also be causes of false-negative results. In the same group of patients, the two false-positives had benign epithelial hyperplasia.

A.   Technical Considerations for Tc-99m Scintimammography

1.   Imaging Equipment

Imaging is performed using a standard gamma camera equipped with a low-energy, high-resolution collimator and interfaced to a computer. This equipment is commonly available in any nuclear medicine department. We use a specially designed breast imaging overlay (Bodfish Research and Design, Inc., Bodfish, CA) with cutouts along the lateral borders, allowing the patient to be placed in a prone position with the breast dependent for imaging (Fig. 1). The detector is brought as close as possible to the surface of the breast being imaged. A symmetric 10% energy window is centered over the 140 keV photopeak [59].

2.   Patient Preparation

A thorough explanation of the procedure by the technologist or physician will decrease patient anxiety and improve patient cooperation. A meticulous medical history and physical examination are performed, including any history of allergic reaction to the radiopharmaceutical agent or problems with the upper-extremity venous system. Recent mammograms and other breast imaging studies should be available for correlation with the scintimammograms (SMMs). A breast examination is essential to describe the location of any palpable masses or skin lesions.

History of any breast injury or surgery should be noted, and SMM should be delayed at least 1 week following cyst aspiration or fine needle aspiration (FNA) cytology and at least 1 month following excisional biopsy or an injury to the breast. This will decrease the possibility of a false-positive result due to inflammation or trauma. The date of the last menstrual period, postmenopausal status, and any use of hormone replacement therapy should be noted. If possible, SMM should not be scheduled the week immediately before or during the menstrual period. A significantly increased incidence of bilateral diffuse MIBI breast uptake, which can obscure focal lesions, has been observed when SMM is performed during this time [60]. Diffuse breast uptake is not specific for menstrual cycle, as it can also be seen in postmenopausal women (Fig. 2).

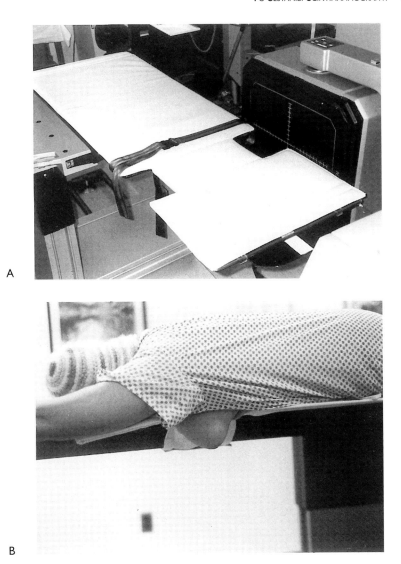

A

B

Figure 1   (A) Imaging overlay and detector positioned for lateral prone dependent-breast imaging. (B) Patient positioned on imaging overlay for lateral image of the left breast.

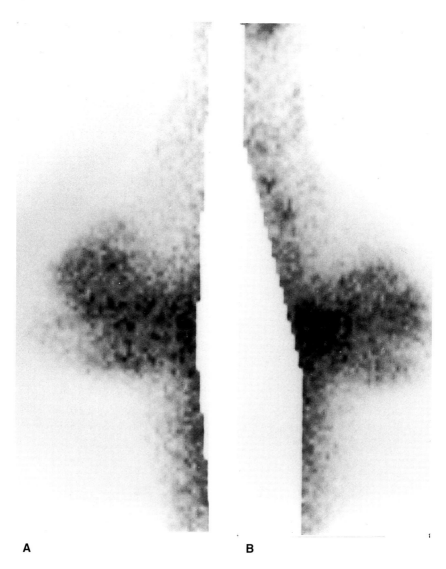

A   **B**

FIGURE 2   Left lateral (A) and right lateral (B) prone dependent-breast scintimammograms of a 35-year-old female acquired 10 min postinjection of 20 mCi ^{99m}Tc-sestamibi show intense bilateral patchy uptake of unknown significance which decreases the diagnostic value of the test. Mammography showed a 2 by 1.5 cm indeterminate mass in the lower inner quadrant of the left breast, as well as a 5 by 4.5 cm phylloides in the retroareolar area of the right breast. Bilateral biopsies showed fibroadenomas and fibrocystic disease with apocrine metaplasia.

3. Patient Positioning

The success of scintimammography relies heavily on accurate positioning. Khalkhali et al. as well as Taillefer et al. have recommended the technique of prone breast imaging using planar lateral views [61,62]. The prone position depicts a natural contour of the breast that is necessary for localization of the lesion. Planar prone breast imaging is more favorable than supine or upright imaging for detection of primary breast lesions, because of the maximum separation of deep breast structures from the high-activity chest and abdominal organs such as the myocardium on the left and the liver on the right side. In addition, relaxation of the pectoralis muscle in prone position enables more favorable imaging of the entire breast, particularly small lesions adjacent to the chest wall. Such lesions could be missed on supine imaging if they are superimposed over the heart or liver.

Anterior upright imaging with the patient's arms raised is used for evaluating the axillary region for metastases. Anterior upright and lateral prone images give complementary information to provide a better diagnostic evaluation of the patient.

Supine scintimammography results in decreased sensitivity and specificity for breast malignancy. Helbich et al. reported 66 women with 75 breast lesions performing ^{99m}Tc-sestamibi scintimammography in supine position obtaining a sensitivity and specificity of 62% and 88%, respectively [63]. This is in contrast to our experience and that of others who have utilized prone dependent-breast imaging [61,62,64–67].

B. Radiopharmaceutical Injection and Radiation Dose

Prior to injection of the radiopharmaceutical, an indwelling intravenous line is placed in the arm contralateral to the known breast lesion. If bilateral lesions are suspected, or if the contralateral breast or axillary region had a prior surgical procedure, the intravenous line is placed in the pedal vein of either foot. Once the intravenous line is placed securely, an intravenous injection of 20 mCi (740 MBq) of Tc-99m sestamibi (Miraluma, Dupont Pharmaceutical Company, North Billerica, MA) is administered, followed by at least 10 cc of saline to clear the tracer from the vessel. Careful placement of the intravenous line and flushing the line with saline will prevent uptake of the radiopharmaceutical in the regional veins or axillary lymph nodes, which makes accurate evaluation of the upper breast and axilla difficult [59]. The total-body absorbed dose from an injection of 740 MBq (20 mCi) of ^{99m}Tc-sestamibi used in scintimammography is approximately 3.3 mSv (330 mrem) [68,69].

1. Image Acquisition

Imaging should begin no later than 10 min after the injection. Each planar view is acquired for 10 min using an acquisition zoom that includes the breast, axilla, and chest wall in the field of view. The first image is a lateral view of the breast with the suspected lesion, followed by repositioning the detector 30° posterior for a posterior oblique view. This view may improve separation of deep lateral lesions from the chest wall. The patient is repositioned and the same views are acquired of the contralateral breast. For postmastectomy patients, the mastectomy side is imaged in the same manner as the intact breast. The study ends with an anterior chest image in the upright position with both arms raised [59].

Some authors advocate the use of radioactive nipple markers in all patients [64]. In our experience routine use of nipple markers has not been helpful. Markers may also be placed on breast abnormalities in either the lateral or anterior view by superimposing a radioactive source on the palpable breast mass abnormality for further clinical correlation. If lesion markers are used, it is important to place them after the patient is positioned for imaging. We have noticed significant alteration of the relationship of the marker to the lesion when the patient is repositioned from upright or supine to prone.

Little has been reported regarding the kinetics of MIBI in breast cancer imaging. Delayed images, obtained >1 hour after injection, may show a rapid washout from the tumor. Waxman et al. have observed an inconsistent pattern of MIBI washout in imaging patients both at early as well as delayed time periods postinjection [64]. In some patients, benign abnormalities may appear to have greater activity 60 to 90 min after injection, whereas tumors may be less active 60 to 90 min postinjection than on the early study. This pattern needs further evaluation to delineate the basis for this finding. Preliminary results of multicenter clinical trials of Miraluma have demonstrated comparable sensitivity and specificity of early and delayed images [65].

2. Image Interpretation

In ^{99m}Tc-sestamibi breast scanning, as well as other oncologic scintigraphic exams, the distinction between positive and negative results depends on the degree of focal radiotracer uptake in the area of suspected tumor location. The normal breast has homogeneous, low-level uptake of ^{99m}Tc-MIBI with no focal findings (Fig. 3). Focal areas of increased uptake of the tracer are interpreted as suspicious for malignancy or probably malignant (Fig. 4). Diffuse or patchy bilateral uptake is observed in about 7% to 10% of scintimammograms, and should not be read as malignancy.

Scintimammography is an objective imaging procedure with high interobserver correlation. The rate of agreement between two experienced nuclear medicine physicians is 97% for primary lesions (kappa = 0.90) whereas the reading of axillary metastasis has a lower interobserver agreement of 74% (kappa = 0.49) [70].

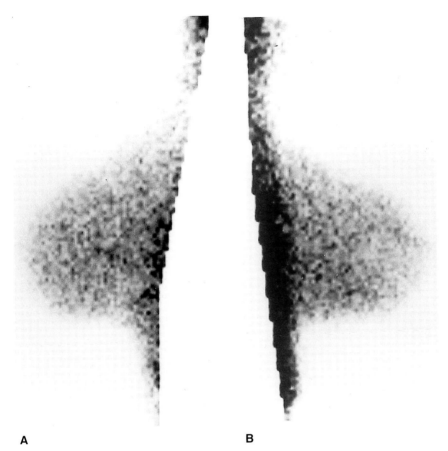

A   **B**

Figure 3   Left lateral (A) and right lateral (B) prone dependent-breast scintimammograms of a 55-year-old female acquired 10 min postinjection of 20 mCi ^{99m}Tc-sestamibi show mild homogenous tracer uptake consistent with a normal study. Mammography of the right breast showed a mammographically malignant mass with microcalcifications which was not palpable on physical examination. A needle localization biopsy showed fibrocystic disease with adenosis and fibrosis, as well as microcyst formation.

IV.   FOCUS POPULATIONS FOR SCINTIMAMMOGRAPHY

Several prospective trials have demonstrated a high diagnostic accuracy of ^{99m}Tc-MIBI in detecting breast cancer (Table 1). The overall sensitivity for the detection of breast cancer ranges from 62% to 96%. The specificity varies from 62% to

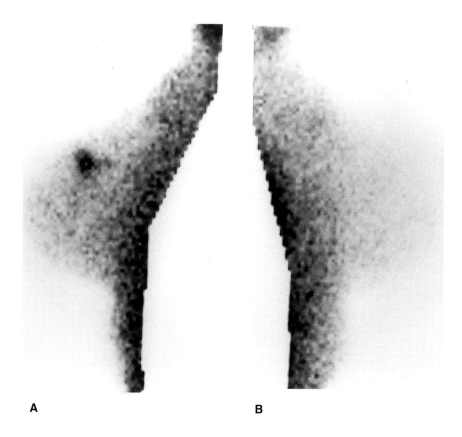

A   **B**

FIGURE 4   Left lateral (A) and right lateral (B) prone dependent-breast scintimammograms of a 57-year-old female acquired 10 min postinjection of 20 mCi ^{99m}-Tc sestamibi show intense focal tracer uptake in the upper left breast. The right breast shows mild homogenous tracer uptake consistent with a normal study. Mammography of the left breast was indeterminate with a few microcalcifications, as well as severe scar and skin thickening in the area of a previous biopsy. Excisional biopsy of the left breast showed ductal carcinoma in situ, comedotype.

100%. As expected, the sensitivity for palpable abnormalities is significantly higher than that for nonpalpable lesions. However, all these studies share the same inclusion criteria bias: the patients are known to have breast pathology by mammogram or physical exam. Scintimammography is not indicated as a screening test in asymptomatic patients.

Mammography is a relatively low-cost, safe test, with overall high sensitivity and widespread availability that should allow it to remain the mainstay of early

TABLE I   Summary of 99mTc Scintimammography (SMM) Prospective Studies
Using Histopathologic Diagnosis as the Gold Standard

Reference	Breast lesions (n)	Palpable: nonpalpable (n)	PPV	NPV	Sensitivity (%)	Specificity (%)
[103]	56	—	88	83	88	83
[63]	75	33:42	73	81	62	88
[63]	73[a]	—	67	91	83	80
Palmedo, 1996 [104]	54	40:14			88 80[a]	
[76]	68	—	—	—	83	84
[66]	66	46:20	94	82	83	93
		46:0			94	91
		0:20			64	100
[105]	27		82	88	82	87
[106]	147		88	93	84	95
[67]	24	0:24	88	56	50	90
[74]	43	43:0			91	62
	13	0:13			60	75
[107]					83	93
[61]	65	44:21			92	94
[70]	153	113:40	81	96	92	89
[75]	41	41:0	93	86	93	86
[108]	673	286:387	74	90	85	81
[109]	38	38:0	100	56	84	100

[a]SPECT.
n = number of lesions; PPV = positive predictive value; NPV = negative predictive value.

breast cancer detection. The results of two prospective multicenter trials sponsored by Dupont suggest that for every 100 patients with palpable lesions that are later shown to be malignant, five will be missed using 99mTc scintimammography [65]. SMM is relatively costly when compared with screening mammography, and because of the high rate of missed cancers among the different prospective studies, the use of MIBI in palpable lesions should not be for purposes of reducing unnecessary biopsies [64]. We have identified several select subgroups of patients that may benefit from this test.

A.   Dense Breast Tissue on Mammography

Mammographic findings are based on anatomic changes in the breast. The differentiation of normality and abnormality is achieved by detecting the pattern of density differences. Despite recent improvements in mammography equipment and technique, the radiographically dense breast remains difficult to image. The problems in imaging the dense breast account for a large percentage of the cases of mammographically "missed" carcinomas [71]. The sensitivity of mammography is limited by the density of the breast tissue [72]. Mammography is best used in women with fatty breasts, such as older women. Sensitivity has been reported to be lowered by 10% or more for women aged 40 to 49 years compared to older women because of increased breast tissue density [17].

Approximately 25% of women have dense breasts [71]. The difficulty in imaging the dense breast is due to several underlying physical characteristics: Breast cancer has X-ray attenuation properties similar to that of dense glandular and fibrous tissue, making its detection more difficult. The lesion is optimally visualized when superimposed or outlined by fat rather than glandular tissue. Routine mammographic screening of the dense breast is more difficult because lesions, if present, are less likely to be detected. The radiographically dense breast produces more scattered radiation, resulting in reduced image contrast. Dense breast frequently has more tissue inhomogeneities and a greater range of attenuation, making it more difficult to optimally expose all areas of the breast. Another factor that increases the difficulty of the interpretation of the mammographically dense breast is the higher exposure needed to achieve adequate film density. A longer exposure time produces increases the probability of motion unsharpness [71].

These limitations could be obviated with scintimammography because the mechanism of uptake is independent of the tissue density. Tc-99m scintimammography is independent of breast density or structural breast distortion and is being investigated for its usefulness in the assessment of breast lesions that are difficult to characterize mammographically [60]. The Dupont multicenter trial of 673 prospectively accrued patients demonstrated a sensitivity of 84% for fatty breasts and 86% for dense breasts [65]. These data support that Tc-99m sestamibi scintimammography was not affected by the density of the breast tissue and may have an advantage over mammography for the clinical management of patients with dense breast and suspected breast cancer (Fig. 5).

B. Symptomatic Breast Masses

Palpable mass abnormalities of the breast are often difficult to evaluate mammographically, especially in patients with fibrocystic changes and dense breasts. The sensitivity of breast examination plus mammography for cancer detection is around 90% in the case of fatty breasts and is significantly less in dense or abnormal breasts [73]. Scintimammography could be very valuable in this diagnostic setting when it is difficult to delineate a palpable abnormality using conventional mammography.

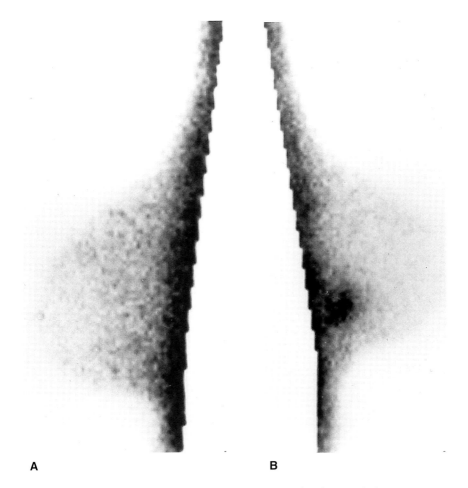

A   **B**

FIGURE 5   Left lateral (A) and right lateral (B) prone dependent-breast scintimammograms of a 35-year-old female acquired 10 min postinjection of 20 mCi ^{99m}Tc sestamibi show an area of intense focal tracer uptake in the lower right breast adjacent to the chest wall. The left breast shows mild homogeneous tracer uptake consistent with a normal study. Mammography was difficult to evaluate due to significantly dense breasts (ACR pattern IV) but showed an indeterminate area of asymmetry in the 3 o'clock location of the right breast. A modified radical mastectomy and axillary lymph node dissection of the right breast showed grade III infiltrating ductal carcinoma with a component of infiltrating lobular carcinoma. No lymph nodes of the 14 dissected were positive for metastatic disease.

When scintimammography was performed in patients with palpable lesions, the sensitivity ranged between 83% and 96% and specificity ranged between 62% and 100%. However, 4% to 16% of malignant palpable lesions will have a false-negative SMM [65,74,75]. One recent report has shown that SMM is 100% sensitive to detect breast cancer in patients with palpable breast lesions [76].

Currently, SMM is not recommended to reduce the number of excisional biopsies in palpable breast masses, and negative results should not delay tissue diagnosis if such an intervention is clinically warranted.

C. High-Risk Patients

Epidemiological studies have established risk factors for breast cancer such as genetic predisposition including BRCA1, BRCA2, and Li Fraumeni syndrome; family history of breast cancer; secondary breast radiation as a result of treatment of other malignancies [77]; use of hormonal contraceptives [78]; prior histological evidence of atypia; and prior history of lumpectomy and radiotherapy [79].

It is estimated that approximately 5% of all women with breast cancer have a germ-line mutation in a gene (BRCA1) localized in chromosome 17q21. Their relatives, if carriers of the BRCA1 mutation, may have an 85% lifetime risk of breast cancer with 50% of the breast cancers occurring prior to age 50 years. Ovarian cancer risk is also elevated in patients with the BRCA1 mutation [80]. A second gene, BRCA2, has been localized to chromosome 13q12-13. BRCA2 confers a high risk of breast cancer and, to a lesser extent, ovarian cancer [81]. Hormonal contraceptives have been shown to increase the risk of breast cancer during the 10-year period immediately following their use [78].

These subsets of patients may benefit from a second surveillance test which needs to be independent of breast density, surgical scars, and radiotherapy changes. SMM has shown to be independent of the mentioned variables [64,65,74]. Further studies are required to establish the role of this promising test in this particular subgroup of patients who are extremely difficult to evaluate and follow up mammographically.

D. Mammographic Abnormalities

The low positive predictive value of screening mammography produces a large number of unnecessary breast biopsies [6,82]. There is a critical need to develop an accurate, noninvasive imaging technique to reduce the number of open surgical biopsies for benign lesions. The detection of a suspicious mammographic abnormality is often followed by a breast biopsy, which is associated with significant physical discomfort and emotional stress [14,83]. The incidence of false-negative scintimammograms for nonpalpable lesions reported in many series precludes the use of this technique in patients with abnormal asymptomatic mammography with the goal of reducing the number of breast biopsies [66,67,74].

The explanation for negative studies in the subgroup of patients without a palpable mass was addressed by Scopinaro et al. [84]. This group suggested that Tc-99m may be a marker of invasiveness; its uptake may be related to angiogenesis and, possibly, to oxidative metabolism of the tumor. Other possibilities for lack of tumor visualization are tumor size, tumor location within the breast, distance of the tumor from the camera, and soft-tissue attenuation in women with large breasts.

Excisional biopsy is currently the most accurate method to determine if a mammographic finding is benign or malignant. However, this procedure costs $1500 to $3000, compared to scintimammography, which is about $600. The risk and cost of performing biopsies are also to be taken in consideration [15]. Although excisional biopsy remains the "gold standard," it exposes the patient to morbidity as well as to psychological and economic costs of a surgical procedure.

E. Breast Cancer Staging

Traditional locoregional management of breast cancer includes axillary dissection. Overall, 30% to 40% of patients with breast carcinoma have pathologically documented lymph node metastases [85–87]. The biologic significance of axillary metastases has not been completely elucidated.

Some investigators have advocated management of patients without axillary dissection, obviating the associated morbidity [88,89]. The determination of the biologic behavior of breast cancer with molecular markers is under investigation, but the available techniques have not proven superior to the determination of the nodal status [89,90]. Radiological techniques, as well as minimally invasive surgical techniques, have been reported previously [7,8]. It is apparent that a noninvasive test to accurately determine the presence of axillary metastases might obviate the need for axillary dissection, which can be followed by the onset of lymphedema, in a significant proportion of patients.

Tc99m-SMM has been used successfully in visualization of primary breast carcinomas as well as lymph node metastasis. Scopinaro et al. suggest that ^{99m}Tc-sestamibi may be a marker of breast cancer invasiveness. Its uptake may be related to angiogenesis and, possibly, to oxidative metabolism of the tumor [84]. A very useful property of ^{99m}Tc-sestamibi is the potential for the assessment of lymph node metastases (Fig. 6). In vitro studies of Maublant et al. show strong concentration of Tc-99m sestamibi in primary breast carcinoma and axillary lymph node metastases, even when images are negative [58]. Several investigators have used SMM to evaluate the axillary regions in patients with breast carcinoma. Comparison of SMM results with histopathology in these patients yielded a sensitivity ranging from 84% to 92% and a specificity ranging from 90% to 94% [61,91,92].

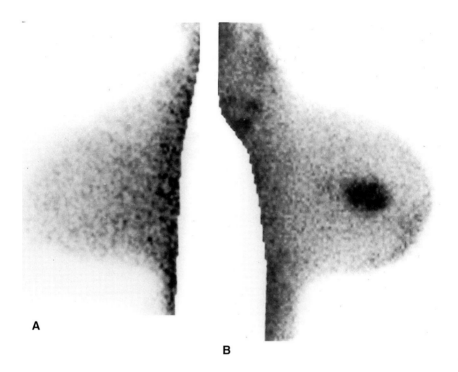

A

B

Figure 6   Left lateral (A) and right lateral (B) prone dependent-breast scintimammograms of a 60-year-old female acquired 10 min postinjection of 20 mCi ^{99m}Tc sestamibi show a large focal area of intense tracer uptake in the right midbreast consistent with primary breast carcinoma, as well as two foci of uptake in the axilla consistent with metastasis to the lymph nodes. The left breast shows mild homogeneous tracer uptake consistent with a normal study. Mammography of the right breast showed a 6 by 5 cm indeterminate mass. An excisional biopsy and axillary lymph node dissection confirmed stage IV infiltrating ductal carcinoma with metasasis to the lymph nodes.

We performed SMM in 31 women who subsequently had axillary lymphadenectomy as part of their standard staging and treatment for breast cancer. The sensitivity, specificity, positive predictive value, and negative predictive value of SMM planar imaging for axillary metastases were 75%, 82%, 88%, and 64%, respectively [93].

The role of axillary dissection is currently in evolution. The value of axillary dissection is advocated on the basis of these premises:

    1.   The importance of axillary metastases as a harbinger of systemic dis-

ease; axillary dissection is used as a means of assessing prognosis to establish appropriate treatment plans for patients with primary breast carcinoma [94].

2. The fact that progressive growth of lymphatic metastases may be the cause of significant mortality.

3. Some animal data seem to indicate that axillary metastases can give rise to systemic metastases. Nevertheless, the therapeutic benefit of a diagnostic axillary dissection is yet unproven.

Clinical evaluation of axillary-node involvement has a high false-positive and false-negative rate. Histological evaluation of the axillary specimen is the gold standard for the assessment of axillary metastasis. Axillary dissection offers no therapeutic benefit to node-negative patients, and it may lead to unnecessary morbidity. The most frequent complications following axillary dissection are wound seroma and infection [95]. Long-term morbidity from axillary node dissection occurs less commonly but may be a source for persistent complaints: mild to severe impairment of arm motion, lymphedema, sensory deficit caused by transection of the intercostobrachial nerves. A further reduction of the morbidity rates by selectively identifying patients who may exhibit a more significant benefit from axillary dissection should be taken into account to preserve an optimal quality of life [96].

Silverstein et al. found an increasing incidence of axillary metastases according to the size of the primary tumor: T1a 3%; T1b 17%; T1c 32%; T2 44%, and T3 60% [97]. Halverson et al. reviewed 178 patients with breast carcinoma no more than 10 mm in size; the incidence of pathological positive lymph nodes was 12.3% [89]. A selective policy of axillary dissection has been proposed by some investigators, based on the low likelihood of axillary nodal metastases in patients with small primary tumors.

A variety of noninvasive techniques for examination of the axilla for the presence of nodal metastases have been previously reported [98,99]. The sensitivity of physical examination is between 35% and 50%, with a specificity of 75% to 97%. CT and MRI have also been investigated, but results have not been very encouraging [74]. Scintimammography seems encouraging in patients with large primary breast cancer to evaluate the axilla. For primary tumors <1 cm, however, the data are unclear.

Since a negative predictive value of 64% is insufficient, future studies are needed to establish whether a combination of the clinical stage, SMM, and possibly sentinel node biopsy would provide a higher reliability in the subset of patients with a negative SMM and a breast mass <1 cm. Based on the available data, SMM is not a reliable test for the detection of axillary metastases in patients with breast cancer, although a high positive predictive value of 88% is encouraging. In conclusion, SMM with its 88% positive predictive value for the detection of axillary metastases can assist the surgeon in assuring a patient's compliance with recommended axillary dissection.

F.   Evaluation of Tumor Response To Chemotherapy

Breast nuclear scanning has been investigated not only for diagnostic purposes but also as a functional imaging technique for evaluation of the susceptibility of the tumor to chemotherapy agents [100]. MIBI has recently been validated as a P-glycoprotein transport substrate that is responsible for multidrug-resistant glycoprotein [54]. The multidrug-resistant P-glycoprotein (Pgp), a M(r) 170,000 plasma membrane protein encoded by the mammalian multidrug resistance gene (MDR1), has been documented in nearly all forms of human cancers [101,102] and could be one of the mechanisms responsible for the lack of sestamibi uptake in tumor cells that express MDR.

V.   FUTURE DIRECTIONS OF SCINTIMAMMOGRAPHY

A.   Breast-Dedicated Imagers

The evidence of some patients with breast cancer and tumors that show high concentration of ^{99m}Tc-sestamibi but normal scintimammograms demonstrates the limitation of the currently used gamma acquisition cameras, which are not specially designed for breast imaging. Dedicated cameras for breast scintigraphy imaging are under development at several sites. Some are equipped with a semiconductor instead of a scintillator and vacuum tubes. The semiconductor camera may eliminate the problem of the dead space, which is typical in the Anger gamma cameras, and can be manufactured in a smaller size, allowing improved resolution by rotation in multiple aspects of the breast without interference from adjacent organs such as the heart and liver. Small cameras using a NaI crystal, which is less expensive than a semiconductor, are also in development. Future development of small detectors for single gamma breast imaging (scintimammography) may allow visualization of tumors located close to the chest wall and those with difficult geometry for the current available larger gamma cameras, as well as improving spatial resolution and detector efficiency. Further information on this subject can be found in the chapter on new instrumentation.

B.   Scintigraphy-Guided Stereotactic Localization of Breast Carcinoma

Our experience with ^{99m}Tc-sestamibi scintimammography allowed us to identify a small subset of patients who present with axillary metastatic adenocarcinoma without mammographic or clinical evidence of primary breast tumor. Further workup with ^{99m}Tc-sestamibi scintimammography demonstrated focal uptake in the ipsilateral breast. This clinical scenario urged us to develop a technique to obtain a surgical specimen for histological confirmation of the suspicious lesion. Mena et al. developed and validated a scintigraphy-guided biopsy device for nonpalpable breast masses identified only by sestamibi scintimammography. A breast phantom was compressed in the cranial and caudal directions by fenestrated paddles. Three freely adjustable radioactive reference lines, each containing about 30 MBq (800 μCi) Tc-99m, were mounted on sliding rulers along x, y, and z axes on the external frame surrounding the breast phantom. The breast phantom was a semi-square-shaped sponge embedded with background activity of 37 MBq (1 mCi). Breast "lesions" labeled with about 11 MBq (300 μCi) of ^{201}Tl were carved out of the same sponge, wrapped in thin plastic film, and placed in various locations within the phantom. Scintigraphy was performed in the anterior and lateral projections, locating the lesion along the x, y, and z coordinates. A 22-gauge needle loaded with 37 MBq (1 mCi) of Tc-99m was introduced into the lesion by real-time visualization of the radioactive biopsy needle. This scintigraphy-guided biplane localization technique successfully localized 90% of all phantom lesions [110].

Stereotactic scintigraphy localization has been used in three patients who demonstrated focal breast uptake by ^{99m}Tc-sestamibi scintimammography. Successful needle localization surgical biopsy was done in all three patients. Breast cancer was demonstrated in two of three patients [111].

VI. SUMMARY

Mammography is the primary imaging modality used for early detection of clinically occult breast cancer. Despite the advances in mammographic techniques, mammography is still limited in both sensitivity and specificity. The low positive predictive value (10% to 30%) demands a second noninvasive test to decrease the number of unnecessary breast biopsies. Scintimammography, approved by the FDA in 1997, has demonstrated in a multicenter trial involving 673 patients an overall sensitivity of 85% and a specificity of 81% [108]. This accuracy decreases significantly for nonpalpable lesions, with a sensitivity of 55% to 72%. Patients believed to benefit from Tc-99m sestamibi scintimammography include patients with dense breasts, patients with architectural distortions or extensive scarring of the breast from prior biopsies, and patients in high risk categories. The potential of needle localization of a scintigraphy focal uptake is important when the only way to detect the breast abnormality is SMM.

At the present time scintimammography with ^{99m}Tc-sestamibi should not be used as a screening test to reduce the number of excisional biopsies indicated by abnormal mammography or the presence of a suspicious palpable breast mass. Mammography remains the procedure of choice in screening asymptomatic women for breast cancer, but scintimammography promises to play an important role as an adjunctive test in detecting malignancies in symptomatic women.

REFERENCES

1. Parker SL, Tong T, Bolden S, Wingo PA. Cancer statistics, 1997. CA Cancer J Clin 47:5–27, 1997.
2. Feuer EJ, Wun LM, Boring CC, Flanders WD, Timmel MJ, Tong T. The lifetime risk of developing breast cancer [see comments]. J Natl Cancer Inst 85:892–897, 1993.
3. Chu KC, Tarone RE, Kessler LG, et al. Recent trends in U.S. breast cancer incidence, survival, and mortality rates. J Natl Cancer Inst 88:1571–1579, 1996.
4. Perdue PW, Galbo C, Ghosh BC. Stratification of palpable and nonpalpable breast cancer by method of detection and age. Ann Surg Oncol 2:512–515, 1995.
5. Bauer TL, Pandelidis SM, Rhoads JE, Owens RS. Mammographically detected carcinoma of the breast. Surg Gynecol Obstet 173:482–486, 1991.
6. Wilhelm MC, Edge SB, Cole DD, deParedes E, Frierson HF. Nonpalpable invasive breast cancer [see comments]. Ann Surg 213:600–605, 1991.
7. Van Dijck JA, Verbeek AL, Beex LV, et al. Breast-cancer mortality in a non-randomized trial on mammographic screening in women over age 65. Int J Cancer 70:164–168, 1997.
8. Van Dijck JA, Verbeek AL, Beex LV, et al. Mammographic screening after the age of 65 years: evidence for a reduction in breast cancer mortality. Int J Cancer 66:727–731, 1996.
9. Baker LH. Breast cancer detection demonstration project: five-year summary report. CA Cancer J Clin 32:194–225, 1982.
10. Tabar L, Fagerberg G, Duffy SW, Day NE, Gad A, Grontoft O. Update of the Swedish two-county program of mammographic screening for breast cancer. Radiol Clin North Am 30:187–210, 1992.
11. Chen HH, Tabar L, Fagerberg G, Duffy SW. Effect of breast cancer screening after age 65. J Med Screen 2:10–14, 1995.
12. Larsson LG, Nystrom L, Wall S, et al. The Swedish randomised mammography screening trials: analysis of their effect on the breast cancer related excess mortality. J Med Screen 3:129–132, 1996.
13. Frisell J, Eklund G, Hellstrom L, Glas U, Somell A. The Stockholm breast cancer screening trial—5-year results and stage at discovery. Breast Cancer Res Treat 13:79–87, 1989.
14. Potchen EJ, Bisesi MA, Sierra AE, Potchen JE. Mammography and malpractice [see comments]. AJR 156:475–480, 1991.
15. Winchester DP. Evaluation and management of breast abnormalities. Cancer 66:1345–1347, 1990.
16. Kopans DB, Moore RH, McCarthy KA, et al. Positive predictive value of breast biopsy performed as a result of mammography: there is no abrupt change at age 50 years. Radiology 200:357–360, 1996.
17. Kerlikowske K, Grady D, Barclay J, Sickles EA, Ernster V. Effect of age, breast density, and family history on the sensitivity of first screening mammography [see comments]. JAMA 276:33–38, 1996.
18. Mann. Giuliano. Arch Surg 118:23–25, 1983.
19. Low-Beer BVA, Bell HG, McCorkle HJ. Measurement of radioactive phosphurus in breast tumors in situ; a possible diagnostic procedure. Radiology 47:492–493, 1946.

20. Low-Beer BVA. Surface measurements of radioactive phosphurus in breast tumors as a possible diagnostic method. Science 104:399, 1946.

21. Baker WH, Nathanson IT, Selverstone B. The use of radioactive potassium (42-K) in the study of benign and malignant breast tumors. N Engl J Med 252:612–615, 1955.

22. Ruffo AH, Lundaburn J. La radioactividad del rubidio y su fijacion en los tejidos normales y neoplasicos. Bol Inst Med Exp 82–92, 1952.

23. Soodee DB, Renner RR, Di Stefano B. Photoscanning localization of tumor, utilizing chlormerodrin mercury. Radiology 84:873–876, 1965.

24. Ito Y, Okuyama S, Awano T, Takahashi K, Sato T. Diagnostic evaluation of ^{67}Ga scanning of lung cancer and other diseases. Radiology 101:355–362, 1971.

25. Jacobstein JG, Quinn JL. Uptake of ^{206}Bi citrate in carcinoma of the breast. Radiology 107:677–679, 1973.

26. Whitley JE. Witcofski RL, Bolliger TT, Maynard CD. Tc-99m in the visualization of neoplasms outside the brain. Am J Roentgenol Radium Ther Nucl Med 96:706–710, 1966.

27. Siegel ME, Friedman BH, Wagner HN. A new approach to breast cancer. Breast uptake of ^{99m}Tc-HEDSPA. JAMA 229:1769–1771, 1974.

28. Cox PH, Belfer AJ, van der Pompe WB. Thallium 201 chloride uptake in tumours, a possible complication in heart scintigraphy. Br J Radiol 49:767–768, 1976.

29. Hisada K. Tonami N, Miyamae T, et al. Clinical evaluation of tumor imaging with Tl-201 chloride. Radiology 129:497–500, 1978.

30. Muller ST, Guth-Tougelids B, Creutzig H. Imaging of malignant tumors with Tc-99m MIBI SPECT. Eur J Nucl Med 28:562, 1987. Abstract.

31. Hassan IM, Sahweil A, Constantinides C, et al. Uptake and kinetics of Tc-99m hexakis 2-methoxy isobutyl isonitrile in benign and malignant lesions in the lungs. Clin Nucl Med 14:333–340, 1989.

32. Blocklet D, Martin P, Schoutens A, Verhas M, Hooghe L, Kinnaert P. Presurgical localization of abnormal parathyroid glands using a single injection of technetium-99m methoxyisobutylisonitrile: comparison of different techniques including factor analysis of dynamic structures. Eur J Nucl Med 24:46–51, 1997.

33. Rauth JD, Sessions RB, Shupe SC, Ziessman HA. Comparison of Tc-99m MIBI and Tl-201/Tc-99m pertechnetate for diagnosis of primary hyperparathyroidism. Clin Nucl Med 21:602–608, 1996.

34. Billotey C, Sarfati E, Aurengo A, et al. Advantages of SPECT in technetium-99m-sestamibi parathyroid scintigraphy. J Nucl Med 37:1773–1778, 1996.

35. Miyamoto S, Kasagi K, Misaki T, Alam MS, Konishi J. Evaluation of technetium-99m-MIBI scintigraphy in metastatic differentiated thyroid carcinoma. J Nucl Med 38:352–356, 1997.

36. Park CH, Kim SM, Zhang JJ, Intenzo CM, McEwan JR. Tc-99m MIBI brain SPECT in the diagnosis of recurrent glioma. Clin Nucl Med 19:57–58, 1994.

37. Tirovola EB, Biassoni L, Britton KE, Kaleva N, Kouykin V, Malpas JS. The use of ^{99m}Tc-MIBI scanning in multiple myeloma. Br J Cancer 74:1815–1820, 1996.

38. Maffioli L, Steens J, Pauwels E, Bombardieri E. Applications of ^{99m}Tc-sestamibi in oncology. Tumori 82:12–21, 1996.

39. Lee VW, Sax EJ, McAneny DB, et al. A complementary role for thallium-201 scintig-

raphy with mammography in the diagnosis of breast cancer. J Nucl Med 34:2095–2100, 1993.

40. Piccolo S, Lastoria S, Mainolfi C, Muto P, Bazzicalupo L, Salvatore M. Technetium-99m-methylene diphosphonate scintimammography to image primary breast cancer. J Nucl Med 36:718–724, 1995.

41. Clyne CA, Perry PM, Gibson A, MacLeod MA. ^{99m}Tc polyphosphate uptake by breast tumours. Br J Surg 65:773–774, 1978.

42. Nishiyama Y, Kawasaki Y, Fukunaga K, et al. [Second phase ^{99m}Tc-HMDP accumulation using three phase bone scintigraphy in a case of primary breast cancer.] Kaku Igaku 33:767–770, 1996.

43. Lind P, Gallowitsch HJ, Mikosch P, et al. Radioimmunoscintigraphy with Tc-99m labeled monoclonal antibody 170H.82 in suspected primary, recurrent, or metastatic breast cancer. Clin Nucl Med 22:30–34, 1997.

44. Schatten C, Barrada M, Mandeville R, et al. Combined use of I-231-labeled BCD-F9 and 4C4 monoclonal antibody with dissimilar specificity for breast cancer: implication for the detection limit of immunolymphoscintigraphy in the assessment of axillary lymph node metastases. Nucl Med Commun 15:422–429, 1994.

45. Piwnica-Worms D, Kronauge JF, Chiu ML. Uptake and retention of hexakis (2-methoxyisobutyl isonitrile) technetium(I) in cultured chick myocardial cells. Mitochondrial and plasma membrane potential dependence. Circulation 82:1826–1838, 1990.

46. Piwnica-Worms DP, Kronauge JF, LeFurgey A, et al. Mitochondrial localization and characterization of 99Tc-sestamibi in heart cells by electron probe X-ray microanalysis and 99Tc-NMR spectroscopy. Magn Reson Imag 12:641–652, 1994.

47. Okada RD, Glover D, Gaffney T, Williams S. Myocardial kinetics of technetium-99m-hexakis-2-methoxy-2-methylpropyl-isonitrile. Circulation 77:491–498, 1988.

48. Mousa SA, Cooney JM, Williams SJ. Relationship between regional myocardial blood flow and the distribution of ^{99m}Tc-sestamibi in the presence of total coronary artery occlusion. Am Heart J 119:842–847, 1990.

49. Piwnica-Worms D, Kronauge JF, Chiu ML. Enhancement by tetraphenylborate of technetium-99m-MIBI uptake kinetics and accumulation in cultured chick myocardial cells. J Nucl Med 32:1992–1999, 1991.

50. Chiu ML, Kronauge JF, Piwnica-Worms D. Effect of mitochondrial and plasma membrane potentials on accumulation of hexakis (2-methoxyisobutylisonitrile) technetium(I) in cultured mouse fibroblasts. J Nucl Med 31:1646–1653, 1990.

51. Delmon-Moingeon LI, Piwnica-Worms D, Van den Abbeele AD, Holman BL, Davison A, Jones AG. Uptake of the cation hexakis(2-methoxyisobutylisonitrile)-technetium-99m by human carcinoma cell lines in vitro. Cancer Res 50:2198–2202, 1990.

52. Crane P, Laliberte R, Heminway S, Thoolen M, Orlandi C. Effect of mitochondrial viability and metabolism on technetium-99m-sestamibi myocardial retention. Eur J Nucl Med 20:20–25, 1993.

53. Delmon-Moingeon LI, Piwnica-Worms D, Van den Abbeele AD, Holman BL, Davison A, Jones AG. Uptake of the cation hexakis(2-methoxyisobutylisonitrile)-technetium-99m by human carcinoma cell lines in vitro. Cancer Res 50:2198–2202, 1990.

54. Piwnica-Worms D, Chiu ML, Budding M, Kronauge JF, Kramer RA, Croop JM.

Functional imaging of multidrug-resistant P-glycoprotein with an organotechnetium complex. Cancer Res 53:977–984, 1993.

55. Horak ER, Leek R, Klenk N, et al. Angiogenesis, assessed by platelet/endothelial cell adhesion molecule antibodies, as indicator of node metastases and survival in breast cancer. Lancet 340:1120–1124, 1992.

56. Visscher DW, DeMattia F, Ottosen S, Sarkar FH, Crissman JD. Biologic and clinical significance of basic fibroblast growth factor immunostaining in breast carcinoma. Mod Pathol 8:665–670, 1995.

57. Cutrone J, Shane-Yospur L, Khalkhali I, et al. Immunohistologic assessment of tc-99m sestamibi uptake in benign and malignant breast lesions. J Nucl Med 1998. In press.

58. Maublant J, de Latour M, Mestas D, et al. Technetium-99m-sestamibi uptake in breast tumor and associated lymph nodes. J Nucl Med 37:922–925, 1996.

59. Diggles L, Mena I, Khalkhali I. Technical aspects of prone dependent-breast scinti-mammography. J Nucl Med Technol 22:165–170, 1994.

60. Diggles L, Mena I, Khalkhali I. Bilateral increase uptake of Tc-99m sestamibi in scintimammography: its correlation with the menstrual cycle. J Nucl Med Tech 111P, 1994. Abstract.

61. Taillefer R, Robidoux A, Lambert R, Turpin S, Laperriere J. Technetium-99m-ses-tamibi prone scintimammography to detect primary breast cancer and axillary lymph node involvement. J Nucl Med 36:1758–1765, 1995.

62. Khalkhali I, Mena I, Jouanne E, et al. Prone scintimammography in patients with sus-picion of carcinoma of the breast. J Am Coll Surg 178:491–497, 1994.

63. Helbich TH, Becherer A, Trattnig S, et al. Differentiation of benign and malignant breast lesions: MR imaging versus Tc-99m sestamibi scintimammography. Radiol-ogy 202:421–429, 1997.

64. Waxman AD. The role of (99m)Tc methoxyisobutylisonitrile in imaging breast can-cer. Semin Nucl Med 27:40–54, 1997.

65. Khalkhali I, Villanueva-Meyer J, Edell SL, et al. Impact of breast density on the diag-nostic accuracy of Tc-99m sestamibi breast imaging in the detection of breast cancer. J Nucl Med 288:74P, 1996. Abstract.

66. Villanueva-Meyer J, Leonard MH, Briscoe E, et al. Mammoscintigraphy with tech-netium-99m-sestamibi in suspected breast cancer. J Nucl Med 37:926–930, 1996.

67. Maffioli L, Agresti R, Chiti A, et al. Prone scintimammography in patients with non-palpable breast lesions. Anticancer Res 16:1269–1273, 1996.

68. Anonymous. Radiopharmaceutical Internal Dose Information Center, July 1990, Oak Ridge Associated Universities. Oak Ridge, TN. 1994; In: Table 4 of DuPont Pharma's (Du Pont Radiopharmaceutical Division, The Du Pont Merck Pharmaceutical Co., Billerica, MA) Cardiolite tc-99m Sestamibi preparation kit. March 1994.

69. Behrman RH. Scintimammography: magic bullet or false promise [letter]. J Nucl Med 36:1929–1930, 1995.

70. Khalkhali I, Cutrone JA, Mena IG, et al. Scintimammography: the complementary role of Tc-99m sestamibi prone breast imaging for the diagnosis of breast carcinoma. Radiology 196:421–426, 1995.

71. Jackson VP, Hendrick RE, Feig SA, Kopans DB. Imaging of the radiographically dense breast. Radiology 188:297–301, 1993.

72. Ma L, Fishell E, Wright B, Hanna W, Allan S, Boyd NF. Case-control study of factors associated with failure to detect breast cancer by mammography [see comments]. J Natl Cancer Inst 84:781–785, 1992.

73. Shapiro S, Venet W, Strax P, Venet L, Roeser R. Ten- to fourteen-year effect of screening on breast cancer mortality. J Natl Cancer Inst 69:349–355, 1982.

74. Palmedo H, Grunwald F, Bender H, et al. Scintimammography with technetium-99m methoxyisobutylisonitrile: comparison with mammography and magnetic resonance imaging. Eur J Nucl Med 23:940–946, 1996.

75. Burak Z, Argon M, Memis A, et al. Evaluation of palpable breast masses with [99mTc]-MIBI: a comparative study with mammography and ultrasonography. Nucl Med Commun 15:604–612, 1994.

76. Palmedo H, Schomburg A, Grunwald F, Mallmann P, Boldt I, Biersack HJ. Scintimammography with Tc-99m MIBI in patients with suspicion of primary breast cancer. Nucl Med Biol 23:681–684, 1996.

77. Bhatia S, Robison LL, Oberlin O, et al. Breast cancer and other second neoplasms after childhood Hodgkin's disease [see comments]. N Engl J Med 334:745–751, 1996.

78. Anonymous. Breast cancer and hormonal contraceptives: collaborative reanalysis of individual data on 53 297 women with breast cancer and 100 239 women without breast cancer from 54 epidemiological studies. Collaborative Group on Hormonal Factors in Breast Cancer [see comments]. Lancet 347:1713–1727, 1996.

79. Jacobson JA, Danforth DN, Cowan KH, et al. Ten-year results of a comparison of conservation with mastectomy in the treatment of Stage I and II breast cancer [see comments]. N Engl J Med 332:907–911, 1995.

80. Miki Y, Swensen J, Shattuck-Eidens D, et al. A strong candidate for the breast and ovarian cancer susceptibility gene BRCA1. Science 266:66–71, 1994.

81. Wooster R, Neuhausen SL, Mangion J, et al. Localization of a breast cancer susceptibility gene, BRAC2, to chromosome 13q12-13. Science 265:2088–2090, 1994.

82. Adler DD, Wahl RL. New methods for imaging the breast: techniques, findings, and potential. AJR 164:19–30, 1995.

83. Cockburn J, Staples M, Hurley SF, De Luise T. Psychological consequences of screening mammography. J Med Screen 1:7–12, 1994.

84. Scopinaro F, Ierardi M, Porfiri LM, et al. [99mTc]-MIBI prone scintimammography in patients with high and intermediate risk mammography. Anticancer Res 17:1635–1638, 1997.

85. Carter CL, Allen C, Henson DE. Relation of tumor size, lymph node status, and survival in 24,740 breast cancer cases. Cancer 63:181–187, 1989.

86. Fowble B, Solin LJ, Schultz DJ, Goodman RL. Frequency, sites of relapse, and outcome of regional node failures following conservative surgery and radiation for early breast cancer. Int J Radiat Oncol Biol Phys 17:703–710, 1989.

87. Haffty BG, Goldberg NB, Fischer D. Conservative surgery and radiation therapy in breast carcinoma: local recurrence and prognostic complications. Int J Radiat Oncol Biol Phys 17:727–732, 1989.

88. Giuliano AE, Barth AM, Spivack B, Beitsch PD, Evans SW. Incidence and predictors of axillary metastasis in T1 carcinoma of the breast. J Am Coll Surg 183:185–189, 1996.

89. Halverson KJ, Taylor ME, Perez CA. Management of the axilla in patients with breast cancers one centimeter or smaller. Am J Clin Oncol 17:461, 1994.

90. Noguchi S, Aihara T, Nakamori S. The detection of breast carcinoma micrometastases in axillary lymph nodes by means of reverse transcriptase-polymerase chain reaction. Cancer 74:1595–1600, 1994.

91. Mansi L, Rambaldi PF, Procaccini E, et al. Scintimammography with technetium-99m tetrofosmin in the diagnosis of breast cancer and lymph node metastases. Eur J Nucl Med 23:932–939, 1996.

92. Lam WW, Yang WT, Chan YL, Stewart IE, Metreweli C, King W. Detection of axillary lymph node metastases in breast carcinoma by technetium-99m sestamibi breast scintigraphy, ultrasound and conventional mammography. Eur J Nucl Med 23:498–503, 1996.

93. Tolmos J, Khalkhali I, Vargas H, et al. Detection of axillary lymph node metastasis of breast carcinoma with technetium-99m sestamibi scintimammography. J Am Surg 1997. In press.

94. Staunton MD, Melville DM, Monterrosa A, Thomas JM. A 25-year prospective study of modified radical mastectomy (Patey) in 193 patients. J R Soc Med 86:381–384, 1993.

95. Ingvar C, Erichsen C, Jonsson PE. Morbidity following prophylactic and therapeutic lymph node dissection for melanoma—a comparison. Tumori 70:529–533, 1984.

96. Jeffrey SS, Goodson WH, Ikeda DM, Birdwell RL, Bogetz MS. Axillary lymphadenectomy for breast cancer without axillary drainage. Arch Surg 130:909–912, 1995.

97. Silverstein MJ, Gierson ED, Waisman JR. Axillary lymph node dissection for Tla breast carcinoma. Is it indicated? Cancer 73:664–667, 1994.

98. Giuliano AE. Sentinel lymphadenectomy in primary breast carcinoma: an alternative to routine axillary dissection. J Surg Oncol 62:75–77, 1996.

99. Giuliano AE, Dale PS, Turner RR. Improved axillary staging of breast cancer with sentinel lymphadenectomy. Ann Surg 222:394–399, 1995.

100. Luker G, Fracasso P, Dobkin J, Piwnica-Worms D. Modulation of the multidrug resistance P-glycoprotein: detection with technetium-99m-sestamibi in vivo. J Nucl Med 38:369–372, 1997.

101. Goldstein LJ. MDRI gene expression in solid tumours. Eur J Cancer 32A:1039–1050, 1996.

102. Correnti M, Cavazza ME, Guedez N, Herrera O, Suarez-Chacon NR. Expression of the multidrug-resistance (MDR) gene in breast cancer. J Chemother 7:449–451, 1995.

103. Tiling R, Sommer H, Pechmann M, et al. Comparison of technetium-99m-sestamibi scintimammography with contrast-enhanced MRI for diagnosis of breast lesions. J Nucl Med 38:58–62, 1997.

104. Palmedo H, Schomburg A, Grunwald F, Mallmann P, Krebs D, Biersack HJ. Technetium-99m-MIBI scintimammography for suspicious breast lesions. J Nucl Med 37:626–630, 1996.

105. Occhiato R, Schillaci O, Broglia L, et al. [Breast scintigraphy with technetium 99m sestamibi, as support to radiologic methods in the study of breast lesions.] Scintigrafia mammaria con 99mTc-SESTAMIBI, come supporto alle metodiche radiologiche nello studio delle lesioni mammarie. Radiol Med (Torino) 91:581–584, 1996.

106. Clifford EJ, Lugo-Zamudio C. Scintimammography in the diagnosis of breast cancer. Am J Surg 172:483–486, 1996.
107. Yuen-Green M, Wasnich R, Caindec-Ranchez S, Davis J. New method for breast cancer detection using Tc-99m sestamibi scintimammography. Hawaii Med J 55:26–28, 1996.
108. Khalkhali I, Villanueva-Meyer J, Edell S, et al. Diagnostic accuracy of Tc-99m sestamibi breast imaging in breast cancer detection. J Nucl Med 37:74P, 1996. Abstract.
109. Kao CH, Wang SJ, Liu TJ. The use of technetium-99m methoxyisobutylisonitrile breast scintigraphy to evaluate palpable breast masses. Eur J Nucl Med 21:432–436, 1994.
110. Mena F, Mena I, Diggles L, Khalkhali I. Design and assessment of scintigraphy guided biplane localization technique of breast tumors: a phantom study. Nucl Med Commun. 17:717–723, 1996.
111. Khalkhali I, Mishkin F, Diggles L, Klein S. Radionuclide-guided stereotactic prebiopsy localization of nonpalpable breast lesions with normal mammograms. J Nucl Med 38:1019–1022, 1997.

13

Using the Sentinel Node Concept to Stage Breast Cancer:

Breast Lymphoscintigraphy and Intraoperative Gamma Probe Sentinel Node Localization

Naomi P. Alazraki and Raghuveer K. Halkur
Emory University School of Medicine and Veterans Affairs Medical Center, Atlanta, Georgia

I. INTRODUCTION

Conventional surgical management of invasive breast cancer includes axillary node dissection to stage the disease. In recent years, surgeons have recognized that in early breast cancer, axillary node dissection shows no tumor spread with increasing frequency. As a result, for noninvasive breast cancer, axillary node dissection has become controversial [1,2] but is still the standard of care for invasive breast cancer with no clinically apparent metastases. As mammographic screening of women and self-examination by women has gained acceptance, earlier diagnosis of early breast cancer has impacted the outcomes of women with this disease. Smaller tumors are found mammographically, and, more frequently, axillary lymph node dissections do not reveal any micrometastases.

The risk of axillary involvement for patients with breast cancer has been studied as a function of tumor size and mode of presentation. For example, in one study [3] for patients with nonpalpable tumors, the risk of axillary involvement was 4% (2/51) for T1a and 7% (6/92) for T1b. For palpable tumors, the risk was 6% (3/50) for T1a, but 23% (33/143) for T1b. based on a survey of reported studies summarized by Recht [4], breast tumors 0 to 0.5 cm were associated with axillary lymph node involvement in 0% to 11% although one report of seven patients indicated 57%, while for tumors 0.6 to 1.0 cm, 7% to 37% with most reporting 17% to 22% associated with axillary lymph node metastases.

Physicians have sought a less invasive approach to staging early breast cancer, so that therapeutically unnecessary axillary node dissections might be obviated [5], saving substantial cost in terms of dollars as well as morbidity [6]. Significant morbidity [4,8,9] associated with axillary node dissection is related to postoperative lymphedema [7] of the involved extremity, neuropathy of the arm [8], seromas [4], painful neuromas, local wound problems, and the need for general anesthesia. The highly successful application of the sentinel node concept to staging melanoma, using radionuclide lymphoscintigraphy and the intraoperative gamma probe, as well as the Vital Blue dye technique by some surgeons, has been adapted for investigation in patients with invasive breast cancer and no clinically apparent metastases.

II. SENTINEL NODE CONCEPT

In melanoma, the sentinel node concept was introduced by Morton [7], using a blue dye (Isosulfan Blue) injected in the operating room intradermally around the tumor in order to stain the sentinel node(s) for visual identification. The sentinel node concept states that the first lymph node to receive lymphatic drainage from the tumor site will show metastases if there is any tumor spread through lymphatics. If the sentinel lymph node is histologically tumor-free, then no lymph nodes in that lymph node basin will harbor tumor metastases.

The sentinel node concept was originally described by Cabanas [8] and applied in patients with penile carcinoma. The lymphatics of the penis drain to a group of nodes, the first of which to receive drainage is the sentinel lymph node. The dominant site of tumor spread in penile carcinoma is to this group of nodes [9]. Cabanas used radiographic contrast lymphangiography to determine that the sentinel lymph node corresponded to the lymph nodes associated with the superficial epigastric vein in the superficial inguinal area. At that time, in the 1970s, no imaging, radiolabeling, or intraoperative localization maneuvers were performed. The sentinel lymph node was found by manual exploration of the expected perisuperficial epigastric vein location. Cabanas reported that in 43 patients with penile carcinoma, 31 with tumor-negative sentinel lymph node biopsies who could be followed up had a 5-year survival rate of 90%. Others [10] found similar predictive accuracy in penile carcinoma of sentinel lymph node biopsies.

More recently, Pettaway et al. [11] reported a retrospective review of 20 patients who underwent extended sentinel lymph node dissection as a regional staging procedure for penile squamous carcinoma between 1985 and 1994. They reported a 25% false-negative rate for the sentinel node approach, but realized that the sentinel node approach used for those 20 patients did not include lymphatic mapping techniques. Therefore, they initiated intraoperative blue dye lymphatic mapping in an investigational setting for penile carcinoma patients. Patients with vulvar cancer have also been studied for applicability of the sentinel node concept using intraoperative Isosulfan Blue dye injected intradermally at the junction of the tumor and normal skin in nine patients. Surgeons found that intraoperative lymphatic mapping is technically feasible in patients with vulvar cancer [12], but further experience is needed. In 1997, DeCicco and co-workers from Milan reported at the Society of Nuclear Medicine meeting [13] that in 15 patients with vulvar cancer and two patients with vulvar melanoma, using scintillation camera imaging and a radioguided approach, identification of the sentinel nodes was easily accomplished without extensive surgical dissection. In three groins a single node metastasis was detected, and in all cases the positive node was the sentinel node. Thus, the sentinel node concept in vulvar cancer may indeed be used in the future to reduce morbidity of complete groin dissection if the sentinel node is tumor-negative.

Most of the recent clinical experience with lymphoscintigraphy and intraoperative gamma probe sentinel node localization has been primarily in malignant melanoma, with several reports in breast cancer. Because axillary lymph node dissection is a basic, routine procedure in breast cancer management of clinically localized disease (Stage I/II), the same rationales applicable for melanoma are relevant in breast cancer. Published experience with the sentinel node concept and lymphatic mapping in breast cancer is considered by most investigators in the field as yet insufficient to presume validation.

III. MELANOMA AND THE SENTINEL LYMPH NODE EXPERIENCE

The melanoma sentinel node experience started with Morton et al. [14,15] and the blue dye lymphatic mapping technique. In 194 of 237 patients with clinical Stage I melanoma, sentinel nodes' basins were delineated by the blue dye; metastases were detected in 40 (21%) of those nodal specimens. They found that nonsentinel nodes were the site of metastases in only two of 3079 nodes from 194 lymphadenectomy specimens (i.e., an identifiable sentinel node/false-negative rate of <1%).

Reintgen et al. [16] presented a validation of the sentinel node approach in melanoma by determining the order of melanoma nodal metastases. In their report of 42 patients, eight had positive sentinel nodes. The sentinel node was the only node with tumor in seven of the eight, providing convincing additional support that nodal metastases from cutaneous melanoma are not random events. The concept of an orderly progression of lymph node metastases in melanoma is quite different from the development of metastases in most other solid malignancies. By showing absence of skip nodal metastases (i.e., no micrometastasis in any node in a lymph node basin whose sentinel node is negative for micrometastasis), the authors present strong evidence of absence of skip metastases, thereby supporting the orderly progression of lymph node metastasis in melanoma. In a 1996 editorial [17], Reintgen argues that with lymphatic mapping and sentinel lymph node biopsy, "the controversy over performing elective lymph node dissection (ELND) for melanoma is now academic and the only reason to perform ELND is when mapping is not possible, because of inadequate nuclear medicine or pathology support. . . . "

Indeed, nuclear medicine physicians have been performing lymphoscintigraphy in melanoma patients for about three decades. In general, the procedure was used in patients when a cutaneous melanoma tumor occurred in a region of uncertain lymphatic drainage, e.g., a midback lesion, an area of overlap between axillary and inguinal drainage.

Recent resurgence of interest in lymphoscintigraphy in melanoma resulted from the popularization of the sentinel node concept in melanoma by the surgeons, primarily Morton et al. [7,14,15] in the U.S., and the availability of a handheld gamma probe for use in the operating room to localize the sentinel node previously imaged on the lymphoscintigram. The final, most compelling component for the success of these technologies is the obvious cost-effectiveness and likely improvement in patient care resulting from the accuracy for staging and elimination of unnecessary lymphadenectomy dissections in patients who did not need those dissections.

IV.   BREAST CANCER STAGING

In breast cancer, axillary lymph node dissection experience has been that most commonly, level 1 axillary lymph nodes (i.e., those lateral to the pectoralis minor) are the nodes involved with tumor spread. In a report from Milan [18], of 539 patients with positive axillary lymph nodes, 519 (96%) had level 1 lymph nodes involved; 58% of these patients showed only level 1 nodes with tumor. Other studies have shown similar data [19,20]. Furthermore, in only 1% of patients with positive lymph nodes were level 2 nodes involved when level 1 nodes were not [18]. Other series have shown level 2 involvement in the absence of level 1 involvement in 2% to 5% [20,21]. But earlier experience cites much higher prevalence of "skip" metastases [19] defined as metastases to level 2 and 3 axillary nodes without involvement of level 1 nodes. Pigott et al. reported that 10% of all women with carcinoma of the breast would be understaged by an axillary node sampling procedure. Based on a retrospective review of 72 patients, 25% had metastatic involvement confined to the upper axillary nodes, of whom 14% had primary lesions <2 cm in size. The fact that no data about clinical or pathological correlation of the skip metastases is available further confounds the issue. However, based on data from several sources [18–21], the risk of a "false-negative" dissection when only level 1 and 2 lymph nodes are removed is very low.

Lymph drainage in the breast was described by Vendrell-Torne et al. [22] based on their studies using colloidal gold. They showed that intramammary injections in all four quadrants of the breast, and in the subareolar region, resulted in different lymph drainage patterns. They reported using radioactive gold-198 colloid (very small particles of about 35 mμ) in 250 normal mammary lymphoscintigraphies. Imaging was performed in 50 cases following 0.3 to 0.5 cc volumes containing 200 μCi injected into the upper out quadrant, 50 cases following injection into the lower inner quadrant, 50 cases following injection into the lower outer quadrant, 50 cases following injection into the upper inner quadrant, and 50 cases following injection into the subareolar area. Scanning was performed at 6, 12, 24, and 48 hours following injection. In an article concerning identification of lymphatic chains for radiation therapy port delineation, Kaplan summarized those data and his experience with radionuclide lymphoscintigraphy in breast cancer patients [23]. From this work [22] we learn that we can expect lymphatic drainage from tumors in the breast to the internal mammary region, regardless of which quadrant of the breast harbors the tumor. Upper outer breast quadrant sites drain to axillary node(s) exclusively in 38% of patients, internal mammary node(s) exclusively in 6%, and a combination of those in 50%, and to supraclavicular node(s) in addition to axillary and internal mammary in 6%.

From Australia, Uren et al. [24] reported on 34 patients with suspected breast cancer who were studied with lymphoscintigraphy using ^{99m}Tc antimony sulfide colloid. They reported unexpected drainage across the center of the breast to axillary or internal mammary nodes in 32% of patients with inner or outer quadrant lesions; drainage to supraclavicular or infraclavicular nodes in 20% of upper quadrant lesions; drainage to ipsilateral axilla in 85% of cases where a single sentinel node was seen. Solin [25] has shown that the frequency of internal mammary node metastases in breast cancer parallels metastases to axillary nodes and correlates with the size of the tumor. Certainly, the implications of drainage to unpredicted lymph nodes for patient surgical management are profound. Current management of breast cancer does not include lymphoscintigraphy to identify lymphatic drainage from the breast cancer site, but does include ipsilateral axillary lymph node dissection for staging invasive breast cancers, regardless of location. Clinical trials to evaluate the therapeutic impact of sentinel node excision and biopsy directed by lymphoscintigraphy to guide lymph node dissection(s) of all nodal beds involved with tumor are under way in the U.S., Europe, Australia, and elsewhere. If the frequency of metastases to axillary, internal mammary, and other nodal groups is proportional to the frequency of lymph drainage to those node groups, then surgical management should probably be modified to

include internal mammary and other nodal bed biopsies and appropriate therapeutic interventions (surgical dissection or radiation). "Surgeons have been ignor-
ing internal mammary node metastases for decades"[26], and the time has arrived
to remedy that oversight. Of course, if the sentinel node biopsy of those nodal
groups is tumor-free, lymph node dissection or radiation of those node beds would
not be warranted.

Data to support application of the sentinel node concept to breast cancer
have been slowly appearing in print. Krag et al. [27] reported 100% sensitivity
and specificity for tumor detection by sentinel node biopsy compared with axillary nodal dissections in 50 patients who had sentinel lymph node biopsy and
regional lymph node dissections use (21 patients had lymph node metastases, and
29 did not) after lymphoscintigraphy and intraoperative gamma probe use guidance. A major problem encountered was the diffusion of radioactivity injected
around the tumor into the breast, which may have precluded identification of a
sentinel node near the tumor site. Some investigators have found that larger volumes of injectate (about eight times the amount used intradermally for melanoma)
are needed to facilitate lymphatic uptake and flow to sentinel node(s), i.e., a total
of about 4 ml of radiocolloid for breast lymphoscintigraphy versus 0.4 to 0.5 ml
for melanoma studies. Thus, some investigators administer about 0.75 to 1.0 ml of
radiocolloid injected in each of four locations surrounding the breast tumor mass
(total 4 cc), using concentrations of about 1 mCi/ml (Fig. 1). The need for these
large volumes of injectate are evident particularly when large colloid particles, as
unfiltered Tc-99m sulfur colloid, ranging from about 200 to 1000 mμ are used
[28,29]. Krag et al.[30] reported an initial pilot study to test the radiolabeled sentinel lymph node technique in breast cancer where smaller volumes (0.5 ml) of
unfiltered Tc-99m sulfur colloid were injected around the breast lesion. Investigators using small colloid particles (i.e., 10 to 90 mμ) are successful with small volumes and lower activity levels (similar to volumes and activity levels used for
melanoma lymphoscintigraphy). Paganelli et al. [31] have obtained high-quality
images and results in identifying and localizing sentinel lymph nodes on images
and using a probe intrasurgically. They use technetium-99m-labeled albumin
microcolloid (Fig. 2) or technetium-99m-labeled nanocolloid (Fig. 3). Figure 4
shows a study from Australia using a smaller particle, technetium-99m antimony
sulfide colloid.

V.   BREAST LYMPHATIC MAPPING TECHNIQUES

At the 1995 Society of Surgical Oncology, Guillano [32] reported data comparing
the yield of metastatic lymph node dissection versus sentinel node biopsy with
lymphatic mapping (blue dye). He reported that sentinel nodes showed tumor in
43% (58/136), whereas the axillary dissections for staging revealed tumor in only

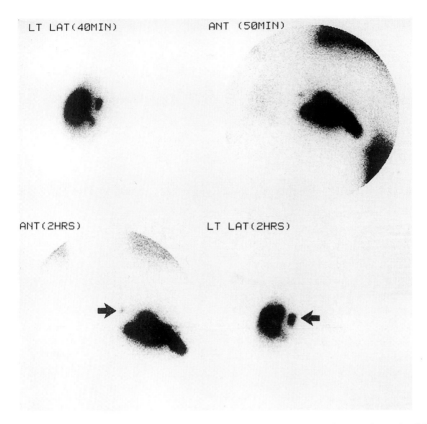

LT LAT(40MIN)   ANT (50MIN)

ANT(2HRS)   LT LAT(2HRS)

FIGURE 1   Tc-99m sulfur colloid, unfiltered, injected in volumes of 1.0 cc in each of four points around the tumor site (total 4.0 cc). Total dose injected was 3.0 mCi. Note large "blob" of activity at tumor site with visualization of an internal mammary sentinel lymph node (arrow, lower left) and an axillary node masked by the blob of activity on anterior views, but imaged on lateral projection (arrow, lower right). Transmission scan using [57]cobalt disc source provides outline of skin surface (image on upper right).

29% (38/133) of his patients. As opposed to using only a blue-dye intraoperative approach to finding the sentinel lymph node, some advantages of lymphoscinti-graphic sentinel node identification preoperatively followed by biopsy are as follows:

    1.   The location of the sentinel node(s) can be identified before any incisions.

    2.   A small incision can be made to excise the sentinel node rapidly and easily.

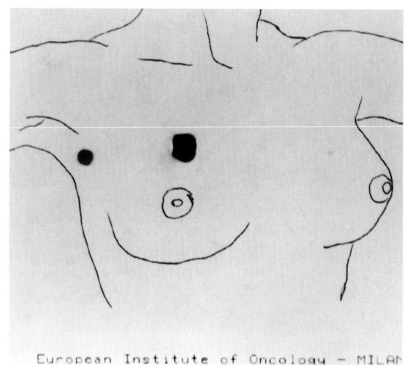

European Institute of Oncology - MILAN

FIGURE 2   Tc-99m albumin colloid particles of 200 to 1000 nm injected subdermally near site of small breast cancer in small volume (0.20 cc) followed by 0.2 ml saline. Total activity used was about 7 Mbq. One axillary sentinel lymph node is seen. Images compliments of Giovanni Paganelli, MD, of the European Institute of Oncology, Milan, Italy.

3.   Staging may be improved over axillary node dissection staging.

4.   Successful identification and excisional biopsy of the sentinel lymph node(s) in the axilla minimize morbidity from axillary node dissection, if axillary node dissection can be avoided, as it can when the sentinel node is tumor-negative. Expense as well as substantial morbidity is thereby saved. Axillary node dissection removes a large bulk of tissue, necessitating drains and limiting physical activity for an extended time. Most women suffer some arm complication from the procedure.

All these, except 1, and often 2, can be achieved either by blue dye or lymphoscintigraphic and gamma probe techniques. But a long learning curve has been experienced and reported by proponents of the blue-dye techniques such that initially there is failure to find a sentinel node in as many as 35% of cases [33].

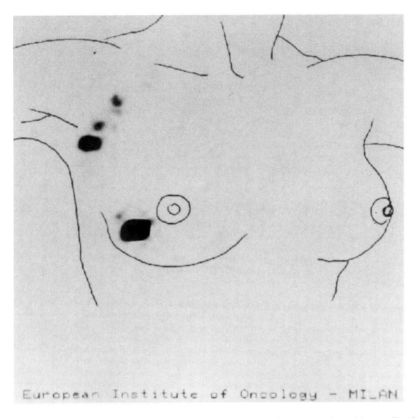

European Institute of Oncology - MILAN

FIGURE 3   Tc-99m albumin (nanocoll) colloid particles of <80 nm injected in small volume (as above) subdermally near the tumor. Three axillary lymph nodes are distinctly visualized. The most inferior and hottest node is certainly a sentinel lymph node. All may be sentinel lymph nodes, if supplied by independent lymph channels, most likely the upper 2 nodes are secondary nodes. Images complements of Giovanni Paganelli, MD, of the European Institute of Oncology, Milan, Italy.

Giuliano et al. [33] reported his first 174 patients for whom Vital dye lymphatic mapping was performed, injecting the dye at the primary breast cancer site intraoperatively (no radioactive tracer or imaging components were included in this study). Axillary lymphatics were identified and followed to the first node (sentinel node), which was excised before an axillary lymph node dissection. In 65.5% (114/174) sentinel nodes were identified. All the missed sentinel nodes occurred among the first 87 procedures. The authors discussed the learning curve and the fact that the surgeon's rate of sentinel node detection increased with experience. Sentinel nodes identified in the last 87 procedures performed were 100%

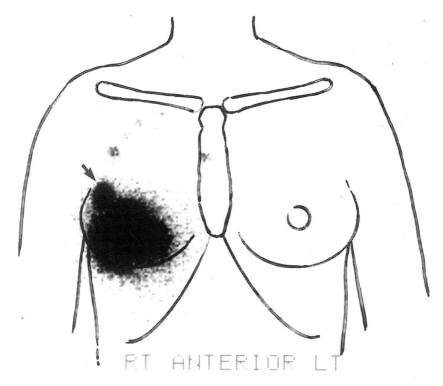

FIGURE 4   Lymphoscintigraphy using ^{99m}Tc-labeled antimony sulfide colloid injected at four sites in small volumes (0.1 ml) surrounding the tumor, using a total dose of 20 Mbq (6.5 mCi). Anterior image shows a single internal mammary sentinel lymph node, one sentinel lymph node in the right axilla (arrow) very close to the injection activity, and four secondary nodes (if separate lymphatic channels had been visualized coursing to those nodes, they would be called sentinel nodes). Dr. Uren interpreted those four as second-tier nodes along the right subclavian chain. He noted the characteristic decrease in intensity as tracer passes on from one node to the next. Images compliments of Drs. Roger Uren and Robert Howman-Giles of Nuclear Medicine and Diagnostic Ultrasound Advanced Nuclear Medicine Services, Camperdown, New South Wales, Australia.

predictive. In 38% of cases where metastases were found, the sentinel node was the only node with tumor. Sentinel nodes were detected in 51 of the first 87 mappings, or 58.6%, and in 72.4% of the last 87 cases.

This is considerably lower than the sentinel node recovery rate when radiocolloid and the gamma probe are used as in Albertini et al. [34]. Albertini et al. reported a prospective trial of 62 patients with newly diagnosed invasive breast cancers in which patients underwent intraoperative mapping using both Vital Blue dye and filtered Tc-99m sulfur colloid to identify sentinel lymph nodes. After removal of axillary sentinel lymph nodes, an axillary lymph node dissection and definitive removal of the primary tumor were performed. Their results showed in 97% of patients, a sentinel lymph node was found and excised; 18 of 62 patients had metastases, and all of their sentinel nodes were tumor-positive. Furthermore, in 12 of these 18 (67%), the sentinel node was the only tumor-positive node found, even after complete axillary node dissection. They concluded that axillary sentinel lymph nodes in breast cancer indeed probably reflect the histology of the remaining axillary lymph nodes. Furthermore, the authors emphasized that this procedure allows the pathologist to focus on one or two nodes, thereby perhaps increasing the yield of micrometastases and the accuracy of staging.

In a reply to a letter written by Dr. Giuliano published in JAMA [35], Drs. Cox and Reintgen [36] wrote that they had performed >200 lymphatic mappings for breast cancer using the combination of Vital dye and radiocolloid localization with a gamma probe. They stated that "the radiocolloid mapping is important to locate the 'hot' spot prior to skin incision and to enable a directed dissection through the axilla. In addition, the radiocolloid mapping allows a quantitative measurement that all sentinel lymph nodes have been removed from the basin." They also pointed out that "To perform lymphatic mapping for melanoma or breast cancer, a surgeon needs good nuclear medicine and pathology support."

Investigators in Milan, on the other hand, are not using blue dye, but solely using lymphoscintigraphy and intraoperative gamma probe localization of sentinel lymph nodes and they report excellent yields in successful identification of axillary sentinel nodes in breast cancer patients [31]. Certainly, the surgical experience in melanoma sentinel node localization with radiocolloid lymphatic mapping appears to have won more widespread acclaim than blue dye. While the same may be true for lymphatic mapping and sentinel node localization in breast cancer, the final conclusions on the comparative efficacy of radiolabeled colloids versus blue dye techniques are not yet written.

Commenting on the improved accuracy of staging using sentinel node localization techniques, Noguchi [37] has pointed out that approximately one-quarter of the axillary dissections reported by Giuliano et al. [33] yielded a sentinel lymph node in level 2 alone (or in level 1 and level 2), whereas most of the sentinel nodes identified by the blue-dye technique were in level 1 of the axilla. Noguchi also advocated preoperative lymphoscintigraphy to more adequately identify sentinel nodes than blue dye alone, pointing to the learning curve reported by Giuliano [33] of detecting the sentinel node in only 59% of the first 87 mapping procedures and 72.4% of the second 87 procedures.

VI. HISTOPATHOLOGY FOR SENTINEL LYMPH NODES

Another aspect of the sentinel node approach which clearly has added to the accuracy of staging is that the pathologist can do multiple sectioning and immunohistochemical staining of one or two sentinel lymph nodes and thereby identify more patients with lymph node micrometastases than is possible with routine histopathologic processing for axillary lymphadenectomies. This is particularly critically important because axillary lymph node metastasis is the strongest correlate with probability of relapse in breast cancer, after potentially curative local therapy has been performed [33].

Noguchi et al. [37] evaluated the effect of intraoperative lymphatic mapping and sentinel lymphadenectomy on the axillary staging of patients with breast cancer. Multiple sections of each sentinel node were examined by hematoxylin and eosin (H&E) and by immunohistochemical staining techniques using antibodies to cytokeratin. One or two sections of each nonsentinel lymph node in axillary lymph node dissections were examined by routine H&E staining alone. They found, for 134 patients who underwent axillary dissections and 162 who had sentinel lymph node excisions followed by axillary dissections, 39 patients (29%) of the axillary dissection group and 68 (42%) in the sentinel lymph node group had metastases. Of these, four (10%) of the axillary dissection group and 26/68 (38%) of the sentinel node group had micrometastases. Thus, they concluded that sentinel node examination with multiple sectioning and immunohistochemical staining increases the accuracy of axillary staging in breast cancer, particularly identifying more micrometastases than routine histopathologic processing of axillary lymph nodes.

This raises the question of the real-life significance of a micrometastasis in an isolated lymph node. Studies have shown that patients in whom serial sectioning [39] immunohistochemical staining [40–42] and/or reverse transcriptase-PCR (polymerase chain reaction) analysis [43,44] detect micrometastases, indeed have poorer survival rates than patients with no micrometastases.

VII. RADIOPHARMACEUTICALS

The radiopharmaceuticals which have been most widely used for lymphoscintigraphy have included: Tc-99m sulfur colloid, Tc-99m nanocolloid, and Tc-99m human serum albumin. The major difference between these agents is the size of the colloid particles or albumin molecule. Tc-99m sulfur colloid has the largest particle size of 0.1 to 2 μm (100 to 2000 nm). Tc-99m antimony sulfide colloid has a much smaller, more desirable particle size of 0.003 to 0.03 μm (3 to 30 nm) [45]. Tc-99m nanocolloid is a labeled albumin colloid with a particle size of about 0.08 μm (80 nm) [46]. Tc-99m serum albumin has a very small size of up to 4 nm (0.004 μm) [47]. Since the rate of colloid transport through lymphatics is a function of colloid particle size, this is a critical factor for performance of lymphoscintigraphy. Particles <4 nm may penetrate capillary membranes and if so, would be unavailable to migrate through lymphatic channels. Furthermore, such capillary blood uptake would add undesirable blood background counts to an image or to counts detected by a gamma probe. Yet, the ideal colloid particle must be sufficiently small to facilitate rapid disappearance from the interstitial space into which it is injected, and transfer into lymphatic vessels. Particles <100 nm (0.1 μm) satisfy the requirement of rapid transfer into lymphatics, and yet are retained for at least many hours in sentinel lymph nodes. Larger colloid particles (500 μm) show a much slower rate of clearance from the interstitial space and therefore slower accumulation into a sentinel lymph node.

Early reports of studies of lymphatic dynamics and lymphatic imaging utilized gold-198 colloid, which has a uniform particle size of 3 to 5 nm [48]. Gold-198 colloid is not used today because of the high radiation dose at the site of injection, related to the physical properties of gold-198 (2.7-day physical half-life with emission of beta particles and a 412-keV gamma photon which is not desirable for imaging). Technetium-99m is a much more favorable radionuclide with minimal radiation dose (6-hour physical half-life and no beta emission) and emission of a 140-keV gamma photon, ideal for imaging. Thus, technetium-99m is utilized today in association with colloid or albumin for lymphoscintigraphy and intraoperative gamma probe work. Table 1 describes lymphoscintigraphic radiopharmaceuticals according to particle size.

In the U.S., the only FDA approved agent for lymphoscintigraphy is Tc-99m sulfur colloid. Tc-99m nanocolloid is used in Europe and other parts of the world, as is Tc-99m antimony sulfide colloid, both of which are more ideal agents for lymphoscintigraphy than the large-particle-size Tc-99m sulfur colloid. Therefore, investigators and practicing nuclear medicine physicians in the U.S. have been using Tc-99m sulfur colloid but have modified its preparation by applying microfiltration, using 0.1-μm and 0.22-μm filters [49,50]. Thus, the injectate is a preparation that is a much smaller, more ideal particle size, i.e., about 50 nm [47,49–51].

In addition to microfiltration, Eshima et al. [51] have described decreasing the heating time and using technetium-99m pertechnetate derived from a generator with a longer time since last elution, as mechanisms to decrease particle size of Tc-99m sulfur colloid. Simply passing the Tc-99m sulfur colloid through a

TABLE 1   Classification of Lymphoscintigraphic Radiopharmaceuticals by Size

Size	Radiocolloid
<4 nm	[99m]Tc human serum albumin
1–15 nm	[198]Au colloid
15–50 nm	[99m]Tc antimony sulfide colloid
~80 nm	[99m]Tc nanocoll (albumin colloid)[a]
>50 nm	[99m]Tc sulfur colloid, depending on filtration and preparation
200–1000 nm	[99m]Tc albumin microcolloid (Albu-res)[a]
200–1000 nm	[99m]Tc sulfur colloid, conventional unfiltered preparation

[a]Available outside the U. S. from Soren-Nycomed/Amersham.

0.22-μm or 0.1-μm filter, or both, appears to give good results as well, and commercial radiopharmacies in the U.S. are using this modification in preparing technetium-99m sulfur colloid for lymphoscintigraphy. The filter retains 10% to 63% of the total activity passed through it, leaving particles of 15 to 50 nm in the injectate [49,52].

A recent report from the Netherlands examined lymphoscintigraphic identification of sentinel nodes in breast cancer using technetium-99m colloidal albumin [53]. Patients were imaged 2 hours and 18 hours after peritumoral injection. Their results showed one to three separate axillary lymph nodes in 33 patients on 2-hour images and in 34 patients on 18-hour images. They concluded that prolonged intranodal retention of Tc-99m colloidal albumin, with its (particle size about 0.08 μm (80 nm) allows successful sentinel node identification in most (92%) patients.

We examined the impact of microfiltration of Tc-99m sulfur colloid on clinical imaging in melanoma cases and found that significantly more visualization of lymphatic channels leading to sentinel nodes was seen on images when 0.22-μm filters were used versus very coarse 5-μm filters [54]. Thus, the finer filtration provided clinically superior studies in visualization of lymphatic drainage pathways and therefore more precise sentinel node identification, with better discrimination between secondary and sentinel lymph nodes.

In contrast, a National Cancer Institute-sponsored multicenter trial (in the U.S.) of sentinel lymph node biopsy in breast cancer versus axillary node dissection utilizes unfiltered technetium-99m sulfur colloid and gamma probe-guided detection in the operating room, with no imaging. One of the trial sites reports sentinel node localization in 97% of patients [55]. The technique used requires a large volume (4 cc) of 1 mCi of unfiltered Tc-99m sulfur colloid injected in four sites into interstitial tissue around the tumor (1.0 cc at each site). If imaging were to be done, a large blob of activity would be seen in the breast, which would make imaging very unsatisfactory, and potentially mask sentinel lymph nodes located close to the tumor site, depending on their location in the breast. These investigators found that large volumes of injectate were necessary to achieve lymphatic uptake of the large unfiltered colloid particle and transport of radiocolloid to sentinel lymph node(s).

VIII. LYMPHOSCINTIGRAPHY AND PROBE LOCALIZATION

A. Injection Technique

In melanoma management, the consensus on performing lymphoscintigraphy is by administering the radiopharmaceuticals in small volume intradermally using a 25-gauge needle at four sites around the primary tumor or the surgical scar [24,56,51]. In breast cancer, European investigators inject using small volumes

(0.25 cc) and lower activity (0.2 mCi) of smaller particles [31,58] subdermally in the vicinity of the breast mass, whereas in the U.S., investigators in a multicenter National Cancer Institute-funded study are injecting into the interstitial tissue around the breast mass [55], using larger volumes (4 cc) and higher activity (1.0 mCi) of larger unfiltered radiocolloid particles.

Investigators in Australia [59] used antimony sulfide colloid particles, and in the Netherlands [53] used albumin colloid particles. Both groups reported satisfactory breast lymphoscintigraphy with smaller volumes and activities, injecting interstitially around the tumor.

B. Imaging

The gamma scintillation camera, which consists of a large NaI crystal detector with an array of photomultiplier tubes and lead collimator, is the device used for lymphoscintigraphy. Dynamic imaging of the lymphatic drainage basin is done continuously at 10 sec frame, starting immediately and for 10 min after the intradermal injections. Imaging continues at 15-min intervals for about 1 hour. Several projections, including obliques as well as anterior and posterior, are obtained of the sentinel node(s). Visualization of a sentinel lymph node is apparent when a distinct focus of activity persists, usually at the end of a lymphatic channel which leads to it. A mark is placed on the skin corresponding to the site of the sentinel node to facilitate intraoperative localization with the probe. Imaging provides visualization of the lymphatic channel(s), which helps to correctly identify the sentinel lymph node(s); the lymph node closest to the primary tumor may not necessarily be the sentinel node in all cases [60]. Occasionally, if the lymphatic channels and sentinel node(s) are not visualized, gentle massaging of the injection site(s) may help promote lymphatic uptake of the tracer, filling the channel(s), and transport of the tracer to the sentinel node(s). In cases of melanoma on the torso, imaging is invaluable to detect drainage to the contralateral axilla or inguinal nodes [50]. The same may be true in breast cancer to identify drainage to the internal mammary chain and/or supraclavicular lymph nodes. Imaging is routinely used by many investigators as a road map to facilitate intraoperative probe localization [50,53,58,59].

C.   Gamma Probes

In 1949 Selverstone et al. used a Geiger Mueller counter and introduced the method of using the intraoperative probe by localizing the margins of an astrocytoma after IV injection of P-32 [61]. The technology has improved greatly since that time. The probe consists of a detector, collimators to focus the detector on identifying the lesion (i.e., improving its resolution) and electronics that will display the findings in digital format and also as an audio signal.

At present the commercially available probes have either NaI (Tl) scintillating crystals (Care Wise) or semiconductor (Cd, Zn, Te) detectors (Neo Probe). NaI (Tl) crystals are sensitive for a wider range of gamma energies but may need a photomultiplier tube which adds to their size. CdZnTe semiconductor detectors do not need a photomultiplier tube and hence are very small, but have lower sensitivity at higher energy levels than the NaI (Tl) crystals.

D.   Intraoperative Use of Gamma Probes: Precautions

Steam, dry heat sterilization, and immersion of the probe in cleaning solution will damage the probe. Electric cautery and X-rays in the vicinity of the probe may interfere with probe readings. A sterile wrapping over the probe as used for intraoperative ultrasound probes provides ideal and easy sterile technique.

Even though the use of probe does not require state or national regulatory commission (NRC) licensing, use and administration of radiopharmaceuticals , as a protective measure of radiation safety practice, must be by authorized users licensed by the NRC or (in agreement states) by the state.

E.   Intraoperative Technique

Once the patient is positioned on the operating table, if preoperative imaging is not performed, the sentinel lymph node is detected by scanning the drainage basin in a gridlike manner to identify the highest tracer concentration as evidenced by the digital or audio reading. If images are available with a skin mark over the site of the sentinel lymph node, then scanning the basin in a gridlike fashion is not necessary. It is important to angle the probe away from the injection site; otherwise there will be significant interference from the radioactivity at the injection site. With the probe placed over the sentinel lymph node (in vivo), counts for 10 sec and a background count level 1 cm away from the sentinel lymph node are recorded. After the sentinel node is excised, the excised tissue is again counted for 10 sec (ex vivo), which usually shows significantly higher counts because of lack of attenuation. Postexcision counts with the probe placed in the sentinel lymph node bed are also measured to assess completeness of excision of the sentinel lymph node. Sometimes a second lymph node may be found very close to the sentinel node and should probably also be excised, as it may be difficult to determine which of two closely positioned lymph nodes is the true sentinel node.

IX.   CURRENT STATUS OF CLINICAL PRACTICE

Based on the recent very important report from Veronesi et al. [58] on lymphoscintigraphic identification of axillary sentinel node(s) in 163 women with operable breast cancer, the predictive value of sentinel node histopathology in patients with small cancers of <1.5 cm size was 100%. Veronesi et al. concluded that lymphoscintigraphy using a relatively small colloid particle (technetium-99m nanocolloid) combined with gamma probe intraoperative localization of axillary sentinel node(s) for excision and biopsy, could be clinically applied "immediately" in small breast cancers as a substitute for axillary dissection. The authors pointed to the need for research into more reliable ways to identify microfoci of metastatic cells to alleviate the problem of intraoperative false-negative results. They identified a false-negative sentinel node reading by frozen section in 17% of cases. This report is in sharp contrast to the NCL multicenter trial methodology, which uses a large colloid particle, no imaging, and relies solely on intraoperative gamma probe detection of sentinel lymph nodes.

Some surgeons remain proponents of the blue dye technique, although the data appearing in print lately may be turning that tide toward radiotracer techniques. The optimum radiopharmaceutical remains unclear as a practical matter in the U.S. The European experience with nanocolloid is clearly satisfactory. Other issues—optimum injection location, volume, and dose of injectate—need further study and validation.

In summary, we have a viable, more conservative management approach to staging breast cancer which is certainly more cost-effective and less invasive than the alternative (axillary dissection). There are ample data and many investigators who believe that sentinel lymph node staging is ready for prime time, i.e., clinical use in patients with small breast cancers. Clearly, the sentinel node approach to staging breast cancer will soon replace axillary lymph node dissection in many women with breast cancer. But the role of this procedure in altering the current surgical conventional management approach of excluding other node groups, i.e., internal mammary and supraclavicular nodes, in the staging for breast cancer remains to be determined.

REFERENCES

1. Cady B. The need to reexamine axillary lymph node dissection. Cancer 73:505–508, 1994.
2. Ruffin et al. J Am Coll Surg 180:245–251, 1995.
3. Silverstein MJ, Gierson ED, Waisman JR, Colburn WJ, Gamagami P. Predicting axillary node positivity in patients with invasive carcinoma of the breast using a combination of T category and palpability. J Am Coll Surg 1995; 180:700–704.
4. Recht A, Houlihan MJ. Axillary lymph nodes and breast cancer: a review. Cancer 76:1491–1512, 1995.
5. Noguchi M. Letter to the Editor. Ann Surg 225:126, 1997.
6. Kissin MW, Querci della Rovere G, Easton D, et al. Risk of lymph-edema following the treatment of breast cancer. Br J Surg 75:580–585, 1986.

7. Morton DL, Wen DR, Foshag LJ, et al. Intraoperative lymphatic mapping and selective cervical lymphadenectomy for early stage melanomas of the head and neck. J Clin Oncol 11:1751–1756, 1992.
8. Cabanas RM. An approach for the treatment of penile carcinoma. Cancer 39:456–466, 1977.
9. Cabanas RM. Anatomy and biopsy of sentinel lymph nodes. Urol Clin North Am 19:2, 1992.
10. Fowler JE. Sentinel lymph node biopsy for staging penile cancer. Urology 23:352, 1984.
11. Pettaway CA, Pisters LL, Dinney CPN, et al. Sentinel lymph node dissection for penile carcinoma: the MD Anderson cancer center experience. J Urol 154:1999–2003, 1995.
12. Levenback C, Burke TW, Gershenson DM, et al. Intraoperative lymphatic mapping for vulvar cancer. Obstet Gynecol 84:163–167, 1994.
13. De Cicco C, Sideri M, Bartolomei M. Sentinel node detection by lymphoscintigraphy and gamma detecting probe in patients with vulvar cancer. J Nucl Med 38(5):33P, 1997.
14. Morton DL, Wen DR, Wong JH, et al. Technical details of intraoperative lymphatic mapping for early stage melanoma. Arch Surg 127:392–399, 1992.
15. Morton DL, Wen DR, Foshag LJ, et al. Intraoperative lymphatic mapping and selective cervical lymphadenectomy for early stage melanomas of the head and neck. J Clin Oncol 11:1751–1756, 1993.
16. Reintgen D, Cruse CW, Wells K, et al. The orderly progression of melanoma nodal metastases. Ann Surg 220:759–767, 1994.
17. Reintgen D. Times are changing (editorial). J Fla Med Assoc 84:(3).
18. Veronesi U, Rilke F, Luini R, et al. Distribution of axillary node metastases by level of invasion: an analysis of 539 cases. Cancer 59:682–687, 1987.
19. Ciatto S, Pacini P, Rosselli del Turco M, Cataliotti L, Cardona G, Carcangiu ML. Patterns of axillary metastases in breast cancer. Radiother Oncol 5:91–94, 1986.
20. Boova RS, Bonanni R, Rosato FE. Patterns of axillary nodal involvement in breast cancer: predictability of level one dissection. Ann Surg 196:642–644, 1982.
21. Chevinsky AH, Ferrara J, James AG, Minton JP, Young D, Farrar WB. Prospective evaluation of clinical and pathologic detection of axillary metastases in patients with carcinoma of the breast. Surgery 108:612–618, 1990.
22. Vendrell-Torne E, Setain-Quinquer J, Domenech-Torne FM. Study of normal lymphatic drainage using radioactive isotopes. J Nucl Med 13:801–805, 1972.
23. Kaplan WD. Lymphoscintigraphy: importance to cancer detection and radiation treatment planning. Radiat Ther Oncol 28:25–36, 1994.
24. Uren RF, Hofman-Giles RB, Shaw HM, et al. Lymphoscintigraphy in high risk melanoma of the trunk: predicinting draining node groups, defining lymphatic channels and locating the sentinel node. J Nucl Med 34:1435–1440, 1993.
25. Solin LJ. Radiation treatment volumes and doses for patients with early stage carcinoma of the breast treated with breast-conserving surgery and definitive irradiation. Semin Radiat Oncol 2:1775–1780, 1995.
26. Giuliano AE. Letter to the Editor. Ann Surg 225:1, 126–127, 1997.
27. West JH, Seymour JC, Drane WE. Combined transmission-emission imaging in lymphoscintigraphy. Clin Nucl Med 18:762–764, 1993.

28. Gulec SA, Moffat FL, Serafini AN, et al. Sentinel node localization in patients with breast cancer. J Nucl Med 38(5):33P, 1997.

29. Shriver C, Balingit AG, Caravalho J, et al. Unfiltered Tc-99m sulfur colloid lymphoscintigraphy and gamma probe in detection of sentinel node in breast cancer patients. J Nucl Med 38(5):33P, 1997.

30. Krag DN, Weaver DL, Aex JC, Fairbank JT. Surgical resection and radiolocalization of the sentinel lymph node in breast cancer using a gamma probe. Surg Oncol 2(6):335–339, 1993.

31. Paganelli G, De Cicco C, Cremonesi M, et al. Gamma probe guided resection of the sentinel node in breast cancer. J Nucl Med 38:(5):33P, 1997.

32. Giuliano AE. Axillary node mapping for breast cancer. Presented at the 48th Annual Symposium of the Society of Surgical Oncology, March 23–25, 1995, Boston, MA.

33. Giuliano AE, Kirgan DM, Guenther JM, Morton DL. Lymphatic mapping and sentinel lymphadenectomy for breast cancer. Ann Surg 220:391–401, 1994.

34. Albertini JJ, Lyman GH, Cox C, et al. Lymphatic mapping and sentinel node biopsy in the patient with breast cancer. JAMA 276:1818–1820, 1996.

35. Giuliano AE. Lymphatic mapping and sentinel node biopsy in breast cancer. Letter to the Editor. JAMA 277:791, 1997.

36. Cox CC, Reintgen D. Reply to: Lymphatic mapping and sentinel node biopsy in breast cancer. Letter to the Editor. JAMA 277:791, 1997.

37. Noguchi M. Letter to the Editor. Ann Surg 225(1):126, 1997.

38. Noguchi M, Koyasaki N, Nagayoshi O, et al. Internal mammary nodal status is a more reliable prognostic factor than DNA ploidy and c-erb B-2 expression in patients with breast cancer. Arch Surg 128:242–246, 1993.

39. International (Ludwig) Breast Cancer Study Group. Prognostic importance of occult axillary lymph node micrometastases from breast cancers. Lancet 35:1565–1568, 1990.

40. Trojani M, de Mascarel I, Bonichon F. Micrometastases to axillary lymph nodes from carcinoma of the breast, detection by immunohistochemistry and prognostic significance. Br J Cancer 55:303–306, 1987.

41. Springall SJ, Rytina ERC, Millis RR. Incidence and significance of micrometastases in axillary lymph nodes detected by immunohistochemical techniques. J Pathol 160:174, 1990.

42. Hainsworth PJ, Tjandra JJ, Stillwell RG, et al. Detection and significance of occult metastases in node negative breast cancer. Br J Surg 80:459–463, 1993.

43. Noguch S, Aihara T, Motomura K, Inaji H, Imaoka S, Koyama H. Detection of breast cancer micrometastases in axillary lymph nodes by means of reverse transcriptase-polymerase chain reaction. Am J Pathol 2:649–656, 1996.

44. Schoenfeld A, Lugmani Y, Smith D, et al. Detection of breast cancer micrometastases in axillary lymph nodes by using polymerase chain reaction. Cancer Res 54:2986–2990, 1994.

45. Product package insert. Antimony sulfide colloid. Cadema Medical Products Inc, Middletown, NY.

46. Product package insert. Solco Nanocoll. Manufacturer SORIN BIOMEDI, Vercelli, Italy.

47. Zinsmeister MS. Lymphoscintigraphy: current techniques and indications. Appl Radiol July:32–39, 1997.
48. Strand SL, Persson BRR. Quantitative lymphoscintigraphy. Basic concepts for optimal uptake of radiocolloids in the parasternal lymph nodes of rabbits. J Nucl Med 20:1036–1046, 1979.
49. Hung JC, Wiseman GA, Wahner HW, Mullan BP, Taggart TR, Dunn WL. Filtered technetium 99m sulfur colloid evaluated for lymphoscintigraphy. J Nucl Med 36:1895–1901, 1995.
50. Alazraki NP, Eshima D, Eshima LA, et al. Lymphoscintigraphy, the sentinel node concept, and the intraoperative gamma probe in melanoma, breast cancer, and other potential cancers. Semin Nuc Med 27(1):55–67, 1997.
51. Eshima D, Eshima L, Gotti N, et al. Technetium-99m-sulfur colloid for lymphoscintigraphy: effects of preparation parameters. J Nucl Med 37:1575–1578, 1996.
52. Gulec SA, Moffat FL, Carrol RG. The expanding clinical role for intraoperative gamma probes. Nucl Med Ann 209–237, 1997.
53. Pijpers R, Meijer S, Hoekstra OS, et al. Impact of lymphoscintigraphy on sentinel node identification with technetium-99m colloidal albumin in breast cancer. J Nucl Med 38(3):366–368, 1997.
54. Goldfarb LR et al. Clinical evaluation of 0.22 micron filtration of Tc-99m-sulfur colloid for lymphoscintigraphic identification of sentinel lymph nodes. In press.
55. Gulec S, Moffat FL, Carroll RG, Serafini AN, Sfakianasis GN, Allen L. Sentinel lymph node localization in early breast cancer: kinetics and technical considerations. J Nucl Med 1997. In press.
56. Mudun A, Murray DR, Herda SC, et al. Early stage melanoma: lymphoscintigraphy, reproducibility of sentinel node detection, and effectiveness of the intraoperative gamma probe. Radiology 199:171–175, 1996.
57. Berman C, Norman J, Cruse CW, et al. Lymphoscintigraphy in malignant melanoma. Ann Plast Surg 28:29–32, 1992.
58. Veronesi U, Paganelli G, Galimberti V, et al. Sentinel-node biopsy to avoid axillary dissection in breast cancer with clinically negative lymph nodes. Lancet 349:1864–1867, 1997.
59. Uren RF, Howman-Giles RB, Thompson JF, et al. Mammary lymphoscintigraphy in breast cancer. J Nucl Med 36:1775–1780, 1995.
60. Taylor A, Murray D, Herda S, Vansant J, Alazraki N. Dynamic lymphoscintigraphy to identify the sentinel and satellite nodes. Clin Nucl Med 21(10):755–758, 1996.
61. Selverstone B, Sweet WH, Robinson CV. The clinical use of radioactive phosphorus in the surgery of brain tumors. Ann Surg 136:643–651, 1949.

14
Atlas on Radionuclide Imaging of the Breast

RAYMOND TAILLEFER and ANDRÉ GAGNON
Centre Hospitalier de l'Universite de Montreal, Montreal, Quebec, Canada

IRAJ KHALKHALI
Harbor-UCLA Medical Center, Torrance, California

PIETRO MUTO
National Cancer Institute, Naples, Italy

HOLGER PALMEDO and HANS J. BIERSACK
University of Bonn, Bonn, Germany

INTRODUCTION

This chapter is divided into 10 sections. The first nine sections will discuss some technical aspects and various scintigraphic patterns observed with radionuclide imaging of the breast performed with 99mTc-sestamibi, by far the most common radiopharmaceutical used in clinical practice for this specific purpose. The last section will present correlative imaging and breast scintigraphy performed with 99mTc-MDP (methylenediphosphonate), another commonly available radiopharmaceutical which can be used for breast imaging in conjunction with bone scintigraphy. Other radiopharmaceuticals (either less or not yet available for clinical use) have already been presented in their specific chapters, so they will not be discussed here.

SECTION I: TECHNICAL ASPECTS

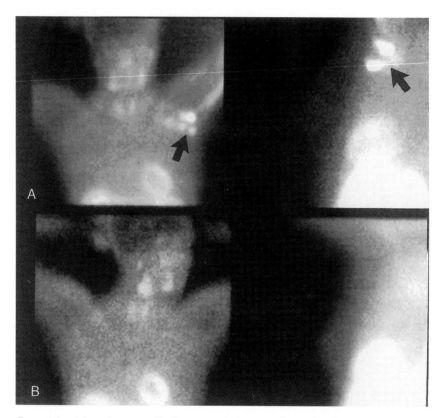

Figure 1.1   After adequate radiopharmaceutical preparation and radiochemical purity verification with a labeling efficiency of more than 95%, 25–30 mCi (900–1100 MBq) of ^{99m}Tc-sestamibi is injected in the antecubital vein of the contralateral arm of the suspected breast lesion. When bilateral lesions are suspected, injection should be performed in a pedal vein. This will eliminate false-positive axillary lymph node uptake due to interstitial injection. Lymph node retention is often seen, even when the injection procedure was thought to be adequate. Ideally, a plastic cannula should be inserted in the vein and the ^{99m}Tc-sestamibi injection should be performed through a three-way stopcock which is then flushed with 10 cc of 0.9% saline solution. This procedure will maximize the delivery of the injected dose. (A) Anterior (supine) and left lateral (prone) thoracic views with a significantly increased uptake of ^{99m}Tc-sestamibi in the left axillary lymph nodes (arrows) following the injection of the radiotracer in the left antecubital vein. A segment of the vein is also seen. There was an extravasation of the radiotracer at the site of injection. (B) The patient was reinjected 2 days later in a pedal vein. There is no more activity in the axillae.

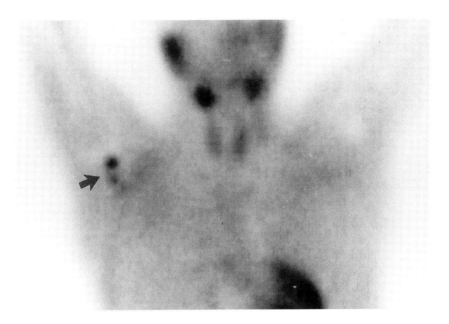

FIGURE 1.2   This patient was injected in the right arm. Although all necessary precautions have been taken to optimize the ^{99m}Tc-sestamibi injection, some right axillary lymph nodes are visualized (arrows). This uptake is caused by some degree of extravasation of the radiotracer at the site of injection and early subsequent uptake by the lymphatic channels and nodes. These nodes should not be described as having positive ^{99m}Tc-sestamibi uptake for metastatic involvement.

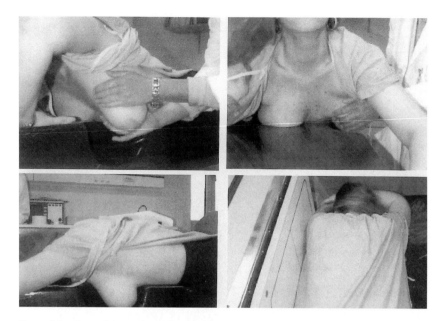

FIGURE 1.3   One of the major difficulty encountered when imaging the breasts with scinti-mammography is the adequate separation of the breast and other adjacent structures. Breast tissue is not well perfused and has an unfavorable count ratio with respect to adjacent organs. Fortunately, the lesion-to-normal breast tissue perfusion ratio is relatively high and allows for good discrimination between lesion and normal structures. The success of scin-timammography relies partially on optimal breast positioning, especially for prone imag-ing. This can be achieved either with a breast cushion or with a special table (Fig. 1.4). This figure shows the use of the breast foam cushion which should be placed flat on the standard imaging table (tomographic or plain imaging table). The side of the cushion with a semi-circular aperture cutout should be positioned close to the edge of the table. Planar views with the breast cushion or on the special table are acquired one breast at the time. The breast to be imaged is placed in the aperture while the other breast lies in the middle of the cushion or table, pressed against the thorax. In this position, the activity from the con-tralateral breast will be kept from interfering with the breast being imaged. First, the patient is asked to lie flat as close as possible to the edge of the positioning device. In this position, the breast is supported in the semicircular aperture. The technologist, using the natural mobility of the relaxed pectoral muscle and the breast, pulls the breast down and laterally such that the breast has a very slight angle with the cushion. Both arms are then placed over the head, making sure that elbows are not lower than the shoulder line. Injection site or vein retention often result in an increased background activity, which is undesirable. This position should be maintained for the duration of the image acquisition. The gamma camera is positioned perpendicular to the patient's back. The surface of the collimator should be as close as possible to the patient's torso.

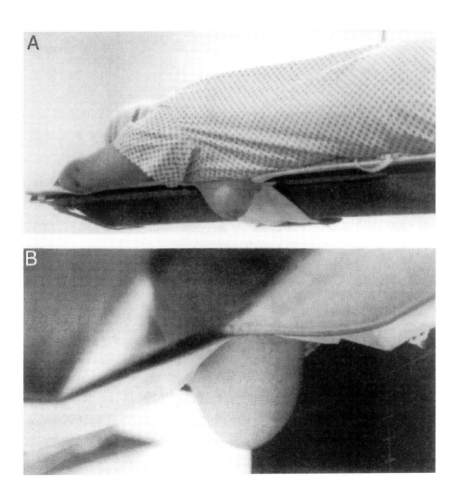

FIGURE 1.4   (A) A table with lateral cutouts can also be used as a breast positioning device. (B) Imaging principles are the same as those for the foam cushion positioning device.

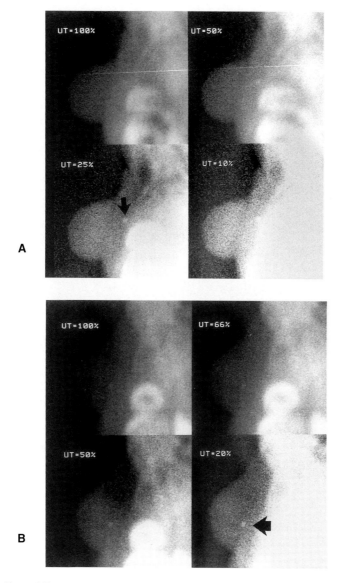

FIGURE 1.5

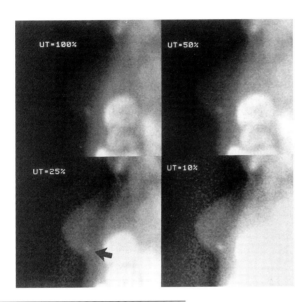

C

FIGURE 1.5   After image acquisition, digital image sets are produced that enhance the breast and axilla contrast from the other structures. The first step is to adjust the upper threshold in order to saturate the pixels over the organs with increased ^{99m}TC-sestamibi uptake. This process should be done for each view, since scintigraphic images of the breast rarely shows similar maximal counts per pixel. It is important to note that the optimal threshold for a given image may vary and depends on different factors such as the location of the tumor and degree of tumoral uptake of the radiotracer. These are three examples (A, B, C) of small primary breast cancers measuring <1 cm in diameter which are more or less easily visualized depending on the upper threshold used to display the images. Small breast lesions, especially those close to thoracic structures or organs, may be barely seen with a high (100%) upper threshold. The opposite may also be true with a very low threshold (10%).

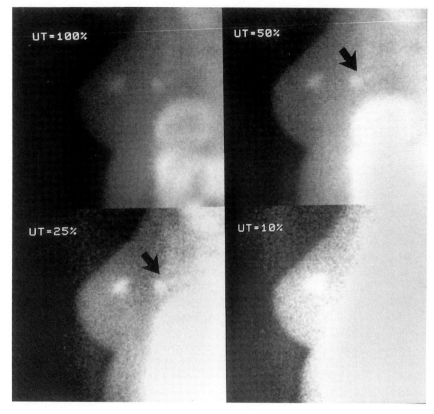

FIGURE 1.6   The discrimination obtained with a specific threshold for a given primary breast cancer will often not be optimal to evaluate metastatic axillary lymph node involvement on the same view. Therefore, a second set of images is sometimes needed in order to better determine the presence or absence of lymph nodes uptake. A too-low threshold may mask axillary lymph node uptake.

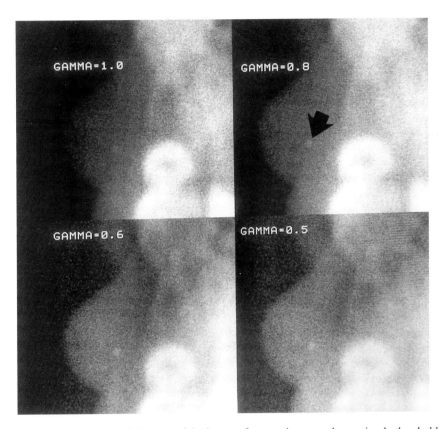

FIGURE 1.7   Scintigraphic images of the breast often require more than a simple threshold adjustment. Contrast enhancement by varying the image gamma factor will allow one to emphasize structures that are in the lower portion of the image color or gray scale (such as the breast and breast lesion with low counting rate). This adjustment is directly affected, like thresholds, by very high maximal pixel counts. Thus, it is important to eliminate organs with high count densities from the field of view. The gamma adjustment allows the users to display images in a nonlinear gray or color scale.

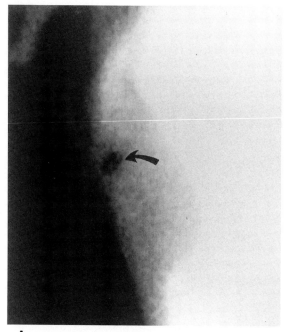

A

Figure 1.8   Although initial studies reporting on the use of radionuclides for detection of breast cancer were performed in supine position, more recent data suggest that prone imaging provides better diagnostic results. Prone imaging allows the breast to be pending according to gravity. Prone lateral thoracic views permit the detection of lesions which are very close to the chest wall or in the projection of the heart or liver (two organs showing very high ^{99m}Tc-sestamibi uptake). Lesions in these locations are rather difficult to detect in the anterior thoracic upright or supine views. On the other hand, anterior supine view is also very useful, especially to better locate a lesion detected on the lateral prone view and also to detect axillary lymph node involvement. In some patients, anterior supine view is very important in detecting internal mammary or cervical lymph node metastatic involvement. Prone imaging will locate a primary breast lesion in either the upper or lower quadrant of the breast. A second view will be necessary to better locate the lesion in the inner or outer quadrant. (A) Lesion in the upper part of the breast with a moderate ^{99m}Tc-sestamibi uptake on the right prone lateral view. On the anterior supine view (B) the lesion is well seen in the upper and inner quadrant of the right breast. Therefore, both views are necessary to obtain optimal diagnostic results.

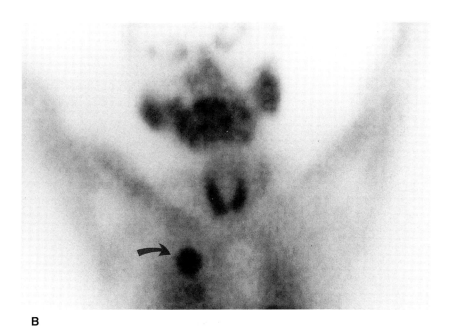

B

FIGURE 1.8

SECTION 2: NORMAL CASES AND VARIANTS

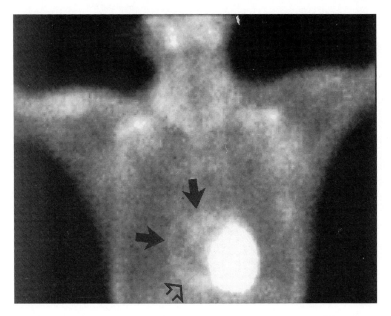

FIGURE 2.1   It is well known from the experience acquired with ^{99m}Tc-sestamibi planar imaging for detection of coronary artery disease that, besides the left ventricle, right atrium (arrow), interatrial septum (arrow), and right ventricle (open arrowhead) can be also well visualized on a ^{99m}Tc-sestamibi study. These normal structures should not be misinterpreted as abnormal lesions on the anterior supine thoracic view.

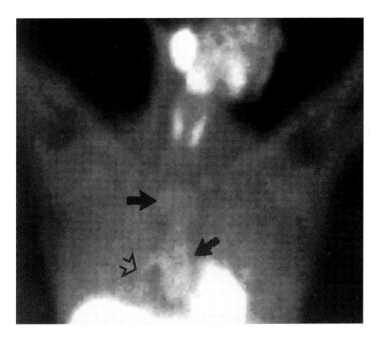

FIGURE 2.2   Bone or medullary uptake of ^{99m}Tc-sestamibi can sometimes be seen in some patients. The radiotracer uptake in these structures may be further enhanced by varying the image threshold. This figure shows a significantly increased ^{99m}Tc-sestamibi uptake in the sternum (arrows) of a patient with chronic anemia. Note that the right atrium is also well seen (open arrowhead). Significantly increased uptake may also be seen in the sternoclavicular joints.

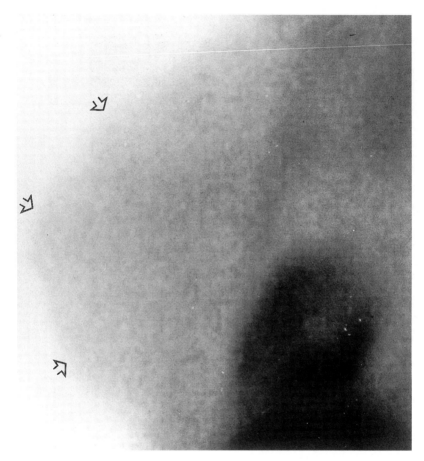

FIGURE 2.3   Normal left thoracic prone view of the breast. The ^{99m}Tc-sestamibi uptake in the breast is uniform and there is no focal or diffuse increased uptake. Although the absolute ^{99m}Tc-sestamibi breast uptake is relatively low, the image display parameters should be adjusted so that the breast contours are well delineated (open arrowheads).

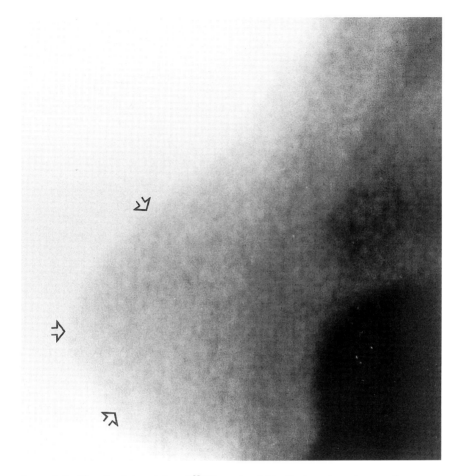

Figure 2.4 The absolute uptake of ^{99m}Tc-sestamibi in the breast can be very low, especially in patients with fatty breasts. In these cases, the threshold of the image should be adjusted in accordance so that the breast contours look more linear and less "patchy."

SECTION 3: BENIGN BREAST DISEASE

Although ^{99m}Tc-sestamibi is most avidly concentrated in breast cancers, increased uptake of the radiotracer can also be detected in various types of benign breast diseases. More extensive clinical experience has lead investigators to recognize some ^{99m}Tc-sestamibi uptake patterns in hyperproliferative fibrocystic breast disease. The following criteria, although not 100% accurate, provide some guidelines in interpreting ^{99m}Tc-sestamibi breast imaging in patients with benign breast disease. Most of the time, fibrocystic disease will be seen on ^{99m}Tc-sestamibi breast scintigraphy as a region or regions of slight to moderate increased uptake, more diffuse than focalized, often bilateral, having contours which are not well delineated and often presenting a "patchy" uptake. Most of the other benign diseases of the breast will not show a significantly increased ^{99m}Tc-sestamibi uptake. Usually, these lesions are not ^{99m}Tc-sestamibi avid. Acute mastitis or juvenile fibroadenomas are exceptions.

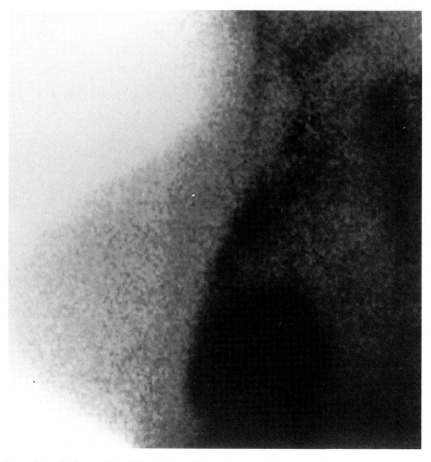

FIGURE 3.1   Patient with a 1.5 × 1.5 cm fibroadenoma of the outer lower quadrant of the left breast. The ^{99m}Tc-sestamibi left prone lateral thoracic view is strictly normal. This is the most frequent scintigraphic pattern of fibroadenoma: a normal study with no significant focus of increased ^{99m}Tc-sestamibi uptake in the breast.

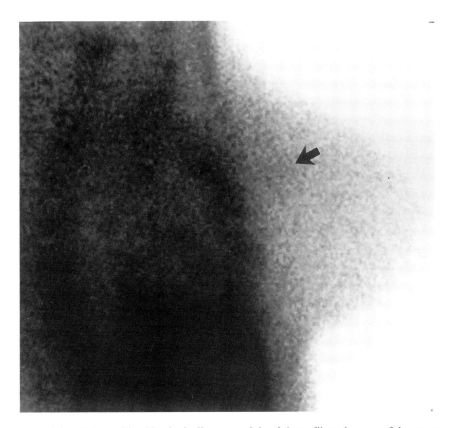

FIGURE 3.2   Patient with a histologically proven 2.0 × 2.0 cm fibroadenoma of the upper quadrant of the right breast. ^{99m}Tc-sestamibi scintigraphy (right prone lateral thoracic view) shows a focus of slightly increased radiotracer uptake in the projection of the fibroadenoma (arrow).

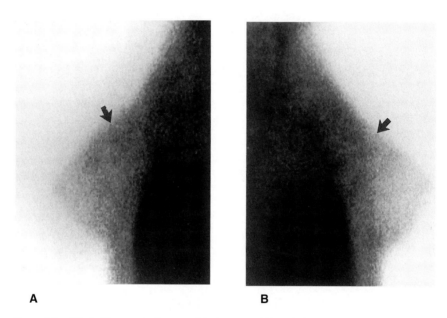

A   **B**

FIGURE **3**.3   Slight fibrocystic disease of the breast. Diffuse bilateral slight increased uptake of [99mTc]-sestamibi, without well-delineated contours, involving mainly the upper quadrants of the breasts (arrows). (A) Left lateral prone view. (B) Right lateral prone view.

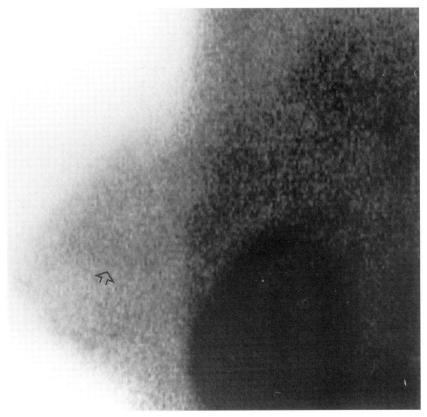

A

FIGURE 3.4   Slight fibrocystic disease of the breast. Same pattern as in Figure 3.3 but with relatively more extensive involvement in both breasts (open arrowheads). (A) Left lateral and (B) right lateral views.

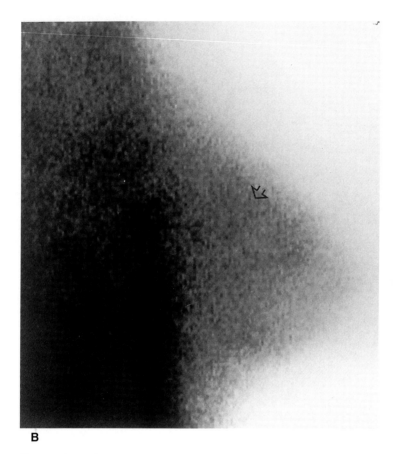

B

Figure 3.4 Continued

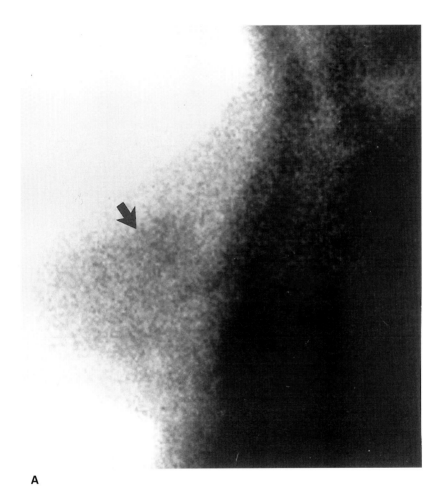

A

FIGURE 3.5   Moderate fibrocystic disease of the breast. Diffuse bilateral and moderate increased ^{99m}Tc-sestamibi uptake without well delineated contours (arrows). (A) Left lateral and (B) right lateral views.

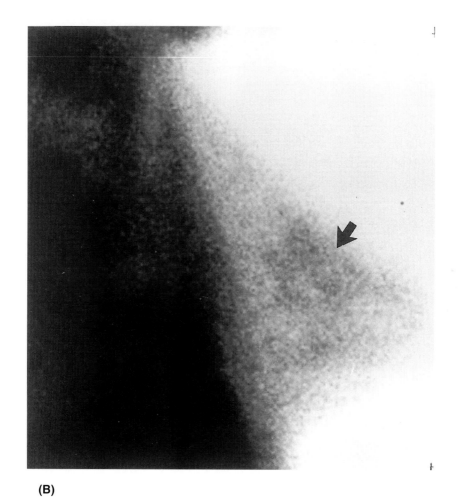

(B)

FIGURE 3.5 Continued

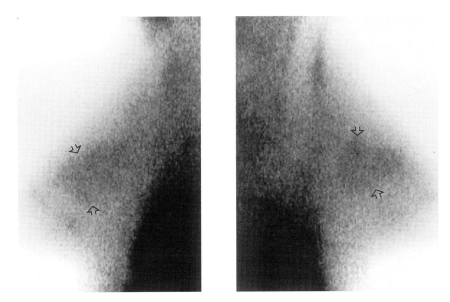

FIGURE **3.6**   Moderate fibrocystic disease of the breast. Same scintigraphic pattern as in Figure 3.5 but the lesions seem to have relatively better delineated contours (open arrowheads).

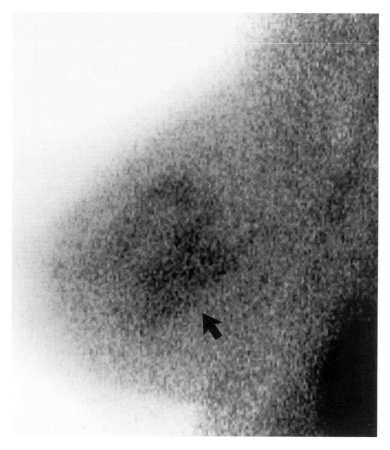

FIGURE **3.7**   Severe fibrocystic disease of the breast. Diffuse and significant bilateral increased uptake of ^{99m}Tc-sestamibi in both breasts (arrows).

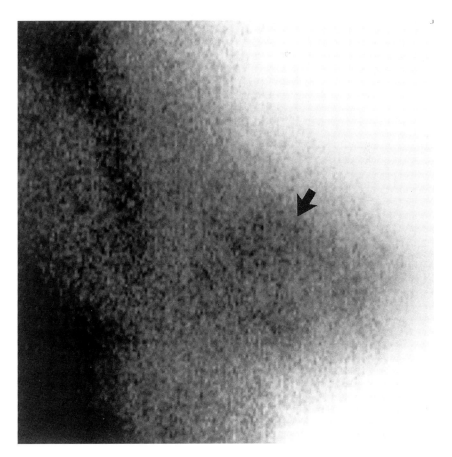

Figure 3.7 Continued

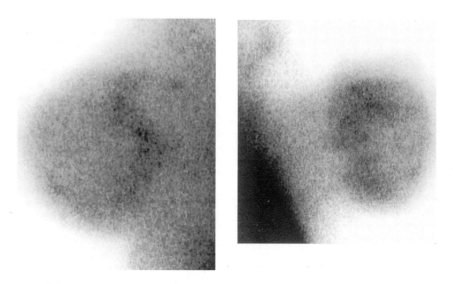

FIGURE 3.8   Extensive involvement of fibrocystic disease of the breasts.

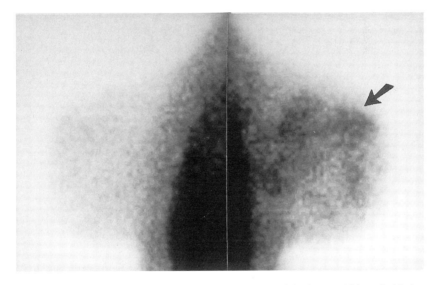

Figure 3.9   Unilateral proliferative fibrocystic disease of the breast. Although this is not usual scintigraphic pattern for fibrocystic disease, a markedly asymmetric or unilateral disease can sometimes be found.

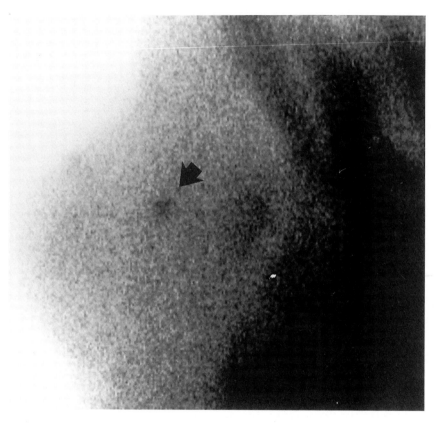

A

Figure 3.10   Fatty necrosis. Prone left lateral thoracic view in a patient with a suspected lesion in the upper part of the breast on mammography. (A) ^{99m}Tc-sestamibi scintigraphy showed a small lesion in the upper quadrant of the left breast (arrow), but this lesion was more posterior in location than the one seen on mammography. It was suggested to repeat the scintimammography. (B) A second ^{99m}Tc-sestamibi was then repeated 3 weeks after the previous one. This second study was completely normal. Two surgical biopsies were then performed on the two locations, and fatty necrosis was found.

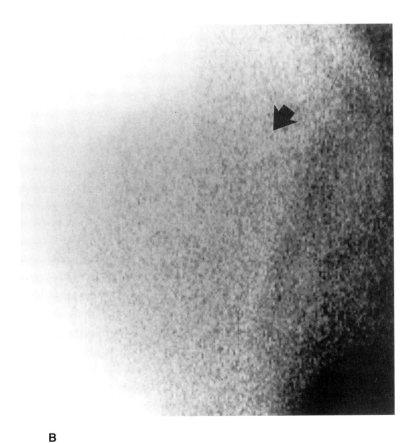

B

FIGURE 3.10   Continued

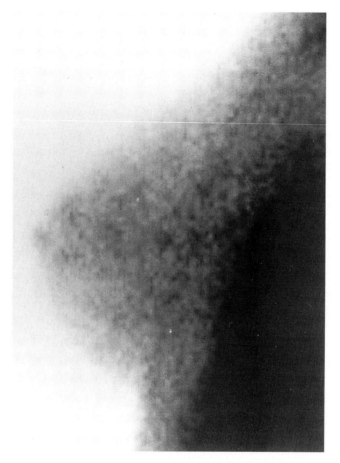

FIGURE 3.11   Chronic mastitis. ^{99m}Tc-sestamibi scintimammography shows a "patchy" uptake of the radiotracer (slight to moderate intensity) in this patient with chronic mastitis.

SECTION 4: FOCAL PRIMARY BREAST CANCER

Contrary to most benign diseases of the breast, primary breast cancers are usually much more well focalized (although there are some exceptions such as inflammatory cancers which are more diffuse); their contours are usually relatively well delineated and unilateral most of the time. The intensity of 99mTc-sestamibi uptake varies from mild to very intense depending on several factors such as size, type, location, and hormonal factors. Furthermore, metastatic axillary lymph node involvement can also be visualized, the detection of which increases the diagnostic confidence for the presence of breast cancer. The following are cases of histologically proven focal primary breast cancers (^{99m}Tc-sestamibi scinti-mammography performed before histological evidence was obtained) without axillary metastatic axillary lymph node involvement.

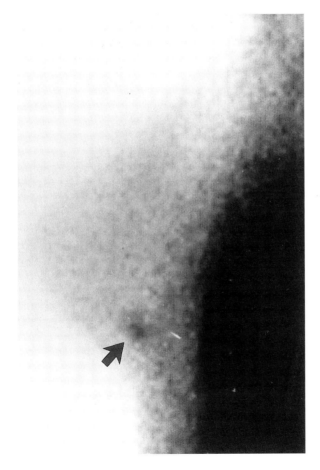

Figure 4.1   Lobular carcinoma of the outer lower quadrant of the left breast (arrow), measuring 1.0×1.2 cm in a patient with palpable mass. Mammography showed a very dense breast tissue.

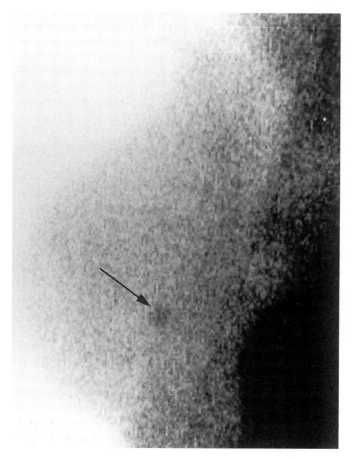

FIGURE 4.2 Ductal carcinoma in situ of the medial lower quadrant of the left breast (arrow), measuring 0.7×0.8 cm.

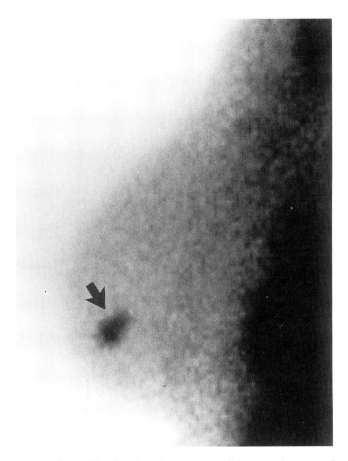

FIGURE 4.3   Infiltrating ductal carcinoma of the outer lower quadrant of the left breast (arrow). The lesion measured 1.0×1.4 cm.

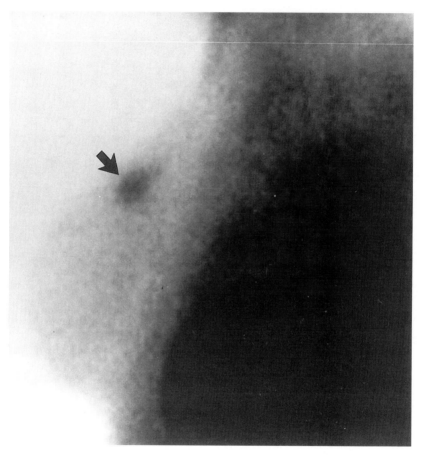

FIGURE 4.4 Infiltrating ductal carcinoma of the inner upper quadrant of the left breast (arrow), measuring 1.5 × 2.0 cm.

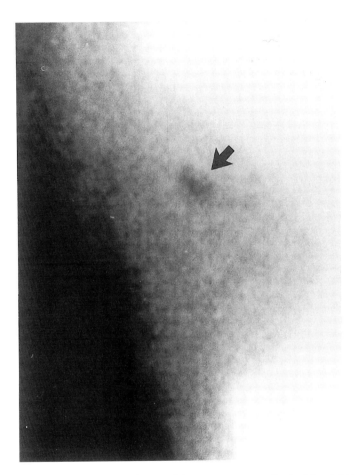

FIGURE 4.5   Lobular carcinoma of the outer upper quadrant of the right breast (arrow). The lesion measured 1.1 × 1.8 cm.

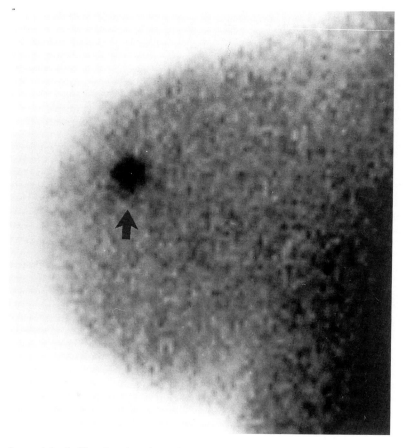

Figure 4.6   Infiltrating ductal carcinoma of the outer upper quadrant of the left breast (arrow) measuring 1.5 × 1.5 cm.

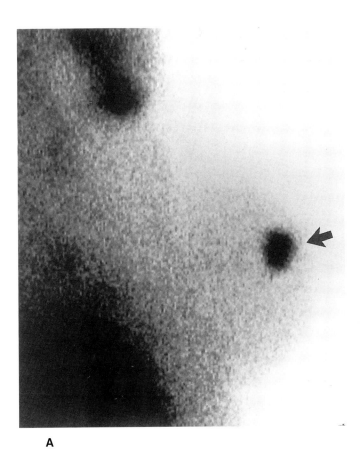

A

FIGURE **4.7**   Primary lymphoma of the breast. (A) Right lateral prone view; (B) anterior supine view. Lymphoma usually presents with a very intense degree of ^{99m}Tc-sestamibi uptake (arrow).

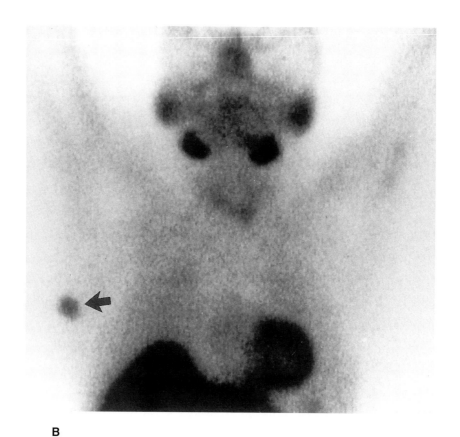

B

Figure 4.7 Continued

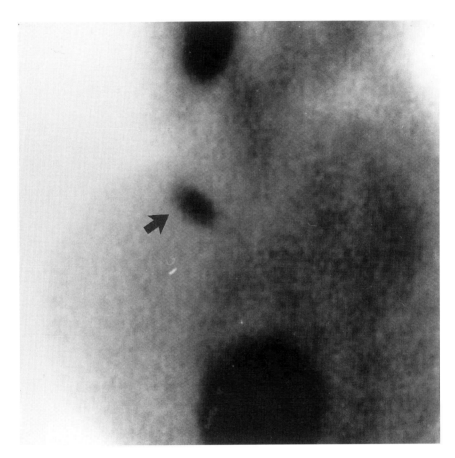

Figure 4.8   Primary lymphoma of the outer upper quadrant of the left breast (arrow), measuring 1.6 × 2.0 cm.

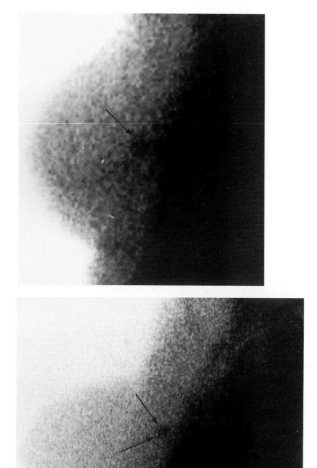

A

B

FIGURE **4.9**   These three different cases illustrate the usefulness of the prone imaging in three patients with primary breast cancers (arrows) very close in location to the chest wall and with either a negative or equivocal mammography. (A) 1.0 × 1.5 cm infiltrating ductal carcinoma of the left breast. (B) 0.8 × 1.0 cm in situ ductal carcinoma of the left breast. (C) 1.5 × 1.5 cm infiltrating ductal carcinoma of the left breast.

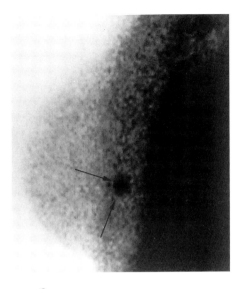

C

Figure 4.9   Continued

SECTION 5: METASTATIC AXILLARY LYMPH NODE INVOLVEMENT

Breast imaging with ^{99m}Tc-sestamibi can also detect metastatic axillary lymph node involvement with an overall diagnostic accuracy of approximately 80–85%. Although this number is too low to advocate the routine use of scintimammography to decide to perform or not an axillary dissection, the presence of increased ^{99m}Tc-sestamibi uptake in the axillary nodes is useful to increase the diagnostic confidence of the test. It is important to note, however, that there is no linear relationship between the number of positive nodes detected on ^{99m}Tc-sestamibi scintimammography and the number of positive nodes diagnosed on histopathology. This is not surprising given the limitation in spatial resolution of the standard gamma camera and the microscopic nature of some lymphatic involvements.

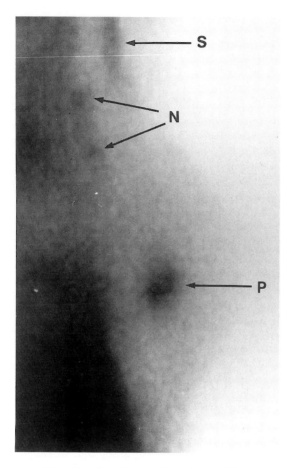

FIGURE 5.1   Right lateral prone thoracic view. The primary (P) breast cancer measuring 2.0 × 2.0 cm is clearly seen. There are also two nodes (N) that are detected in the axilla. These foci of uptake are different from that more superficial (S), corresponding to skin folds or sometimes excessive sudation. This later uptake is linear and superficial whereas the nodes are more deeply seated in the axilla and rounded in shape. Four out of 20 removed nodes were positive for metastatic involvement.

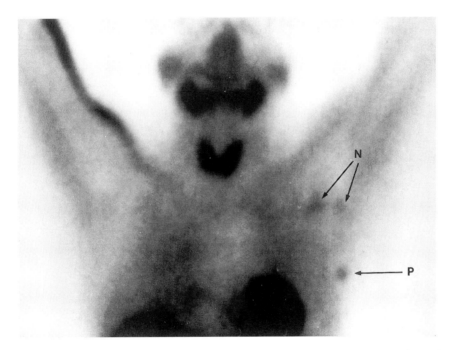

FIGURE 5.2   This patient had an infiltrating ductal carcinoma of the outer upper quadrant of the left breast (P). On the anterior supine thoracic view, at least two nodes (N) are clearly visualized. Persistent increased ^{99m}Tc-sestamibi uptake is also seen in the right vein arm (see Section 1). Five out of nine removed nodes were positive for metastatic infiltration.

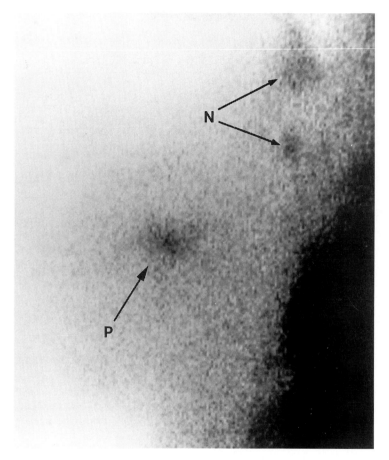

FIGURE 5.3   A primary (P) left breast cancer (infiltrating ductal carcinoma) measuring 1.6 × 2.1 cm was found in this patient. Many foci of significantly increased ^{99m}Tc-sestamibi uptake were also detected in the ipsilateral axilla. Fourteen metastatic axillary lymph nodes were found.

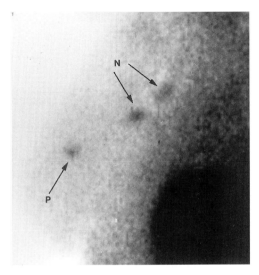

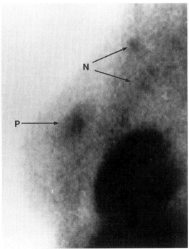

FIGURE 5.4   Four different patients with primary breast cancer (P) and metastatic axillary lymph node involvement (N).

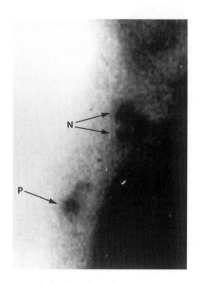
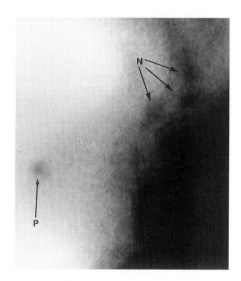

FIGURE 5.4   Continued

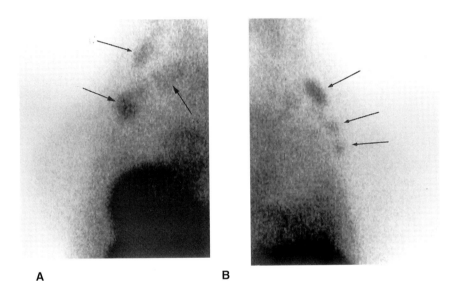

A   **B**

FIGURE 5.5   This patient was referred for a scintimammography because of bilateral suspicious lesions on mammography. ^{99m}Tc-sestamibi was therefore injected on the left pedal vein. The study (A, left lateral view; B, right lateral view) did not show any focus of increased ^{99m}Tc-sestamibi uptake in breast parenchyma. However, several bilateral foci of ^{99m}Tc-sestamibi uptake were detected in both axillae (arrows). This finding, in addition to the absence of breast lesion, suggested the presence of lymphoma with bilateral axillary involvement. This diagnosis was confirmed with a biopsy of some nodes. Follow-up and one breast biopsy did not reveal any breast cancer.

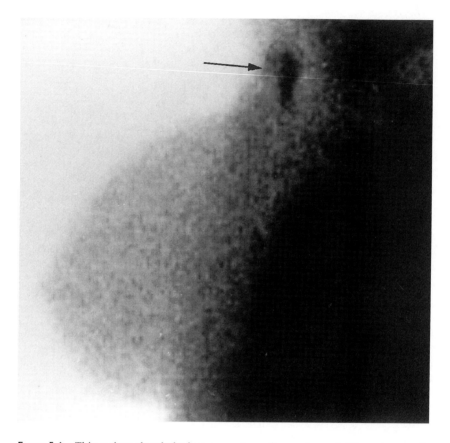

FIGURE 5.6   This patient already had a tumorectomy for a primary left breast cancer but refused to have an axillary dissection because of the possible side effects. ^{99m}Tc-sestamibi scintimammography was performed to evaluate the status of the left axilla. The study clearly detected a focus of significantly increased ^{99m}Tc-sestamibi uptake in the left axilla (arrow). Based on this result, the patient finally accepted to have the axillary dissection, which confirmed the presence of five positive metastatic nodes.

SECTION 6: EXTENSIVE PRIMARY BREAST CANCER

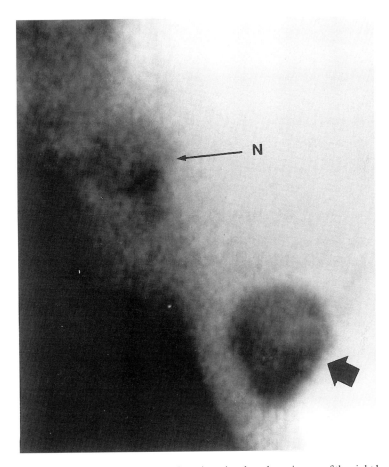

FIGURE 6.1   Patient with a 6.0 × 7.0 cm invasive ductal carcinoma of the right breast (arrowhead) with necrotic center (showing less intense ^{99m}Tc-sestamibi uptake). Positive axillary uptake of the radiotracer is also seen (N). Seven nodes were found histologically positive for metastatic disease.

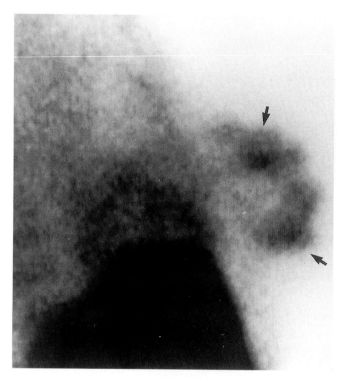

A

FIGURE 6.2 Patient with an inflammatory cancer of the right breast involving almost the entire parenchyma (arrow). It has a multilobulated appearance and heterogeneous ^{99m}Tc-sestamibi uptake. (A) right lateral prone view; (B) anterior supine view.

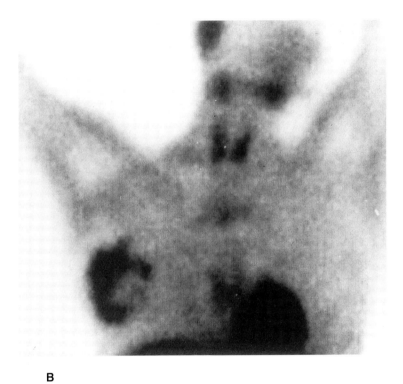

B

FIGURE 6.2   Continued

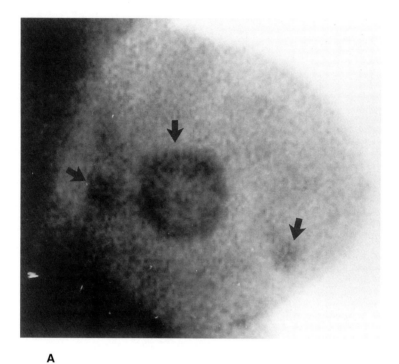

A

Figure 6.3 Patient with a multifocal invasive ductal carcinoma of the right breast. Both right lateral (A) and anterior (B) views show at least four or five sites of significantly increased ^{99m}Tc-sestamibi uptake (arrows). One of them, the larger one, has a necrotic center with relatively decreased uptake in its center.

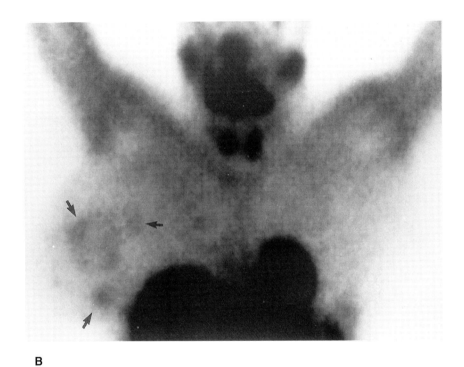

B

FIGURE 6.3   Continued

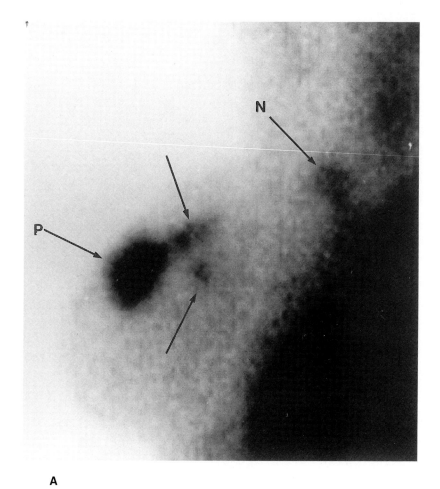

A

Figure 6.4   The following three different cases (A, B, C) show a similar scintigraphic pattern: an intense increased ^{99m}Tc-sestamibi uptake in the primary breast cancer (P or arrowhead) and local invasion where the extension of the tumor is relatively linear and well delineated (arrows). Furthermore, in cases A and B, axillary metastatic lymph node involvement is well seen (N).

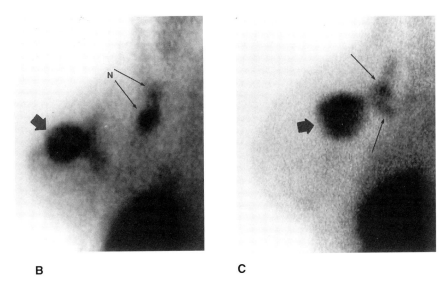

B   C

FIGURE 6.4   Continued

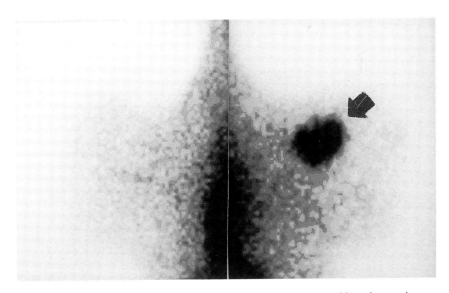

FIGURE 6.5   Patient with a phylloides tumor with parts of sarcoma and invasive carcinoma of the upper outer quadrant of the right breast. The ^{99m}Tc-sestamibi uptake within the primary breast tumor is very intense.

SECTION 7: PROSTHESIS

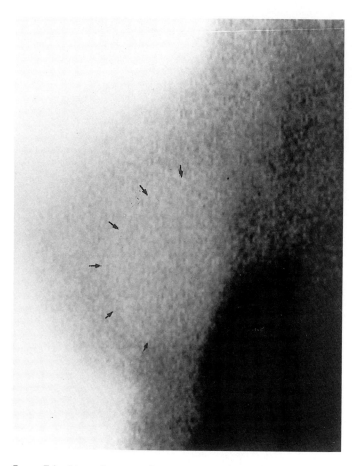

FIGURE 7.1   Normal aspect of mammary prosthesis. The mammary prosthesis is usually easily recognized. The prosthesis does not concentrate ^{99m}Tc-sestamibi and therefore creates a relatively "cold" defect (arrows) in comparison to the rest of the normal breast parenchyma. The normal parenchyma will show a slight and diffuse increased uptake of the radiotracer, as seen in normal patients.

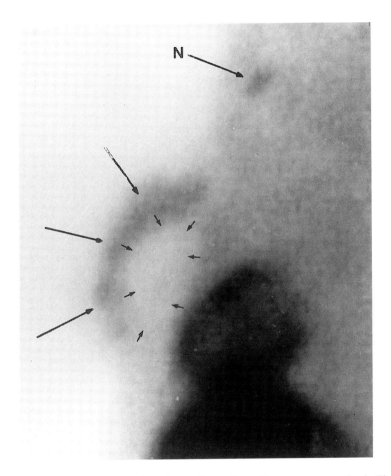

FIGURE 7.2   Invasive ductal carcinoma in a patient with mammary prosthesis. The "shadow" of the mammary prosthesis is well seen (small arrows). The upper part of the breast parenchyma overlying the prosthesis show a significantly increased ^{99m}Tc-sestamibi uptake which is irregular (arrows). Furthermore, an axillary focus of increased uptake is also detected (N). An invasive ductal carcinoma and positive axillary metastatic lymph node involvement were found in histopathology.

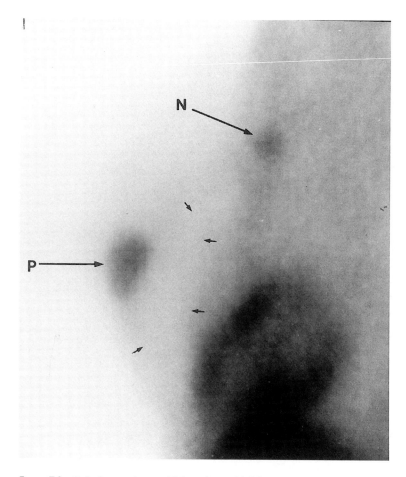

Figure 7.3   Lobular carcinoma. This patient with bilateral mammary prosthesis had a palpable nodule in the periareolar region. ^{99m}Tc-sestamibi scintimammography (left lateral view) shows an increased uptake in the retroareolar region (arrow), corresponding to the palpable nodule. The "shadow" of the mammary prosthesis is well seen (small arrows). Furthermore, an axillary node is also detected (N). Histology confirmed the diagnosis of a breast cancer (lobular carcinoma) with axillary metastatic involvement.

SECTION 8: PRE- AND POSTCHEMOTHERAPY ASSESSMENT

^{99m}Tc-sestamibi scintimammography is currently being investigated as a marker of tumor viability or as a marker of the presence of the P-glycoprotein 170 in tumors overexpressing the MDR-1 gene in patients submitted for chemotherapy for breast cancer. It is too soon to draw conclusions on the clinical impact of such findings in humans and on the role of ^{99m}Tc-sestamibi scintimammography in this particular situation, but preliminary clinical experience seems to demonstrate a good correlation between the presence of ^{99m}Tc-sestamibi uptake and the presence of tumor cells in the breast before and after chemotherapy.

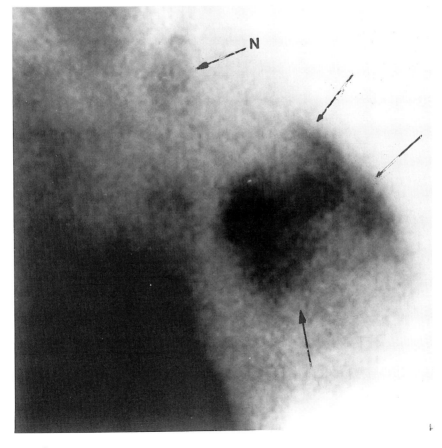

A

Figure 8.1

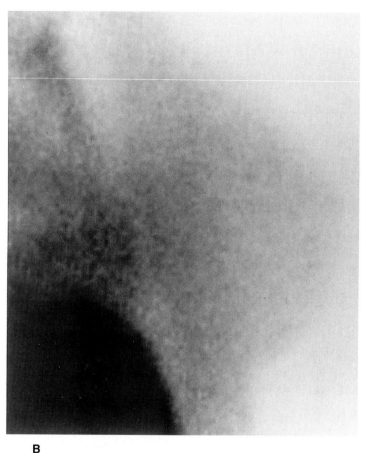

B

FIGURE 8.1   Patient with a diffuse invasive ductal carcinoma of the right breast. (A) ^{99m}Tc-sestamibi scimtimammography (right lateral view) performed before chemotherapy shows a very intense radiotracer uptake (arrows) involving almost half of the breast with metastatic axillary lymph node involvement (N). (B) A second ^{99m}Tc-sestamibi study was performed after chemotherapy. There is only a faint and diffuse uptake of the radiotracer in the upper quadrants of the right breast.

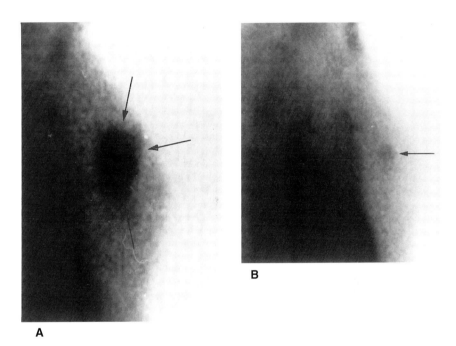

A

B

FIGURE 8.2   This patient had a large invasive ductal carcinoma of the right breast. ^{99m}Tc-sestamibi scintimammography was performed before (A) and after (B) chemotherapy. Although the size of the primary breast tumor decreased (arrows), tumoral ^{99m}Tc-sestamibi activity persisted after chemotherapy.

SECTION 9: MISCELLANEOUS

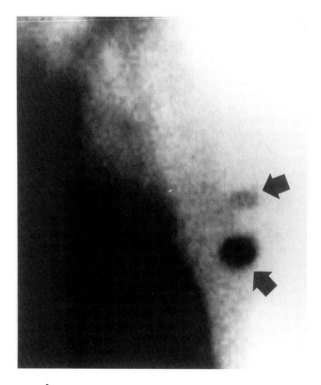

A

FIGURE **9.1**   Bifocal lobular carcinoma. This patient with a palpable nodule of the right breast had a mammography which showed a suspicious lesion of the outer inferior quadrant of the right breast. ^{99m}Tc-sestamibi scintimammography (A, right lateral view; B, anterior view) detected two lesions in the right breast (arrows). Histopathology showed that the two lesions were a bifocal lobular carcinoma which were partially missed on mammography.

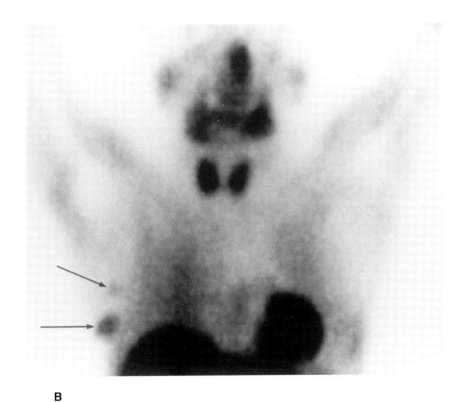

B

FIGURE 9.1   Continued

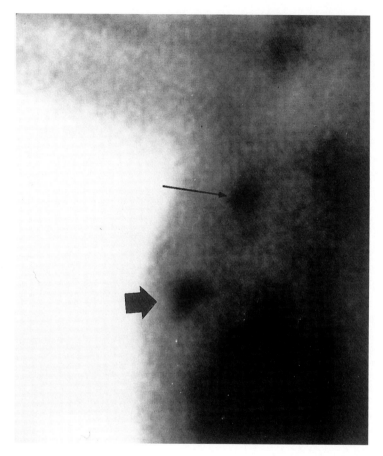

FIGURE 9.2 Recurrent disease. This patient had a left mastectomy 8 years ago. ^{99m}Tc-sestamibi scintimammography was performed because of a palpable lesion at the site of the scar. The study showed an intense focus of increased uptake at the site of the palpable lesion (arrowhead) and also an axillary uptake (arrow). A recurrent invasive ductal carcinoma and metastatic axillary lymph node involvement were found.

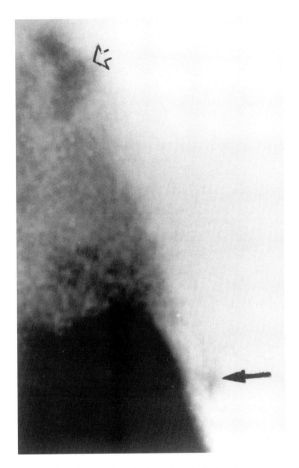

FIGURE **9.3**   This patient had a palpable lesion in a very small right breast which could not be imaged by mammography. ^{99m}Tc-sestamibi scintimammography showed a small focus of increased uptake in the lower quadrant of the right breast (arrow) with axillary uptake (open arrowhead). Histology confirmed the presence of an invasive ductal carcinoma and axillary metastatic lymph node involvement.

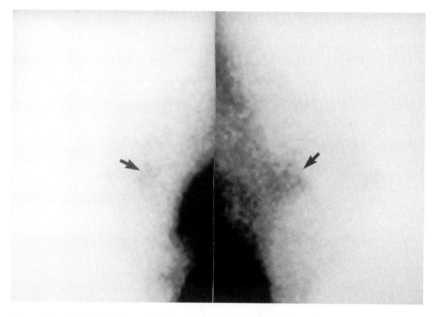

Figure **9.4** Myeloid leukemia. This patient had a palpable mass in the outer upper part of the right breast. The left breast did not show any palpable abnormality. The patient had received local irradiation because of a cutaneous infiltration from acute myeloid leukemia 2 months before. Mammography and ultrasonography were indicative of fibrocystic disease. ^{99m}Tc-sestamibi scintimammography showed a focal accumulation in the middle of the right breast (arrow) close to the chest wall. A second focus was also found in the center of the left breast (arrow). Histopathology revealed an infiltration of myeloid leukemia in both breasts.

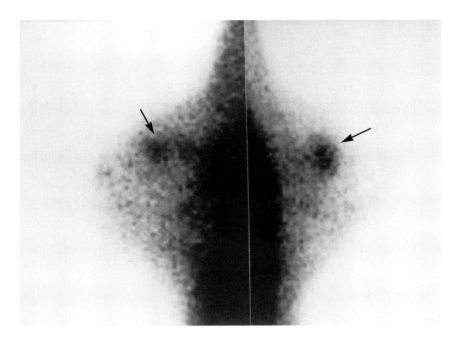

FIGURE **9.5**   Bilateral breast cancer. This patient had a palpable mass in the upper part of the right breast. Mammography showed a suspicious opacity in the right breast. ^{99m}Tc-sestamibi study detected a focal uptake in the upper quadrant of the right breast (arrow) and also a second focus of increased uptake (arrow) in the upper quadrant of the left breast. Histopathology revealed an invasive ductal carcinoma in the right breast measuring 2.6 cm and an invasive ductal carcinoma in the left breast with a lesion diameter of 1.5 cm. Although the uptake was bilateral, the contours of the lesions were relatively well delineated, the lesions were more focalized, and the uptake was intense, suggesting that these lesions were malignant and not only benign.

SECTION 10: ^{99M}TC-MDP SCINTIMAMMOGRAPHY

As seen in Chapter 9, ^{99m}Tc-MDP can also be used for detection of primary breast cancer in conjunction with whole-body bone scintigraphy. The following eight cases illustrate the scintigraphic pattern of some breast lesions with this commonly used radiopharmaceutical.

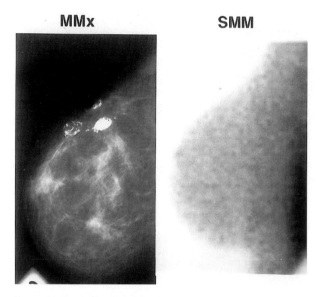

MMx   **SMM**

Figure 10.1   Benign calcification. This patient had previous recurrent episodes of breast inflammation, especially during breastfeeding. The lateral view mammography (MMx) shows many and massive calcifications in the upper quadrants of the left breast, suggestive of a benign lesion. ^{99m}Tc-MDP scintimammography (SMM) of the left breast is normal, and there is no focus of increased uptake in the breast. Clinical follow-up confirmed the benign nature of these calcifications. As with ^{99m}Tc-sestamibi SMM, benign calcifications will not show increased radiotracer uptake.

MMx **MMx** **SMM**

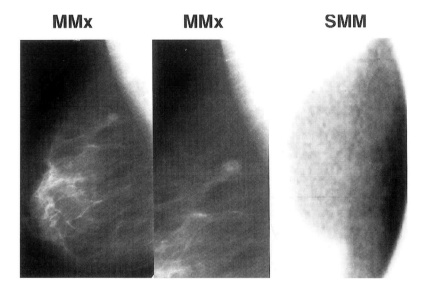

FIGURE 10.2   Fibroadenoma. This patient was investigated for a palpable mass located in the upper-outer quadrant of the left breast. The lateral view mammography and relative zoom magnification show an area of moderately increased density, with irregular margins, located in the area of the palpable lesion. ^{99m}Tc-MDP scintigraphy (SMM) of the left breast was normal. Histology diagnosed a fibroadenoma. ^{99m}Tc-MDP, as with ^{99m}Tc-sestamibi, usually will not concentrate within a fibroadenoma.

MMx   MMx   SMM

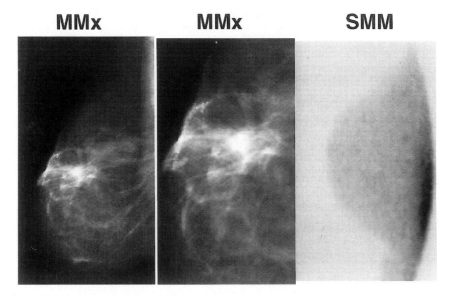

FIGURE 10.3   Chronic mastitis. This patient was medically treated 15 years ago for an abscess of the left breast. She was investigated for a recent skin retraction and increased thickness in the same area. Mammography and magnification show an opacity with irregular margins, with suspicion of skin infiltration, located in the breast. No ^{99m}Tc-MDP uptake was observed in the left breast. Chronic mastitis was diagnosed on histopathology.

MMx   **MMx**   **SMM**

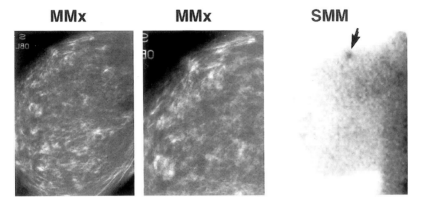

Figure 10.4   Invasive ductal carcinoma. Left lateral mammography and relative magnification show a small spiculated opacity in the superior quadrant of the left breast in this patient without clinical evidence of palpable lesion. ^{99m}Tc-MDP scintigraphy of the left breast detected a small focus of increased uptake (arrow) corresponding to the lesion seen on mammography. Histology confirmed the malignity of the lesion (invasive ductal carcinoma), which measured 0.6 cm.

MMx   **SMM LAT.**   **SMM ANT.**

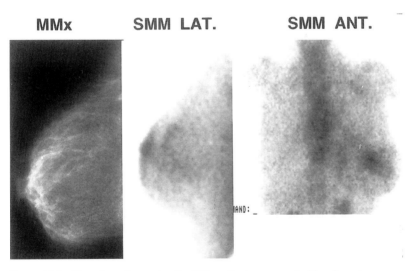

Figure 10.5   Ductal carcinoma in situ. This patient was enrolled in a breast cancer screening program. Mammography showed an increased thickness in the retroareolar region of the left breast, without associated mass or microcalcifications. Left lateral and anterior views of the left breast on scintimammography show a clear, diffuse and intense ^{99m}Tc-MDP uptake in the periareolar region (arrow). A ductal carcinoma in situ was found on histopathology.

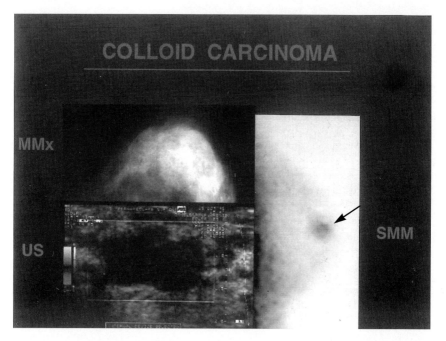

FIGURE 10.6   Colloid carcinoma. This patient presented with a palpable nodule located posterior to the nipple, in the right breast. The nodule was not clinically suspicious for cancer, given its soft consistency and mobility. Mammography of the right breast shows a dense breast with consequent poor ability in detecting pathologic findings. Ultrasound color Doppler shows a hypoechoic nodule with irregular borders without posterior acoustic attenuation, characterized by a single vascular pole. This finding was not evident for breast cancer, but suspicious for fibroadenoma. ^{99m}Tc-MDP scintimammography detected a focus of increased uptake in the retroareolar region (arrow). Histology diagnosed a colloid carcinoma.

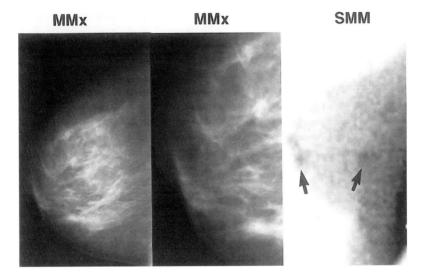

MMx   MMx   SMM

FIGURE 10.7   Bifocal invasive ductal carcinoma. This patient presented with a palpable nodule located in the area under the left nipple. Left lateral mammography and relative magnification show an area of moderately increased density located in the subareolar region. ^{99m}Tc-MDP scintigraphy detected two foci of increased uptake (arrows). The first corresponded to the lesion detected by mammography; the second one was located more posteriorly, very close to the chest wall. This second lesion was missed by mammography. A bifocal invasive ductal carcinoma was found on histopathology. The relative largest diameters were 0.6 and 0.5 cm.

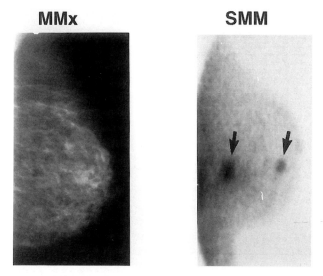

FIGURE 10.8 Bifocal lobular carcinoma. This patient had a palpable nodule located posteriorly in the right breast. Right lateral mammography shows an area of increased density
located posteriorly to the areolar region, classified as with intermediate risk for breast cancer. [99mTc]-MDP scintimammography showed two foci of increased uptake (arrows). The
first was also recognized by mammography, but the second, deeply located, was not detected
by mammography. A bifocal lobular carcinoma was diagnosed on histology, having largest
diameters of 1.0 and 2.2 cm.

15

Health Technology Assessment and Policy for Radionuclide Imaging of the Breast

FRANK J. PAPATHEOFANIS
The Institute for Biomedical Engineering and University of California School of Medicine, La Jolla, California

I. ADOPTING NEW MEDICAL TECHNOLOGY

The importance of cost to the diffusion of new diagnostic imaging technology can be traced back to the adoption of the X-ray tube in the United States almost a century ago. Records from Pennsylvania Hospital and other hospitals founded by the growth and expansion of the American railway system indicate that very detailed accounts of expense and utilization patterns concerning X-ray equipment were kept starting about 1900 [1]. Although the public quickly came to regard X-ray machines and the images they produced as examples of the achievement of "modern" science, turn-of-the-century hospital administrators were soon sensitized to the potential fiscal implications of this adoration and the impact it would have on bottom-line institutional profitability. Interestingly, the effectiveness of this technology was not a question. The meaning of X-ray images did not exist, so no comparisons could be drawn to competing modalities or alternative technologies. X-ray images soon replaced surgical exploration and some comparisons emerged. Nonetheless, the spread of X-ray imaging was so rapid and so involved that it left a legacy that is of interest to students of cost-effectiveness analysis that will never by duplicated again.

Paradoxically, in several ways, the current landscape of medical technology adoption and diffusion is not unlike that of the 1900s. Physicians and scientists provide exhilarating new discoveries from the laboratory and clinic. Public and media attention contribute the interest and fuel the sustained desire to see many technologies emerge. Payers challenge the usefulness, cost, and effectiveness of any new technologies. Manufacturers attempt to provide responsible products while maintaining profitability and shareholder loyalty. In the latter part of the century, however, government regulation has emerged as a vital force in determining which technologies are introduced into the marketplace, and when such introduction occurs. More importantly, payers have sought to scrutinize and choose which technologies they will reimburse regardless of governmental approval of the safety and efficacy of the technology. The adoption of a new technology now faces the conditions imposed by payers, something not anticipated even 5 years ago. Payer decision making has become a vital step in the diffusion of a new technology because it represents the major element of the type of market-driven health care system seen presently in the United States.

II. HEALTH TECHNOLOGY ASSESSMENT

A. Definition

Several important tools have emerged for decision makers to call upon for the evaluation of new health technology. Health technology assessment (HTA) has gained special prominence in this regard because it combines the rigor of biostatistical methodologies with a semiquantitative analysis of specific clinical settings and patient indications. Moreover, HTA has evolved toward outcomes, effectiveness, and appropriateness research as the boundaries between these lines of inquiry have become more and more obscured. Although technology assessment began receiving attention in the 1970s as an approach for considering the social impact of medical technologies, it was not until the mid-1980s that analyses derived from private and public sector HTA programs were integrated into clinical practice guidelines that the field properly matured and became an indispensable part of health care policy research efforts.

The Institute of Medicine defines technology assessment broadly as "any process of examining and reporting on medical technology used in health care, such as safety, efficacy, feasibility, and indications for use, cost and cost-effectiveness, as well as social, economic, and ethical consequences, whether intended or unintended" [2]. This definition applies to drugs, techniques, procedures, equipment, and combinations thereof. The very practical definition of technology assessment is that it is a process of evaluating new or existing technology to formulate a conclusion regarding the role of a particular technology in relation to its adoption and widespread diffusion in clinical practice.

The information that is utilized to perform technology assessment is derived from clinical trials [published in peer-reviewed journals, preferably; or, unpublished patient registry data], manufacturers' databases (PMA applications, etc.), federal and other regulatory information, and expert opinions provided by national consensus panels and specialty society position statements. The appropriateness of a medical technology is also determined by including factors such as provider and patient preferences, overall value, and ethical considerations. Clearly, the overall goal of HTA is to evaluate the impact of the proposed technology on the overall quality of life, which goes far beyond the notion of safety and efficacy.

B.   Health Technology Assessment Organizations

Many groups perform HTA, and a recent analysis identified over 125 active programs worldwide [3]. The funding sources and motivations behind these groups may be used to classify them in order to gain a better understanding of the HTA process. Likewise, the distribution or dissemination of the results obtained by these groups is another way of categorizing them that offers some insight into their methods and motivations.

Provider associations such as the American Medical Association (AMA), American College of Physicians (ACP), and University HealthSystem Consortium (UHC) generally have the interests of physicians or hospitals in mind and perform HTA on behalf of and for the use of their primary membership or constituency. The AMA tends to poll member physicians for their insights regarding the safety and efficacy of new technologies. The Diagnostic and Therapeutic Technology Assessment (DATTA) program is the AMA's primary formal HTA group. The results of polls and DATTA analyses are often published in the Journal of the American Medical Association (JAMA) and receive considerable attention from physicians and patient advocacy groups. The ACP operates in a very analogous manner and performs HTA formally through its Clinical Efficacy Assessment Project (CEAP). ACP position papers are often published in the Annals of Internal Medicine. UHC includes over 70 academic and affiliated medical centers as its members. It forms an effective group purchasing organization (GPO) at one level but also provides its membership with timely, useful HTA of important new technologies. UHC prepares HTA monographs and disseminates these reports to member institutions as well as other entities.

Third-party payers have emerged as a very strong force in determining the diffusion of new technologies because of their role in reimbursement and related fiscal matters. Where Food and Drug Administration (FDA) approval once represented the make-or-break point of a new or emerging technology, payer acceptance and reimbursement now redefine the path a new technology must take before it is accepted by providers. The national Blue Cross and Blue Shield Association (BCBSA) formed the Technology Evaluation Center (TEC) to perform HTA to facilitate decisions regarding insurance coverage. The TEC program utilizes a set of defined HTA criteria (Table 1) to provide consistent evaluation of many different technologies [4]. The strength in this approach is the uniformity of assessment

TABLE I   Blue Cross and Blue Shield Association Technology Assessment Criteria

1.	The technology must have approval from the appropriate government regulatory bodies.
2.	The scientific evidence must permit conclusions concerning the effect of the technology on health outcomes.
3.	The technology must improve the net health outcomes.
4.	The technology must be as beneficial as any established alternatives.
5.	The improvement must be attainable outside the investigational setting.

objectives, but many critics have argued that the TEC criteria are too inflexible and do not account for nuances in health outcomes data derived from the application of different technologies. AETNA, CIGNA, and other major payers in the United States also have HTA programs in place but largely rely on the decisions and analyses performed through the BCBSA TEC program to guide them in their clinical policy development and formulation.

Major federal programs in HTA include the FDA, the Agency for Health Care Policy and Research (AHCPR), and the Center for Health Care Technology (formerly the Office of Health Technology Assessment). The latter program advises the Health Care Financing Administration (HCFA) in making Medicare decisions concerning coverage for new technologies. The AHCPR recently designated 12 evidence-based clinical practice centers throughout the United States and Canada to also participate in HTA for determining national reimbursement and clinical practice policy. Almost every nation in Europe and Asia with a national health program has a national HTA program as well. The Canadians, especially, have established a leadership role in HTA by developing effective networks for analysis and dissemination of research findings.

Several private organizations also undertake HTA on a contractual basis and disseminate their results through proprietary reports; open, peer-reviewed publications; and other routes. ECRI (formerly Emergency Care Research Institute) publishes its results in a number of newsletters. Applied Technology Assessment (ATA) has emerged as a leader in modeling and product pipeline development of new and emerging technologies which anticipates the needs of payers. Several university-based programs also undertake HTA and generally disseminate their results in the open literature.

C. Technology Assessment Methods

A variety of analytical tools and approaches are utilized in HTA, but all of the methods require solid data for successful execution [5]. Consequently, an evaluation of data quality is often an important part in undertaking any HTA. A thorough review of primary medical and scientific literature is a basic step in this direction and forms the most important link between assessors and investigators. Multidisciplinary consensus panels often include representatives with specific expertise in a technology under evaluation. These experts are also generally familiar with the literature in their field. When such experts cannot be identified within HTA programs, outside experts are used. These experts are important members because of their perspective and ability in assisting other members in formulating appropriate technology assessment questions.

For diagnostic imaging technology evaluation, statistical analysis (hypothesis testing and confidence interval analysis), as well as quantitative measures such as sensitivity, specificity, and predictive values are often key components of successful HTA. Meta-analysis and other similar modeling tools have gained favor in HTA because they allow combinations of data sets to be analyzed. These approaches often yield more robust statistical findings because they increase comparable sample size and permit registration of substantially more outcomes measures than individual studies.

The analysis of health outcomes is the cornerstone of HTA because it permits the comparison of the performance of a new or emerging technology against established or recommended standards of care. Accordingly, clinical guidelines and practice parameters represent an attempt to utilize outcome assessment to evaluate new medical technology. Decision analysis, based on outcomes and closely related to the formulation of clinical practice guidelines, is an important, practical tool for HTA; likewise, the information obtained from HTA can be utilized to formulate increasingly representative decision analyses.

A basic framework for conducting HTA is illustrated in Figure 1. This framework utilizes a fundamental approach that can be applied to any technology. The initial steps involve identification of an important new technology that requires HTA. Priorities for performing HTA are varied but include (1) regulatory or payment decision needs, (2) large number of potential patients involved, (3) scientific or public controversy, and (4) high burden of morbidity or mortality. Once a problem formulation has been developed, data collection must be performed to establish a suitable pool of information on which to base comparisons. This central part of any HTA effort requires the collection of data on the proposed technology as well as established alternatives identified in the initial stages of the assessment. The final steps of the HTA process are generally interpretive and analytical in nature. The data must be consolidated, synthesized, and interpretable in its entirety. The evidence regarding the proposed technology must be interpreted in view of existing alternatives, setting the context for a dissemination of findings and recommendations that are based on a comparative analysis. Finally, the impact of implementing the decision that emerges from the HTA process should be monitored closely. New information and reinterpretation of existing information must

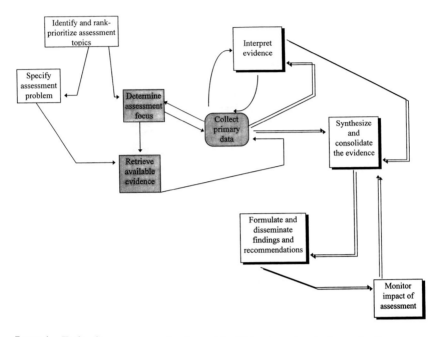

FIGURE 1   Technology assessment pathway identifying key steps in the evaluation process.

be added to the body of evidence, and reassessment is a potential loop that cycles through the HTA process until the technology is ultimately accepted or discarded.

III.   ASSESSMENT OF RADIONUCLIDE IMAGING OF THE BREAST

The model outlined in Figure 1 serves as a format for performing HTA of radionuclide imaging of the breast and is used as a template for this analysis.

A.   Identify and Rank-Prioritize Assessment Topics

Radionuclide imaging of the breast is an important technology for assessment because of the large number of patients who are diagnosed and die from breast cancer. In 1997, it is estimated that 181,600 Americans will be diagnosed with breast cancer; 44,190 women and men will die of the disease [6]. Another reason why radionuclide imaging of the breast warrants assessment is that early detection of breast cancer by X-ray mammography (XRM) and self-examination is highly controversial. For example, although mammography possesses good sensitivity, its specificity and positive predictive value (PPV) for nonpalpable disease is low, and many biopsies yield no evidence of malignancy. Both mammography and ultrasound (US) are utilized in attempts to distinguish benign from malignant breast tissue, but the diagnosis can only be made unequivocally with tissue biopsy. Radionuclide imaging of the breast has been proposed as a complementary procedure to mammography and justifies assessment because of the controversy surrounding noninvasive assessment of breast lesions.

B. Specify Assessment Problem

Does the available evidence permit conclusions about the diagnostic performance of radionuclide imaging of the breast in distinguishing between benign and malignant breast lesions among patients with suspicious mammograms or palpable disease?

C. Determine Assessment Focus

The major goal of differentiating between benign and malignant breast lesions is to improve patient selection for biopsy. Radionuclide imaging of the breast is proposed to reduce the number of unnecessary biopsies and the inconvenience and pain associated with performing those biopsies. Also, does the use of radionuclide imaging of the breast to guide decisions about performing biopsies improve health outcomes? Similarly, if the predictive value of radionuclide imaging of the breast is high, it can also reassure patients of the absence of disease. Alternatively, if a patient refrains from biopsy of an undetected malignancy based on a false-negative radionuclide imaging of the breast, the patient may miss the treatment benefits associated with identifying early-stage disease. This represents a negative health outcome (harm). These considerations must be in light of comparisons to mammography and ultrasound as well as other scintigraphic techniques utilized for breast imaging (^{201}Tl, ^{111}In pentetreotide [Octreoscan], and ^{99m}Tc IMMU-4 [CEA-scan]).

D. Retrieve Available Evidence

A literature search of the Medline database from 1990 to September 1997 was performed utilizing the key words "breast neoplasms," "malignancy," "scintigraphy," "radionuclide imaging," and "diagnostic imaging." Additionally, bibliographies of relevant articles were used to assure complete retrieval of appropriate primary articles. Abstracts of papers presented as national meetings over the specified interval were also reviewed. Tables of contents of recent and current relevant publications in print were also reviewed. This search retrieved 37 relevant articles.

E.   Collect Primary Data

The data reported in all relevant articles identified by the search indicated above were reviewed. Primary data were collected from reports that included patient selection information, detailed patient historical information, detailed information on imaging and data acquisition parameters, appropriate data analysis (diagnostic performance: sensitivity, specificity, positive predictive value, negative predictive value), tissue biopsy or other "gold standard" comparison data, and negative health outcome information. These study selection criteria were used to refine the search for appropriate data for evaluation, and the results of the application of these requirements identified a final set of 27 references for analysis.

F.   Interpret Evidence

A key consideration in the use of radionuclide imaging of the breast is whether these methods can be used to differentiate between benign and malignant lesions and whether use of radionuclide imaging of the breast alters whether biopsy is performed in a manner that improves net health outcomes. Direct evidence would have to compare equivalent, matched patient groups evaluated with and without radionuclide imaging of the breast. The groups would be followed to observe differences in biopsy referral rates over specified time intervals. However, this type of evidence is lacking. Instead, this analysis must rely on diagnostic performance data from studies which correlated radionuclide imaging of the breast results with biopsy findings and attempted to infer whether the results would influence biopsy decisions. The desired finding, consequently, is a very high negative predictive value (NPV). In other words, if the recommendation is against biopsy based on radionuclide imaging of the breast results, the probability of a false-negative result (i.e., undetected malignancy) must be very small to justify the advantages of not undergoing biopsy (reassurance, pain, inconvenience).

Table 2 summarizes the pooled data according to radionuclide imaging of the breast technique. The largest body of evidence involves the use of ^{99m}Tc sestamibi (Miraluma) [7–20]. Several studies were pooled because they appeared to be serial updates, and overall pooled data are indicated. Overall, the quality of study methods was very good with excellent uniformity of data acquisition. At least three views were taken of each breast (lateral and anterior) in all of the included studies. The dose of radiopharmaceutical was 20 mCi in 10, 20 to 30 mCi in two, and 25–30 in one study. Additionally, one study reported results based on 13.5 mCi whereas two studies utilized 15 mCi.

The most common patient selection criterion was suspicion of breast cancer based on XRM or physical examination, or both. Nine studies included a mixture of patients with suspicious XRM both palpable and nonpalpable lesions. Four studies included only patients with palpable masses whereas two included only

TABLE 2   Summary of Pooled Data on Differentiating Benign from Malignant Breast Lesions with Various Radionuclide Imaging of the Breast Techniques

Technique	Reference studies	Patients (n)	Sensitivity	Specificity	PPV	NPV
MIBI-SPECT	2	134	0.830 (0.828–0.833)	0.807 (0.796–0.821)	0.721 (0.667–0.774)	0.888 (0.865–0.907)
MIBI-planar	14	833	0.854 (0.5–1.00)	0.892 (0.688–1.00)	0.876 (0.667–1.00)	0.873 (0.563–0.960)
Tl-201-SPECT	1	39	1.000	0.954	0.944	1.000
Tl-201-planar	5	301	0.879 (0.529–0.957)	0.906 (0.75–0.958)	0.930 (0.818–0.981)	0.841 (0.778–0.920)
Octreoscan-SPECT	2	39	0.839 (0.76–0.938)			
Octreoscan-planar	1	50	0.750			
CEA-Scan-SPECT	1	12	0.889	0.917	0.889	0.917
Oncoscint-SPECT	1	16	1.000	1.000	1.000	1.000

MIBI, ^{99m}Tc-sestamibi; PPV, positive predictive value; NPV, negative predictive value. Range of values indicated in parentheses.

patients with nonpalpable disease. Seven studies included within subject comparisons between ^{99m}Tc sestamibi and other imaging tests including XRM US, and magnetic resonance imaging.

When all 14 studies involving 833 patients were pooled, the sensitivity is 85.4% and the specificity is 89.2% for planar radionuclide imaging of the breast. The pooled NPV is 87.3%, indicating that in patients with negative scans on radionuclide imaging of the breast 12.7% would still be at risk of malignancy if the test is used to recommend against biopsy.

Seven studies reported the results of ^{201}Tl radionuclide imaging of the breast, of which five utilized planar and one single-photon emission tomography (SPECT) techniques [16,21–25]. The sensitivity estimate of results from 301 patients is 87.9% with a specificity of 90.6% and pooled NPV of 84.1%. Given these performance characteristics, if a ^{201}Tl radionuclide imaging of the breast study result was utilized to decide whether a biopsy should be performed, 15.9% of patients with negative scans would still be at risk for malignancy.

Three studies utilized ^{111}In pentetreotide for breast imaging, two SPECT and one planar [26–28]. These data are insufficient to permit conclusions on the performance of the technique because they did not include benign disease in their study groups. All of the data were obtained from patients with confirmed malignancies, instead. One small study included the use of ^{99m}Tc IMMU-4 (CEA scan) and another the ^{111}In-labeled B72.3 monoclonal antibody (Oncoscint), and although encouraging results were obtained, one study by itself is insufficient to permit conclusions about the diagnostic performance of the test.

G. Synthesize and Consolidate Evidence

An important comparison between radionuclide imaging of the breast and XRM offers some valuable insight into the utility and proposed application of the new technique. A recent study of XRM in a cross-sectional study population of 28,271 women indicated that for those aged 50 and older the sensitivity of initial screening mammography was initially high but decreased with length of follow-up after mammography: 98.5% for 7 months of follow-up, 93.2% for 13 months, and 85.7% for 25 months [31]. For women <50 years, sensitivity also decreased with increasing length of follow-up: 87.5% for 7 months, 83.6% for 13 months, and 71.4% for 25 months. For women <50 years, breast density did not affect sensitivity—81.8% for those with primarily fatty breasts versus 85.4% for those with primarily dense breasts. It was lower (68.8%) among women with a family history of breast cancer. XRM sensitivity is highest among women aged 50 years and older who have primarily fatty breast tissue (versus dense tissue). In younger women, factors other than breast density appear to play a role in the accuracy of XRM. Consequently, a role for radionuclide imaging of the breast exists if it allows the identification of disease in radiographically "silent" tissue. One possible explanation based on the findings in patients with first-degree relatives with diagnosed breast cancer is that the rate of tumor growth is faster in some breasts. An agent that detects metabolically active disease (e.g., related radiopharmaceuticals) may have an improved chance of localizing in such tissues. Such increased localization should improve diagnostic performance for such techniques.

For women <50 years, the sensitivity of XRM was in the range of 83% to 87% at a follow-up period of 1 year. Comparable, age-selected or age-matched data cannot be extracted from the radionuclide imaging of the breast literature. However, overall, the sensitivity of ^{99m}Tc sestamibi radionuclide imaging of the breast is quite comparable to XRM at 85% for planar imaging. Consequently, the techniques offer comparable results in that population. Important comparisons are required, however. For instance, it would be useful to compare the performance of radionuclide imaging of the breast in age-matched groups, and directly with XRM. It would also be useful to compare radionuclide imaging of the breast in dense and fatty tissue breasts in a more rigorous manner. Additionally, radionuclide imaging of the breast should also be compared to XRM more directly in the same patients, and direct comparisons of performance characteristics should be based on such data.

H.   Formulate and Disseminate Findings and Recommendations

The analysis of published results reviewed above indicates that radionuclide imaging of the breast has comparable performance to XRM in patients <50 years old. Radionuclide imaging of the breast results suggest that it may serve as an adjunctive technology in cases where XRM is negative, but strong clinical suspicion of patient history suggests otherwise. Additional comparative data would improve the power of any analysis performed to compare radionuclide imaging of the breast to XRM for younger women. Importantly, if these data consistently demonstrate positive findings in patients with negative XRM, radionuclide imaging of the breast may quickly be adopted as an adjunctive procedure for the patient populations indicated above. Additional data from patients with benign disease are needed for radionuclide imaging of the breast to conclusively demonstrate comparability and, in some settings, superiority to XRM. Additional negative studies will adjust the diagnostic performance characteristics of radionuclide imaging of the breast in such a manner as will result in improved sensitivity. Moreover, future studies should include a ratio of 70:30 benign:malignant lesions in their analysis of performance because this is a much more representative disease severity ratio to base decisions upon. Studies that only report the results of patients with known malignancy serve limited utility in the formulation of diagnostic pathways incorporating radionuclide imaging of the breast.

Diagnostic algorithms based on radionuclide imaging of the breast can be constructed from the above analysis. This is an area of ongoing research in several programs. Several routes are available for the dissemination of these results. Clinical pathways should be published in appropriate oncology and diagnostic imaging literature that is covered by non-nuclear-medicine specialists as well as nuclear medicine physicians. Regional cooperative oncology groups (SWOG, ECOG, etc.) should be informed of such analyses, and the results should be made available to their memberships. In this manner, dissemination of the outcomes of HTA will be hastened and will reach appropriate decision makers in a timely manner.

I. Monitor Impact of Assessment

This is probably one of the most challenging aspects of HTA, and one where very little information and guidance is available. A significant impact will become known when the number of radionuclide imaging of the breast studies performed increases. Likewise, the adoption and incorporation of clinical pathways utilizing radionuclide imaging of the breast will be another measure of adoption. The entrance of radionuclide imaging of the breast into main-line practice may also be gauged when referring physician specialists begin to include radionuclide imaging of the breast data in their publications and other information that may be used to educate other physicians. Finally, patient advocacy groups that become public champions of radionuclide imaging of the breast and request that their providers make the study available will be one further measure of a successful and productive impact.

IV. TECHNOLOGY POLICY AND RADIONUCLIDE IMAGING OF THE BREAST

Technology assessment is a process for determining which technologies work best, and under what conditions, in a manner that patients care about. The managed competition model will most likely be the starting place for discussions of technology policy in a climate of reform. Government and private sectors have yet to address the importance of health technology policy from the perspective of technology and outcomes analysis because their focus has been cost-driven. Cost containment has also been the focus of nongovernmental health plans which have largely fallen behind in adoption of new high-end technologies and services. Health plans, however, are in an optimal position for testing new technologies because of the recent trend to decentralize decisions about capital equipment purchases.

The adoption and diffusion of radionuclide imaging of the breast will have to take advantage of private sector efforts to understand new technologies. These efforts are based on outcomes research and analysis. Although the data accumulated so far strongly suggest a role for radionuclide imaging of the breast in the evaluation of breast disease, additional data comparing radionuclide imaging of the breast to XRM, cost-effectiveness analysis, and decision analysis for utilization of radionuclide imaging of the breast will greatly enhance its likelihood for adoption into main-line diagnostic pathways and practice patterns.

REFERENCES

1. Howell JD. Technology in the Hospital. Baltimore: Johns Hopkins University Press, 1995.
2. IOM (Institute of Medicine). Assessing Medical Technologies. Committee for Evaluating Medical Technologies in Clinical Use, Division of Health Sciences Policy, and Division of Health Promotion and Disease Prevention. Washington, D.C.: National Academy Press, 1988.
3. Perry S, Gerdner E, Thamer M. The status of health technology assessment worldwide. Int J Technol Assessment 13:81–98, 1997.
4. Gleeson S. Blue Cross and Blue Shield Association initiatives in technology assessment. In: Adopting New Medical Technology (Institute of Medicine). Washington, D.C.: National Academy Press, 1994.
5. OTA (Office of Technology Assessment). Tools for evaluating health technologies: five background papers, BP-H-142. Washington, D.C.: U.S. Government Printing Office, 1995.
6. Parker SL et al. Cancer statistics, 1997. CA Cancer J Clin 47:5–27, 1997.
7. Palmedo H et al. Technetium-99m-MIBI scintimammography for suspicious breast lesions. J Nucl Med 37:626–630, 1996.
8. Hekbich TH et al. Differentiation of benign and malignant breast lesions: MR imaging versus Tc-99m sestamibi scintimammography. Radiology 202:421–429, 1997.
9. Khalkhali I et al. Scintimammography: the complementary role of Tc-99m sestamibi prone breast imaging for the diagnosis of breast carcinoma. Radiology 196:421–426, 1995.
10. Taillefer R et al. Technetium-99m-sestamibi prone scintimammography to detect primary breast cancer and axillary lymph node involvement. J Nucl Med 36:1758–1765, 1995.
11. Burak Z et al. Evaluation of palpable breast masses with ^{99m}Tc-MIBI: a comparative study with mammography and ultrasonography. Nucl Med Commun 15:604–612, 1994.
12. Kao CH, Wang SJ, Yeh SH. Technetium-99m-MIBI uptake in breast carcinoma and lymph node metastases. Clin Nucl Med 19:898–900, 1994.
13. Moretti JL et al. Primary breast cancer imaging with technetium-99m sestamibi and its relation with p-glycoprotein overexpression. Eur J Nucl Med 23:980–986, 1996.
14. Lam WW et al. Role of MIBI breast scintigraphy in evaluation of palpable breast lesions. Br J Radiol 69:1152–1158, 1996.

15. Villanueva-Meyer J et al. Mammoscintigraphy with technetium-99m-sestamibi in suspected breast cancer. J Nucl Med 37:926–930, 1996.

16. Maurer AH et al. Limitations of craniocaudal thallium-201 and technetium-99m-sestamibi mammoscintigraphy. J Nucl Med 36:1696–1700, 1995.

17. Cliffford EJ, Lugo-Zamidio C. Scintimammography in the diagnosis of breast cancer. Am J Surg 172:483–486, 1996.

18. Maffioloi L et al. Prone scintimammography in patients with non-palpable breast lesions. Anticancer Res 16:1269–1273, 1996.

19. Tiling R et al. Comparison of technetium-99m-sestamibi scintimammography with contrast-enhanced MRI for diagnosis of breast lesions. J Nucl Med 38:58–62, 1997.

20. Lu G et al. ^{99m}Tc-MIBI mammoscintigraphy of breast masses: early and delayed imaging. Nucl Med Commun 16:150–156, 1995.

21. Rebollo AC et al. Evaluation of palpable breast masses with ^{201}Tl scintigraphy. Br J Radiol 68:1052–1057, 1995.

22. Cimitan M et al. The use of thallium-201 in the preoperative detection of breast cancer: an adjunct to mammography and ultrasonography. Eur J Nucl Med 22:1110–1117, 1995.

23. Ozdemir A et al. Ti-201 scintigraphy, mammography and ultrasonography in the evaluation of palpable and nonpalpable breast lesions: a correlative study. Eur J Radiol 24:145–154, 1997.

24. Lee VW et al. A complementary role for thallium-201 scintigraphy with mammography in the diagnosis of breast cancer. J Nucl Med 34:2095–2100, 1993.

25. Waxman AD et al. Thallium scintigraphy in the evaluation of mass abnormalities of the breast. J Nucl Med 34:18–23, 1993.

26. Chiti A et al. Axillary node metastasis detection in breast cancer with ^{99m}Tc-sestamibi and ^{111}In-pentetreotide. Tumori 83:537–538, 1997.

27. Bajc M, Ingvar C, Palmer J. Dynamic indium-111-pentetreotide scintigraphy in breast cancer. J Nucl Med 37:622–626, 1996.

28. van Eijck CHJ et al. Somatostatin receptor scintigraphy of primary breast cancer and its predictive value in the follow-up comparison with CEA and CA 15-3. J Nucl Med 35:21P, 1994. Abstract.

29. Gulec SA et al. Detection of breast carcinoma by Tc-99m labeled Fab′ fragment of the anti-CEA antibody. Proc Am Assoc Cancer Res Annu Meeting 36:219, 1995.

30. Lamki LM et al. Indium-111-labeled B72.3 monoclonal antibody in the detection and staging of breast cancer: a Phase I study. J Nucl Med 32:1326–1332, 1991.

31. Kerlokowske K et al. Effect of age, breast density, and family history in the sensitivity of first screening mammography. JAMA 276:33–38, 1996.

16

Radionuclide Imaging of the Breast Using a Solid-State Gamma Camera

WILLIAM L. ASHBURN
Digirad Corporation, San Diego, California

I. INTRODUCTION

Hal Anger, in the early 1960s, may not have envisioned that one day the gamma scintillation camera would be called upon to image the breast. Yet today, scinti-mammography is performed using gamma camera technologies that have changed relatively little over the past 35 years. The introduction of solid-state radiation detector arrays for nuclear medicine imaging presents the opportunity for improvements in gamma camera design, most notably the performance and physical dimensions of the imager head.

II. CONVENTIONAL GAMMA SCINTILLATION CAMERAS

The fundamental principle underlying most gamma scintillation camera designs remains the same. Individual gamma ray photons emitted from the patient enter the detector through one of the parallel holes in the collimator and produce a momentary weak flash of light (scintillation). The intensity of the scintillation is proportional to the loss of photon energy in the thin sheet of sodium iodide crystal. The scintillation is converted into an electrical signal by an array of 37 or more photomultiplier (PM) tubes positioned behind the crystal. The location of the scintillation event in the crystal, hence the location in the body from which the gamma ray was emitted, is determined by a weighted average of the intensities of the output signals from the three or more PM tubes closest to the event. The sum of the PM tube outputs (pulse height) is used to calculate the energy of the photon detected by the crystal.

Although well suited for routine organ imaging, there are a number of physical characteristics of the typical gamma scintillation camera that make it somewhat less than ideal for breast imaging. The PM tubes must be placed slightly beyond the outer edge of the crystal in order to detect and correctly position gamma photons that produce a scintillation near the outer edge of the crystal. This creates a "dead space" (nonimaging zone) of up to several inches between the crystal and the side of the detector head. Moreover, the presence of PM tubes and their associated electronics increases the thickness of the detector head and adds considerable weight by virtue of the amount of lead shielding required.

III. PROBLEMS WITH SCINTILLATION CAMERAS

As a result of the dead space and thickness of the detector head inherent in conventional gamma scintillation camera designs, it is difficult if not impossible to image the breast from its medial aspect, close to and tangential to the curved shape of the chest wall. It is well known that increasing the distance between a focal accumulation of radioactivity in tissue and the detector surface causes a decrease in object contrast; therefore it is less detectable. This could create a problem in the case of medially located lesions identified on X-ray mammography or palpable masses in an inner quadrant of the breast. Likewise, there is the concern that a small radiopharmaceutical accumulation in a malignant lesion might go undetected if it is located deep within the breast or next to the chest wall.

IV. SOLID-STATE GAMMA CAMERAS

A solid-state, multicrystal gamma camera operates on a different principle than a conventional scintillation camera. Although standard collimators are used, there are no PM tubes. The detector head including the collimator can be made as thin as 3 in. In addition, the useful imaging area can be extended to within 0.5 in. of the leading edge of the detector head; this essentially depends on the thickness of the surrounding lead shielding. As a consequence, the advantages of the solid-state design makes it easy to image a variety of organs in which it is important to place the detector as close as possible to the object in order to achieve maximum image resolution. It is particularly well suited for breast imaging since, because of its size, the solid-state detector head can be placed close to the organ in virtually any position. As illustrated in Figure 1, the detector head can be placed against the

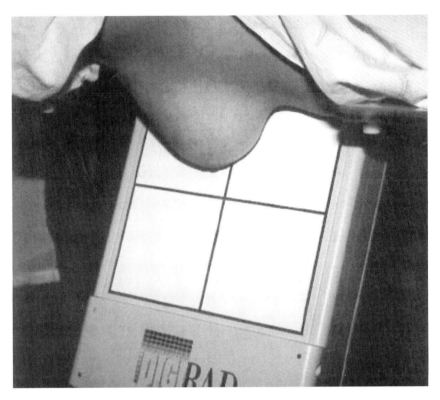

FIGURE I   Digirad 2020*tc* Imager head positioned on the medial side of the patient's left breast. The detector edge is placed against the sternum and angled tangential to the chest wall to detect uptake deep within the breast.

sternum between the breasts and angled tangential to the chest wall to produce an image from the medial aspect of the breast.

V.   PRINCIPLE OF A SOLID-STATE MULTICRYSTAL GAMMA CAMERA

The principle behind a solid-state multicrystal gamma camera is that the radiation detector consists of a matrix ("pixelated array") of cadmium-zinc-telluride (CZT) crystals rather than one NaI crystal [1,2]. The loss of energy of a gamma ray photon entering an individual crystal is converted directly into an electrical signal.

This is different from what occurs in a conventional gamma scintillation camera in which the photon energy loss in the NaI crystal produces a scintillation which is detected as light by the PM tubes and converted back to an electrical signal. Consequently, there are inherent signal-to-noise advantages in a solid-state imaging device, with the potential for improved image contrast.

The first commercial solid-state imager approved by the U.S. Food and Drug Administration for marketing as a general-purpose planar gamma camera is the Digirad 2020*tc* Imager. In this instrument, the solid-state crystal detectors are arranged in a grid pattern of 64 by 64 elements, each approximately 3.1 × 3.1 mm, for a total of 4096 pixels. This provides a useful field of view (UFOV) of 21.6 × 21.6 cm. (8.4 × 8.4 in.). Modules, consisting of 1 × 1 in. arrays of 64 elements, are placed close together in rows and columns to form a contiguous imaging array. As a result, tiled arrays of detector modules can be configured in the future to create virtually any size or shape imaging head.

Positioning the photon interactions (events) in a multicrystal solid-state gamma camera is a function of assigning a digital address to each detector element. Therefore, the x and y positions of each event are known to within the dimension of individual detector elements. As a result, the full-width half-maximum (FWHM) intrinsic spatial resolution is essentially equal to its full-width tenth maximum (FWTM). This is different than in the case of Anger-type scintillation cameras, in which an array of PM tubes is used to approximate the position of scintillation within the NaI crystal. The result is a weighted gaussian approximation in which the FWTM spatial resolution of a conventional scintillation camera is greater than the FWHM, leading to greater uncertainty as to the position of the photon event within the detector, thus the location in the body where it originated.

VI.   IMPROVED ENERGY RESOLUTION

Another advantage of using CZT as the radiation detector material in the solid-state imager is improved energy resolution. Whereas the best single NaI crystal scintillation cameras may have a FWHM energy resolution of approximately 10% at 140 keV, CZT detectors typically have a FWHM of 8% or better at the energy of technetium-99m. The improved energy resolution could allow the technologist to select a narrower energy window, the intent being to minimize the likelihood that gamma rays scattered within the soft tissues will be recorded as true, unscattered events. When a photon undergoes Compton scatter in tissue, it changes direction and in the process loses some of its energy. A narrower energy window is used to improve lesion-to-background contrast by eliminating undesired Compton scatter from the image. This improvement in signal-to-noise ratio is particularly desirable in breast imaging because of the great amount of extraneous photons originating in adjacent breast tissues or outside the breast, e.g., the chest wall and heart.

VII. COLLIMATORS

Collimators are required for both conventional scintillation and solid-state gamma cameras. Collimator choices include: parallel hole, slant angle, converging, single as well as multiple pinholes in order to imager closer to the organ, e.g., chest wall, achieve better resolution, create magnified views, or produce limited angle tomography.

High-resolution, parallel-hole collimators are most commonly used for breast imaging. To achieve maximum lesion detection, it is necessary that the collimator surface of the detector be placed as close as possible to the organ or at least to the part of the organ in which there may be an abnormality. This is particularly true in the case of breast imaging in which the lesion-to-background tissue concentration (ratio) of radiopharmaceutical is typically quite low (perhaps 5:1 or less). An important concept to remember is that lesion size per se is less an issue than is the radiopharmaceutical concentration in the abnormality compared with the uptake in surrounding normal (background) tissues. Even a relatively poor gamma camera might be able to detect a drop of radioactivity on a needle tip when there is little or no surrounding background radioactivity and minimal scattered activity.

One advantage of the smaller size of the solid-state detector is that by placing the collimator much closer to the organ, e.g., the breast, one can use a low-energy, all-purpose (LEAP) parallel-hole collimator rather than the high-resolution collimator. In general, the increase in count rate sensitivity associated with a LEAP collimator can be as much as twice that of a high-resolution collimator. The increase in count rate might be used to (1) reduce the recording time per view, (2) obtain better counting statistics for the same period of time, (3) lower the radiopharmaceutical dose administered to the patient, or (4) narrow the energy further in order to maximize Compton scatter rejection, or a combination of these. The tradeoffs have yet to be defined.

VIII. BREAST COMPRESSION

Breast compression is essential in X-ray mammography. The radiographic technique depends on transmission of relatively low kvP X-rays through as uniform a thickness of breast tissue as possible. However, the degree of compression used during the brief X-ray exposure in standard X-ray mammography is probably unsuitable for gamma camera imaging.

There are theoretical advantages for advocating at least some degree of breast compression in spite of the longer recording times required for gamma camera breast imaging [3]. The most compelling reason is the opportunity to decrease the relative thickness of the normal breast tissue surrounding an abnormal accumulation of radiopharmaceutical in a malignant lesion, which presumably is less compressible than the normal tissue. This would be expected to increase lesion-to-background count density, thus enhance lesion contrast and improve detectability. Another argument in favor of compression is stabilization of the breast during imaging.

One disadvantage to breast compression may be the unrecognized entrapment of skin folds between the detector and the compression device. This might lead to artifacts in the final image. Because the technologist can visually control positioning of the comparatively thin head of the solid-state camera, the chance for this type of artifacts is probably reduced.

IX. ADDITIONAL VIEWS

Although the first commercial solid-state gamma camera is not designed or marketed with the intent of being a breast imager, the field of view and physical size of the instrument are well suited for this application, being only slightly larger than the film cassette of a standard X-ray mammogram unit. Because of its somewhat similar dimensions it would seem logical to try to obtain comparable routine projections. However, because of the differences in breast compression techniques mentioned earlier, it is unlikely that perfect coregistration between the X-ray mammogram and the nuclear study would be possible. Even so, it would be possible to approximate the standard craniocaudal and medial-oblique projections.

Currently, the prone position with the breast dependent is the most popular method to ensure that as much of the breast as possible will be included within the camera's field of view. This position is usually facilitated by using a special bed or mattress with an attached cutout for the breast. Imaging is usually limited to one lateral view of each breast. However, this view alone, without additional views, could possibly fail to detect small abnormal uptake in the inner aspect of the breasts (Fig. 2) or adequately evaluate a palpable mass in a location some distance away from the collimator surface (Fig. 3). The same may be true for lesions that are very close to the chest wall. As mentioned earlier, when using a standard large-field-of-view gamma scintillation camera with its associated large "dead space," there are few options for additional views. Although useful to evaluate the axilla, the anterior view of the left breast may be of limited value due to the superimposition of radiopharmaceutical uptake the heart. Posterior-oblique views may be useful for detecting lesions close to the chest wall in the outer quadrants of the breast, but may miss medial accumulations.

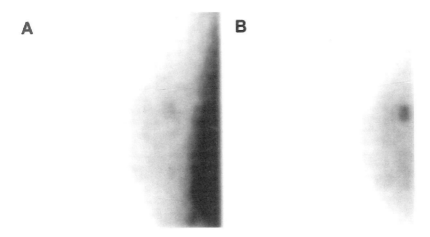

FIGURE 2 A 50-year-old woman with an abnormal finding in the medial aspect of the left breast on X-ray mammography. Panel A: Lateral view of the left breast. Panel B: Medial view of the same breast. Exposure time was for 10 min for studies obtained with the solid-state imager. Note the significantly higher lesion-to-background contrast of the Tc-99m sestamibi in the biopsy-proven cancer on the medial view versus the standard lateral view.

Additional views of the breast might include any that optimally examine all quadrants including the axilla. Obviously, due to relatively long acquisition times (typically 10 min/view) compared to X-ray mammography, one must for practical reasons choose the one or two routine views that image the most common sites in which lesions might occur. In X-ray mammography, additional projection or magnified views are commonly obtained to help clarify suspicious densities. Similarly, the small size of the solid-state gamma camera lends itself well to obtaining additional views appropriate to the findings on the standard views or according to the location of a palpable mass. A magnified image of a suspicious area using a converging collimator might be appropriate in selected cases.

As mentioned earlier, the medial view of the breast could become a routine projection with a solid-state gamma camera. The smaller size and reduced thickness of the imager would appear to be well suited for placement between the breasts and up against the sternum. To further add to the value of the medial view, the detector can be angled so that its field of view is tangential to the chest wall.

Unfortunately, not all commercial bed cutouts for prone breast imaging are wide enough to accommodate the width of the available solid-state detector head. The cutouts can be widened if precautions for safety are considered, but there are other possible patient positions that would permit dependent breast imaging. The technologist could instruct the patient to lean forward with arms folded and sup-

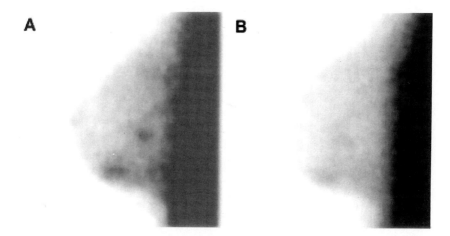

FIGURE 3   A 72-year-old patient with dense breasts and a suspicious finding in the midportion of the left breast on X-ray mammography. Panel A: Lateral view of the left breast imaged with the solid-state gamma camera using a LEAP collimator. Panel B: Same lateral view imaged with a conventional scintillation camera, using a high-resolution collimator. Exposure time was for 10 for both studies. Note the higher lesion-to-background contrast achieved with the solid-state gamma camera in spite of using a LEAP collimator. Tc-99m sestamibi uptake was also noted in the inferior portion of both breasts, assumed to be a benign artifact. Higher contrast may be due to the excellent energy resolution of solid-state detectors plus the intrinsic advantages of a "pixelated" multicrystal imager. These images are reproduced from Digirad's Web site: www.digirad.com.

ported on a table in front. The detector head then could be positioned easily between the breasts and angled tangential to the chest wall, as mentioned, to obtain a medial view. Obviously, not all patients will be able to bend at the waist to the degree necessary to allow medial imaging.

Other views are possible with the patient standing or seated. One can angle the detector towards the patient's feet or toward the head in order to obtain superior-inferior or inferior-superior views, respectively. This takes advantage of the minimal dead space of the solid-state detector head (Fig. 4). In the inferior-superior view, care must be taken to turn the patient's head to avoid extraneous radioactivity from being included in the field of view.

X.   OTHER POSSIBLE APPLICATIONS OF THE SOLID-STATE IMAGERS

There is increasing interest in using gamma cameras to assist in the localization of suspicious lesions for biopsy. Khalikhali et al. at the Harbor-UCLA Medical

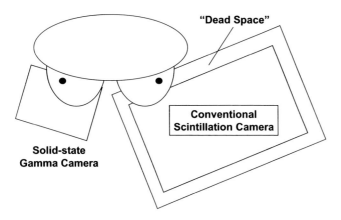

FIGURE 4   The typical "dead space" (nonimaging zone) of a conventional gamma scintillation camera may be 2 in. or more. This precludes placing the detector edge close enough against the chest wall to detect abnormal uptake deep in the breast in all projections. By comparison, the minimum dead space of the solid-state gamma camera is 0.5 in.

Center [4] have successfully used a technique in which two or more images are acquired, at right angles, to define the location of the radiopharmaceutical accumulation in the lesion to be biopsied. By using a grid that includes one or more radioactive line sources, accurate needle placement is facilitated.

Clinical investigators have used gamma camera imaging to locate sentinel nodes in cases of melanoma and breast cancer using a variety of injection techniques [5]. It seems likely that in the future, stereotactic nuclear medicine techniques will emerge for real-time image-guided biopsy of the sentinel node or of the primary breast lesion itself. Radioactive-tipped needles and/or lead-attenuating markers have been used in the past to help identify radioactive accumulations during surgical procedures, such as during the insertion of nonopaque catheters and during a biopsy procedure [6]. The small "footprint" of the solid-state imaging camera may prove useful for such procedures in the operating room.

In this chapter, we have discussed the application of a small, solid-state, general-purpose gamma camera for breast imaging. It possible that other gamma camera imaging techniques will prove to be useful for breast imaging. Pani et al. [7] advocate the use of Position Sensitive PM tubes and advanced scintillation crystals such as YAP:Ce and CsI.

ACKNOWLEDGMENTS

The author would like to express his appreciation to Iraj Khalikhali, M.D., and Linda Diggles, CNMT, at Harbor-UCLA, and Michael Kipper M.D., and Linda

Krohn, CNMT, at Tri-City Hospital Outpatient Nuclear Medicine, in Vista, CA, for their assistance in acquiring the breast images. Thanks also to Mr. Liem Le at Digirad for his technical assistance and Mr. Robert Diggles of Bodfish Research & Design, Inc. for providing a modified breast imaging table suitable to accommodate the larger width of the Digirad 2020*tc* Imager head.

REFERENCES

1. Butler JF, Friesenhahn SJ, Apotovsky A, et al. $Cd_{1-x}Zn_x$ Te detector imaging array. Proceedings of the Society of Photo Instrumentation and Electronics (SPIE), Newport Beach, CA, Feb. 14–15, 1986; pub. SPIE, Bellingham, WA, 1993: 30–37.
2. Butler JF, Friesenhahn SJ, Lingren C, et al. CdZnTe detector arrays for nuclear medicine imaging. Conference Record, IEEE Nuclear Science & Medical Imaging Conference, Nov. 1993, 93CH3374-6, 1 1993: 565–568.
3. Pani R, Scopinaro F, Pellegrini R, Soluri A, Weinberg IN, De Vincentis G. The role of Compton background and breast compression on cancer detection in scintimammography. Anticancer Res 17:1645–1650, 1997.
4. Khalikhali I, Mishkin FS, Diggles LE, Klein SR. Radionuclide-guided stereotatic prebiopsy localization of nonpalpable breast lesions. J Nucl Med 38:1019–1022, 1997.
5. Uren RF, Howman-Giles RB, Thompson JF, et al. Mammary lymphoscintigraphy in breast cancer. J Nucl Med 36:1775–1780, 1995.
6. Green JP, Ashburn WL, Hurwitz SR, Halpern SE. Sealed sources of Tc-99m inserted into standard biopsy needles and catheters: use in anatomic localization of external radionuclide imaging. J Nucl Med 14:743–746, 1973.
7. Pani R, Scopinaro F, Pellegrini R, et al. Single tube gamma camera for scintimammography. Anticancer Res 17:1651–1654, 1997.

Index